CHILDREN, ETHICS, AND MODERN MEDICINE

Medical Ethics

DAVID H. SMITH AND ROBERT M. VEATCH, EDITORS

Mary Anderlik. *The Ethics of Managed Care: A Pragmatic Approach*

Norman L. Cantor. *Advance Directives and the Pursuit of Death with Dignity*

Norman L. Cantor. *Legal Frontiers of Death and Dying*

Arthur L. Caplan. *Am I My Brother's Keeper? The Ethical Frontiers of Biomedicine*

Arthur L. Caplan. *If I Were a Rich Man Could I Buy a Pancreas?*
And Other Essays on the Ethics of Health Care

James F. Childress. *Practical Reasoning in Bioethics: Principles, Metaphors, and Analogies*

Cynthia B. Cohen, ed. *Casebook on the Termination of Life-Sustaining Treatment*
and the Care of the Dying

Cynthia B. Cohen, ed. *New Ways of Making Babies: The Case of Egg Donation*

Roger B. Dworkin. *Limits: The Role of the Law in Bioethical Decision Making*

Larry Gostin, ed. *Surrogate Motherhood: Politics and Privacy*

Christine Grady. *The Search for an AIDS Vaccine: Ethical Issues in the Development*
and Testing of a Preventive HIV Vaccine

A Report by the Hastings Center. *Guidelines on the Termination of*
Life-Sustaining Treatment and the Care of the Dying

Paul Lauritzen. *Pursuing Parenthood: Ethical Issues in Assisted Reproduction*

Joanne Lynn, M.D., ed. *By No Extraordinary Means:*
The Choice to Forgo Life-Sustaining Food and Water, expanded edition

William F. May. *The Patient's Ordeal*

Richard W. Momeyer. *Confronting Death*

Thomas H. Murray, Mark A. Rothstein, and Robert F. Murray, Jr., eds.
The Human Genome Project and the Future of Health Care

Jennifer A. Parks. *No Place Like Home? Feminist Ethics and Home Health Care*

Susan B. Rubin. *When Doctors Say No: The Battleground of Medical Futility*

David H. Smith, Kimberly A. Quaid, Roger B. Dworkin,
Gregory P. Gramelspacher, Judith A. Granbois, and Gail H. Vance.
Early Warning: Cases and Ethical Guidance for Presymptomatic Testing in Genetic Diseases

Lois Snyder and Arthur L. Caplan. *Assisted Suicide: Finding Common Ground*

S. Kay Toombs, David Barnard, and Ronald Carson, eds.
Chronic Illness: From Experience to Policy

Robert M. Veatch. *The Patient as Partner: A Theory of Human-Experimentation Ethics*

Robert M. Veatch. *The Patient–Physician Relation: The Patient as Partner, Part 2*

Leonard Weber. *Business Ethics in Healthcare*

Robert F. Weir, ed. *Physician-Assisted Suicide*

Children, Ethics, and Modern Medicine

RICHARD B. MILLER

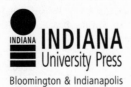

INDIANA
University Press

Bloomington & Indianapolis

Publication of this book is made possible in part with the assistance
of a Challenge Grant from the National Endowment for the
Humanities, a federal agency that supports research, education,
and public programming in the humanities.

This book is a publication of

Indiana University Press
601 North Morton Street
Bloomington, IN 47404-3797 USA

http://iupress.indiana.edu

Telephone orders   800-842-6796
Fax orders   812-855-7931
Orders by e-mail   iuporder@indiana.edu

Library of Congress Cataloging-in-Publication Data

Miller, Richard B.
   Children, ethics, and modern medicine / Richard B. Miller.
      p. cm. — (Medical ethics)
   Includes bibliographical references and index.
   ISBN 0-253-34222-8 (cloth : alk. paper)
   1. Pediatrics—Moral and ethical aspects. 2. Medical ethics.
   3. Children—Diseases—Treatment—Moral and ethical aspects.
   [DNLM: 1. Ethics, Clinical. 2. Pediatrics. 3. Ethics, Medical.
   WS 21 M649c 2003] I. Title. II. Series : Medical ethics series.
   RJ47 .M55 2003
   174'.2—dc21
                                                    2002014748

1 2 3 4 5 08 07 06 05 04 03

For my mother,
Lucille Dean Miller

Oh! mystery of Man, from what a depth
Proceed thy honours! I am lost, but see
In simple childhood something of the base
On which thy greatness stands
            —Wordsworth, *The Prelude,* bk. 11

CONTENTS

ACKNOWLEDGMENTS

The remotest origin of this book dates to my childhood in the early 1960s, when I was admitted to a hospital in Hawaii to undergo a traumatic diagnosis for a possible heart tumor. No less now than at the age of nine, I believe that adults' care of children involves special virtues and duties, many of which were lacking in my experience as a pediatric patient and research subject. More recently, this book finds its beginnings in the early 1990s, when Jim Wind (then of the Lilly Endowment) approached my colleague, David H. Smith, and me about the possibility of developing an alternative research model for professional ethics, one that draws from lay experience in professional contexts. The main goal was to see what normative implications we could draw after studying professionals and the persons they are supposed to serve, integrating various features of cultural anthropology and ethnography into ethical inquiry. With the support of the Lilly Endowment and the Poynter Center at Indiana University, Smith and I embarked on a pilot project in 1991–92 that assembled an interdisciplinary seminar of Indiana University faculty to read and discuss various approaches to professional ethics, focusing on the merits and limits of ethnography as a research tool. That project was followed up by a three-year national seminar, "Religion, Morality, and Professional Life," for which Smith and I brought together scholars from around the country to theorize and carry out ethnographic approaches to ethical issues in education, journalism, the ministry, law, and medicine.

Throughout these seminars, my thoughts focused on children and medicine, working on the intuition that pediatrics was a field relatively unexplored in biomedical ethics. In 1997–98, I continued this line of work as a fellow in the Program in Ethics and the Professions at Harvard University, an incomparable intellectual experience under the direction of Dennis Thompson. Guided by weekly seminars and by conversations with philosophers, political theorists, medical anthropologists, and health care providers in the Boston area, I drafted the main contours of this work and carried out a significant amount of the field research that informs it. A subsequent grant from the Lilly Endowment under the rubric of "Religion, Ethnography, and Professional Life" provided release time to continue research and writing in 1998–99, enabling me to bring this project closer to completion.

Numerous critics have read drafts of this book, or parts therein, and have provided helpful (and sometimes extensive) commentary. Listing their names here does little justice by way of thanking them, and over time, I hope to express my gratitude more directly. For reading all or parts of this manuscript, thanks go to Byron Bangert, Alexandra Berkowitz, Barry Bull, Jeff Burns, Deborah Chung, David Cockerham, Peter de Marneffe, Mark Graham, Gwakhee Han, Laura Hartman, Lisa Lehmann, Sebastiano Maffettonne, Terence Martin, Jr., David McCarty, Heather McConnell, Christine Mitchell, Ann Mongoven, Douglas Ottati, Julie Pedroni, Richard Pildes, John Reeder, Walter Robinson, Ken Ryan, William Schweiker, Lisa Sideris, David H. Smith, Dennis Thompson, Robert Truog, Charles Wilson, and Mark Wilson. Heather McConnell and Kathryn Bryan provided invaluable research assistance. Judith Granbois and Karen Hellekson carefully pored over my prose, finding countless places for improvement. Paul Lauritzen and Jennifer Girod not only read an earlier manuscript but passed along lengthy suggestions for revision. David Smith patiently watched as this book become longer and more focused; I cannot thank him enough for his sage and supportive counsel. Kellie Hindman attended to numerous last-minute details. Marilyn Grobschmidt of Indiana University Press provided encouragement and editorial guidance. My colleagues in the Department of Religious Studies, always a source of intellectual stimulation and goodwill, assumed added responsibilities while I was on research leave in 1997–99. Craig Dykstra of the Lilly Endowment provided grant support that released me from department duties for the second of those two years. To all of these individuals, I am extremely grateful.

Books benefit from formal as well as informal dialogue, and for the latter I am indebted to many friends and colleagues. For many conversations—spirited and leisurely—I thank Maria Antonaccio, Ginny and Nigel Biggar, Jeff Wolin, Betsy Stirratt, Oscar Kenshur, Margot Gray, Ash and Kim Nichols, and Chuck Garrettson.

Several parts of this book grew out of fieldwork in different medical settings, and to those who enabled me to observe their practices, clinics, or hospitals I cannot express thanks enough. This work would not have been possible were it not for several special individuals who took it upon themselves to open their doors to me and, in the process, to challenge me intellectually and psychologically. In order to maintain confidentiality, I will not mention their names or their institutions here, but they enabled me to immerse myself in contexts in ways that are unimaginable to most scholars in the academy today. I trust that each of these persons in Bloomington, Indianapolis, and Boston knows who he or she is, and knows that my appreciation is no less profound for being unspecified here.

I presented a few parts of this book at the invitation of various persons and institutions, and I want to thank them for the opportunity to develop my ideas. To Edward Vacek and John Reeder I am grateful for invitations to present a draft of Chapter 9 to students at Boston College and Brown University, respectively, in winter 1998. I presented a revised draft of that chapter at a special session on religion and bioethics at the annual meeting of the Association for Professional and Practical Ethics in March 2000. At the invitation of Gabriel Palmer-Fernandez, I presented Chapter 10 in a plenary session of the Regional Meeting of the Society for Health and Human Values at Youngstown State University in April 1998. I presented Chapter 6 at a conference on religion and the professions, supported by the Lilly Endowment, in February 2000. In May 2000, I presented a paper on "Ethical Challenges in Pediatric Medicine," outlining the main argument of this book, at a meeting of the Southern Indiana Pediatricians that was organized by Sandy DeWeese. To all of these persons and groups, I am grateful.

In what seems like a former life, I spent the summers of 1977–81 working with young people at a community swimming pool that was nestled in an enchanted hollow on the grounds of Camp Calvert in Leonardtown, Maryland. Overlooking the quiet, pacific estuary of Breton Bay, the Ryken Pool brought together a community of children and adolescents so diverse in age, background, and ability as to defy description. Memories of those magical times, now twenty years past, often visited me like a muse as I developed this project. For their hard work, spirited humor, and generous affection, thanks go to Bruce, Brian, and Pam Abell; Molly, Margaret, and Joan Bowes; Mary Farquhar; Kelly and Belle Mattingly; Megan and Patrick O'Neil; Andrew, Jordan, and Molly O'Neill; Karla and Blaine Sommerville, and the redoubtable Apryl Yates. No less cherished are memories of those who made that youthful utopia possible: Debbie Beasley, Dave Cooley, Shelly Cabana, and Jerry Murphy.

My deepest thanks go to Barbara Klinger and Matthew Miller. Without their enduring patience, affection, wit, zeal for adventure, and commitment to care, I would never have been able to envision this project or enjoy some of the goods that I hope to describe in the pages that follow.

R.B.M.
Bloomington, Indiana
June 2002

CHILDREN, ETHICS,
AND MODERN MEDICINE

Introduction

THE PEDIATRIC PARADIGM (AND ITS REVISIONS)

This is a book about medical ethics and the care of children, focusing on parental and professional responsibilities toward patients who are young and ill. Two controversies from my home in southern Indiana—one well known, the other less so—help to focus ideas. In 1982, the case of Baby Doe brought national attention to Bloomington when parents refused life-saving surgery for their baby, born with Down syndrome, to correct his esophageal blockage. After Bloomington Hospital challenged that decision, the Monroe County Circuit Court decided in the parents' favor. In 1998, in nearby Morgantown, the parents of twelve-year-old Bradley Hamm opted to treat his pneumonia with prayer rather than antibiotics. That decision went medically and legally uncontested, and Bradley, like Baby Doe, died from a correctable problem. In both cases, parents were given absolute decision-making authority, contrary to the apparent medical interests of their children. Did the parents do the right thing? Was it right to grant them this degree of authority? What were the responsibilities of medical professionals working with these families? Surprisingly, there is little sustained discussion in bioethics that helps to answer these questions.

I hope to correct for that oversight in these pages. Drawing on research in medical ethics and participant observation in various pediatric medical settings, this book will develop moral norms for professional and parental responsibility in the care of children. My goals are to define basic norms that should shape family and professional responsibility in pediatrics and deepen our understanding of those norms by connecting them to important cases in American law or to moral cases that materialized in my hospital fieldwork. In the process, I will clarify duties and virtues that shape how adults ought to direct their energies toward young patients in need of care.

Why has bioethics devoted so little attention to questions in pediatrics? In part the answer lies in the synergism between the politics and ethics of biomedicine. Starting in the 1960s, bioethics sought to give voice to the patients' rights movement—to define and defend a basic set of protections to ensure that professionals will respect adult patients as persons. In the process, bioethics developed guidelines for primary care providers, medical researchers, and specialists to treat patients and research subjects humanely. Focusing on such problems as legal and moral issues regarding informed consent in medical treatment and research; genetic testing; patient confidentiality; organ procurement, distribution, and transplantation; and treatment of previously competent or dying patients, bioethics focuses considerable attention to the rights of adults as free and equal persons. A central goal is to defend individual autonomy—the right of patients to decide on treatment, regardless of whether such decisions advance their medical welfare. Patients' rights provide individuals with protections against others' power, interventions, or collective interests; the norm of patient autonomy constrains what health care providers may do for a patient's medical benefit.[1] Such rights are generally seen in negative terms—that is, as rights to refuse unwanted treatment or not to be deceived by health care professionals. Adult medicine is thus structured by a strong presumption against paternalism.

Lost in that synergism of rights and norms are the many interests of the voiceless, perhaps because it has been assumed that a framework for adult, competent patients could be expanded to subsume young children and other noncompetent patients. I believe that in the case of children and young adolescents, this assumption is wrong—that adult and pediatric medical ethics differ sufficiently to warrant a separate analysis for the latter. Grafting pediatric ethics to the adult paradigm is a mistake for at least two reasons. First, most children generally lack the level of self-determination that is assumed for adults. Accordingly, professionals may presume to protect or promote children's welfare with fewer limits on their authority than in adult contexts—at least during their patients' early years. Second, family members are principally responsible for guarding their child as a needy and developing human being; the patient is a member of a social unit rather than a freestanding agent. That fact complicates professional responsibility by requiring medical providers to triangulate their commitment to patient welfare with the opportunities and constraints provided by the child's needs and the family's commitments and background. Pediatric care providers must forge a *therapeutic alliance* with the patient and his or her family, and they must advocate for the patient's basic interests when that alliance has broken down or cannot be established.

At the risk of oversimplifying, we can distinguish between two models of medical ethics: the adult and the pediatric paradigm. In the former, *the norm of respect for autonomy has general priority to the norm of beneficence.* Professionals are expected to respect an adult patient's autonomous wishes to refuse treatment, even if those wishes are not in that patient's medical interests. Generally with adults, what poses as beneficent treatment must be acceptable on the patient's own terms. In the latter, *the norm of beneficence has general priority to the norm of respect for autonomy.* With children, care providers may often act in ways that subordinate respect for autonomy, such as it is, to the value of patient benefit. Children are generally not free to make decisions that put themselves at considerable risk; adults may discount a child's decision in order to protect that child's current or future welfare.

Like most paradigms, these are very broad, and in the pages that follow, I will amend the pediatric model in important ways.[2] For now, note that it is subject to three revisions: the social revision, the interventionist revision, and the developmental revision. The first revision reminds us that children exist in a social unit and that pediatric care must thus accommodate the value of parental autonomy and family privacy—very different ideas from patient autonomy and individual privacy, as I will argue. The second revision is meant to amend the first: When parents or guardians fail to protect the basic interests of their children, outsiders may justifiably intervene in a family's domestic affairs. The final revision qualifies both. It reminds us that children develop powers of self-determination as they mature, and this fact must affect all interactions between adults and young people.

The priorities that distinguish adult from pediatric care are a function of different ideas about freedom, responsibility, and rights of vulnerable persons in relation to others with power. In adult medicine, the patient's rights movement developed in response to the question, "Whose life is it, anyway?" That question, made famous by Brian Clark's play in the late 1970s, focuses attention on who should finally be responsible in adult medical decision making.[3] One effect of modern bioethics has been to shift authority away from medical professionals to patients who must bear the consequences of a medical decision. With adults, the answer to the question, "Whose life is it, anyway?" is this: "Theirs." Today, the modern bioethics movement urges medical professionals to adopt the "first language" of individualism when thinking about adult patients, however much those patients might see themselves not as isolated and freestanding, but as socially embedded or connected to a wider web of family and communal ties.[4] Viewed as self-determining agents, adult patients are expected to be responsible for themselves. They must shoulder the effects of treatment and thus should be free to decide whether to encumber themselves with that treatment. In that way, modern bioethics enshrines a commitment to human dignity—the capacity of individuals to be free and responsible.

With children, matters are different. The general answer to the question, "Whose life is it, anyway?" is this: "Ours." That is to say, children's welfare is not a matter that they alone are finally expected to determine, for they have done little to prepare for such responsibilities, and their ability to make such determinations is often in the process of developing. Because of their physical, emotional, and intellectual limitations, children rely on others to advance their welfare and development. Children's well-being is thus a social duty, encumbering others to protect their interests and to nurture their understanding of self-care.

The notion that children occupy a special stage in life, with peculiar wants and needs, is hardly a venerable one in Western thought and culture. The social historian Philippe Aires notes that Western consciousness did not embrace the special characteristics of childhood until the early modern period. Before the seventeenth century, Aires observes, "No one thought of keeping a picture of a child if that child had either lived to grow to adulthood or had died of infancy. A surviving child had simply passed through a phase of which there was no need to keep a record. A dead child, since it had died so early in life, was not worthy of remembrance." Aires continues: "There were far too many children whose survival was problematical. . . . One had several children in order to keep just a few. People could not allow themselves to become too attached to something that was regarded as a probable loss."[5] With advances in medicine over the past two hundred years—developed in part because of high infant mortality rates—children became less a matter of "probable loss."[6] Many cultures began to see that childhood was a special stage in life and that children could (and should) be attended to in order to grow up as happy, healthy adults.

More to the point, if children's lives and welfare are—or have become—a matter of social obligation, then approaching pediatric medical ethics in terms of patients' rights does not fully capture the moral contours of family and professional obligations in pediatric settings. This point is especially true if we view patients' rights in negative terms—as protections against unwanted treatment or medical power. In Chapter 2, I will thus argue that it is more fitting to approach children in terms of the category of moral *responsibility*, which includes, but goes beyond, protecting children's rights.[7]

The belief that a child's life is, in some sense, "ours" raises the question, "Who should be included among those who are implicated in a child's well-being?" Who is the group to whom the possessive pronoun primarily refers? Over the course of Western thought and practice, various institutions have been proposed as principally responsible for a child's welfare, ranging from the nuclear family to the state. I will argue that the duty to care for a child falls first to a child's parents or guardians. That claim might seem counterintuitive, given the two examples with which I began this introduction, and I will sharpen it soon. A mixture of philosophical reasons and social conventions provide grounds for assigning the duty to care first to a child's parents or those who agree to guard that child's basic interests.

This point means, among other things, that strong reasons exist to honor family privacy and parental autonomy, values that enshrine a family's right to govern itself and regulate its internal affairs. Hence one reason to amend the pediatric paradigm. Parents need a good measure of freedom to nurture their offspring according to their values and commitments. Social responsibility is often less effective when it is supervised by outsiders. In more technical moral terms, there is a strong presumption in favor of respecting parental authority and family privacy. Families resemble sovereign states: secure, more or less, within their own borders to regulate domestic affairs. In domestic life and international relations, there are many things that some persons or groups can, but ought not, do for others' good. Like the ethics of global relations, the ethics of pediatric care is structured by a strong presumption against (but not absolute prohibition of) intervention.

Liberal, Western societies assign great latitude to parents, allowing them to raise their children according to distinct values and customs. The modern family takes many forms, sizes, and shapes. Some families are two-headed households, but many are not. Heterosexual and homosexual couples raise children, often outside the institution of marriage. What constitutes a family is further complicated by the high rates of divorce, remarriage, and the role of grandparents or extended family members in the rearing of children. Seeking to cover traditional and nontraditional arrangements, I will presume a definition of *family* as an intimate social unit in which one or more adults is responsible for raising at least one nonemancipated child.

In ideal circumstances, honoring a family's values does not conflict with the ethics of professionals who might be required to treat a sick child. But the right of family privacy is not absolute; it is contingent on whether parents or guardians respect their child's fundamental needs. When those needs are neglected, it may be necessary for others to help. An ethics of pediatric care should be designed to address ideal and nonideal circumstances alike, defining the contours of a therapeutic alliance and the grounds for rescuing persons in need.[8] Hence the second amendment to the pediatric paradigm. If a child's life and welfare are, in some sense, "ours," then parents or guardians should not enjoy absolute sovereignty over their children. As in the international arena, so too in domestic affairs: Interventions may be justified to protect basic rights from despotic authority. In this way, a pediatric care provider may resemble an international leader: When alliances falter, each may be called on to rescue the innocent.

Families differ, and so do children. Children's differences reveal themselves not only when we compare one child with another, but when we consider the developmental changes that each child undergoes during a normal lifetime. Children have life histories in which they discover (unevenly, to be sure) increasing powers of self-sufficiency and independence. Accordingly, adults must calibrate their expectations of a young persons' competence to the age and maturity of those within their care. Beneficence is prior to patient autonomy when adults interact with infants, children, and early adolescents. But as children grow and develop, priorities change. Hence the third amendment to the pediatric paradigm. At a critical juncture in a youth's development, we must shift the moral balance so that respect for autonomy has general priority to the demands of beneficence. In fact (as we shall see), pediatricians treat a phenomenal range of patients, from newborns to early (and sometimes fully mature) adults.

ETHICS-DISTANT AND ETHICS-NEAR

I have mentioned that this book is informed by participant observation in medical contexts, and I wish to make a few remarks about that experience and its place in a work on medical ethics. Here we do well to note another synergism, this one between clinical immersion and detached reflection as they inform the methodology of bioethics.

David J. Rothman's social history of biomedicine, *Strangers at the Bedside: A History of How Law and Bioethics Transformed Medical Decision-Making,* provides an instructive starting point. Rothman notes that modern bioethics arose in order to replace "bedside ethics," which was done by "teaching by example, by role modeling, by students taking cues from practicing physicians." On that model, "students were not to learn ethics by studying principles but by watching senior physicians resolve individual situations and then doing likewise."[9] Rothman observes that many medical schools long resisted the formal teaching of ethics "not because they believed that ethics could not be taught, but because it had to be taught at the bedside, by starting with the individual case."[10]

Bioethics replaced this approach in the late 1960s in response to scandals in research settings or moral and legal questions surrounding the proper care of defective newborns, persons in need of organ transplantation, or patients at the end of life. Those controversies eroded trust in the medical profession and the model of education on which it relied. Accordingly, lawyers, theologians, philosophers, and policy makers collaborated in the courts, in governmental or university medical centers, or in public policy forums, seeking to develop directives to guide the conduct of medical professionals—directives that were stated in clear principles and grounded in common morality. In that way, medical ethics moved away from the bedside and into public policy and law.

The downside of this development is that, in order to produce guidelines that are general enough to cover different situations, bioethics acquired a detached and abstract quality. The literature of much bioethical writing reflects what anthropologist Clifford Geertz calls an "experience-distant" as opposed to an "experience-near" perspective.[11] Lost from the former perspective are some of the real-life dimensions of medical care, those more finely grained aspects of professional experience that characterize the everyday lives of medical practitioners. And it is about this abstract, detached quality of bioethics that social theorists complain. Sociologist Daniel F. Chambliss writes, for example, that "much of bioethics assumes that people are autonomous decision makers sitting in a fairly comfortable room trying logically to fit problems to given solution-making patterns. The whole business is almost deliberately unreal—intellectually challenging but not very useful." Experience is different, Chambliss observes: "Inside hospitals . . . decisions are driven not by academic problem-solving techniques but by the routines of life in a professional bureaucracy."[12] Medical decision making is collective, not individual, involving a clash of interests and perspectives.

For medical anthropologist Arthur Kleinman, the problem with conventional bioethics is not that it is uninformed by sociology but that it ignores the personal challenges of patient suffering. Kleinman writes that "by and large the contextually rich, experience-near illness narrative is not privileged" in bioethics. Patients' experience is "reinterpreted (also thinned out) from the professional bioethical standpoint in order to focus exclusively on the value conflicts that it is held to instantiate."[13] Absent in the literature are "lay perspectives and everyday life experiences that might generate a deeper critique of that medical–moral domain and the economic interests with which it is inextricably held."[14] Chambliss and Kleinman thus call for a more "experience-near" approach to bioethics, one that draws from and critically addresses the power struggles of medical professionals and the illness experiences of those they treat.[15]

Today, the challenge of bioethics is to build on its advances in law and policy while heeding those who call for a more on-the-ground approach to bioethical writing. Stated differently, the challenge is to tack back and forth between an "ethics-distant" and an "ethics-near" orientation, a distinction that parallels Geertz's distinction (as noted above) in the social sciences. Following that distinction, we can say that an ethics-near approach immerses the researcher in the moral immediacies and vernacular traditions of individuals and institutions. The idea is for ethical inquiry to capture the lived features and complexities of moral experience, focusing on individual and corporate commitments, motivational wellsprings, aesthetic sensibilities, power relationships, and felt needs in everyday life. An ethics-distant approach, in contrast, abstracts from the particulars of experience to craft impersonal principles as guides for social criticism. Typically, the goal is to construct a set of normative standards that are free of complicity in any specific account of the good life, an impartial set of requirements that privilege no single tradition or point of view.

The respective danger of each orientation, taken in isolation, is to privilege either vernacular customs or detached, impersonal perspectives. To correct this problem, Geertz recommends deploying experience-near and experience-distant concepts dialectically, enabling each concept to restrain the other. As Geertz notes, intellectuals must produce "an interpretation of the way a people lives which is neither imprisoned within their mental horizons, an ethnography of witchcraft as written by a witch, nor systematically deaf to the distinctive tonalities of their existence, an ethnography of witchcraft as written by a geometer."[16]

The challenge to ethicists, no less than to anthropologists, is artfully to move in the intermediate space between personal and impersonal perspectives, deploying each in what is now famously known as a reflective equilibrium.[17] Seen in that way, ethics-near approaches draw on ethics-distant theories to discipline and illuminate what is discovered about local knowledge. In my view, ethicists must deploy features of ethics-distant orientations as diagnostic tools for lifting up and refining salient features that emerge from our attention to moral particulars, and to translate ethics-near orientations into an idiom that speaks more generally to different lay and professional audiences. At the same time, ethics-distant concepts are illumined and enriched as they are brought to bear on real-life cases. In the synergism between immediate experience and detached reflection, general and local knowledge, insights travel in both directions.

Toward the goal of building an experience-near perspective into pediatric ethics, I immersed myself in various pediatric settings as part of my research for this book. In 1993, I observed a pediatric primary care provider's daily practice in a small town setting. Later in 1993, and in 1997–98, I entered into the world of two pediatric intensive care units, in the Midwest and on the East Coast, respectively, seeking to acquaint myself with questions and issues that arise in acute care settings. In the Midwest, I made rounds for five weeks with attending physicians and residents at a city hospital and in a pediatric burn unit. This experience led me to write an article that commented on professional practices and identities, and the challenges of coordinating care in theaters of tragedy.[18] On the East Coast, I spent a year in a large children's research hospital, where I participated in that hospital's ethics committee; made rounds in its intensive care unit (ICU); initiated numerous conversations with physicians, nurses, chaplains, counselors, parents, and patients; and discussed some of my ideas and arguments with hospital personnel.

I immersed myself in these settings on the premise that ethnographic experience would open a range of perspectives and illness narratives that are typically bleached out of bioethical writing. The most important and instructive context was the East Coast children's hospital. In this work, I will refer to several cases and conversations that draw from my research in that hospital, to which I have assigned the pseudonym Baylin Pediatric Medical Center. That pseudonym is meant to provide confidentiality of patients and professionals there. In fact, I have revised the identities and names of all persons whom I interviewed for this book, with one exception: Joyce Roush, the first nondirected organ donor on record, who provided explicit permission to disclose her identity.

As a participant observer for six months in Baylin's ICU, I arose early each morning, took two long bus rides across town, and found myself sitting in conference rounds at 8:00 A.M., those rounds providing a ten-minute organizational prelude to medical rounds in the ICU. Making rounds in the ICU lasted forty-five minutes to two and a half hours as I accompanied an attending physician (rotating biweekly), a clinical fellow, a collection of residents (rotating monthly), nurses, respiratory therapists, and other specialists who tracked the daily developments of each medical patient on the floor. It was a grueling, nightmarish regimen. In addition to observing children who were suffering from near drowning, attempted suicide, tonicoclonic seizures, cystic fibrosis, AIDS, severe cardiac distress, parental abuse, or genetic illnesses that impaired their mental or motor capacities, I was quickly forced to decode changes in a patient's condition by interpreting information about bilirubin levels, heart rates, electrolyte levels, tidal volumes, fluid retention, blood gases, lung mechanics, neurological activity, pain control, reactions to medications, renal function, necrotizing digits, red and white blood cell counts, sodium levels, bowel sounds, infection status, and antibiotic regimens—data often communicated through brief acronyms and in-house jargon. After rounds, I typically sought solitude to gain some perspective on all that I had absorbed, to grapple with my own anguish and grief, and to make sense of my notes before returning to the ICU with a veneer of composure in order to interview parents or speak with house staff about how a patient or family was faring.

With this participant observation, I hoped to probe the more fine-grained features of professional and patient experience—to work my way into the interstices of everyday life in medical contexts—in order to see how affected persons cope with chronic or acute problems. I wanted to know, among other things, what personal, religious, and cultural resources professionals and families rely on to address the challenges of childhood illness, trauma, and suffering. With that knowledge, I presumed, I could then chart the intimate geography of pediatric medical ethics, commenting on real persons, concrete circumstances, and the actual idioms that inform personal experience and professional practice. One aim was to develop a reflexive ethnography for medical ethics, a form of social criticism that pays close attention to moral particulars by coordinating ethnographic study in medical settings with insights from recent developments in casuistry and interpretation theory.

That aspiration was only partly fulfilled. In the process of immersing myself in specific medical contexts, I came to discover that ethnography does not guarantee attention to particularity. In fact, my immersion led me to discover some enormous differences between adult and pediatric medical ethics. I have mentioned several of those differences in this Introduction: the need for an approach that subsumes, but goes beyond, the language of rights; the fact that the patient is a dependent member of a social institution (the family), with its own conditional authority in decision making; and the need for adults (parents and professionals) to adjust to children's increased competence and maturity as they move from infancy to late adolescence and the age of majority. Perhaps most notable is the fact that medical professionals in the field of pediatrics act with fewer presumed limits on their commitment to care than is typically the case in adult contexts. As I have suggested, what medical ethicists understand as the tension between beneficence and autonomy plays itself out in terms that are quite different from the paradigm of adult medical care. In many ways, the "pediatric patient as person" only faintly resembles the patient who is presumed in adult settings. My immersion led to a grand epiphany about how and to what extent pediatrics differs from adult medical care, leading to an epistemological shift in my research and reflection. In addition to moving through some of the interstices of professional experience and patient suffering, I came to the conclusion that an alternative framework is needed for thinking about social responsibility in pediatric medical ethics.

This book is, in part at least, an attempt to articulate and develop the various transformations I underwent during my ethnographic research. Clinical immersion, I came to discover, does not only (or perhaps primarily) allow for an intimate geography of everyday life. It rather holds the promise of transforming the researcher, affecting a researcher's patterns of seeing and hearing. That transformation may involve either large or small epiphanies. Expecting only the latter, I experienced both.

In what follows, I hope to coordinate two sets of insights—local and general knowledge, and small and grand revelations—about the proper medical care of children. As I have indicated, my attention to local knowledge led to a grand epiphany about children, social responsibility, and medicine. My more general ideas are found in Chapters 2 to 5, often in connection with practical cases. In those chapters, I develop *practical moral contours* for pediatric medical ethics. There, I attempt to lift up and refine core features of pediatric role morality, providing voice and reason to what children's care providers invoke when expressing "common complaint" about professional and parental practice.[19] Those chapters are followed by a more direct discussion of *cases* in Chapters 6 to 10, in which I move closer to the ground of professional and lay experience. Although this book is not a work of sociology or anthropology in any strict sense, it aims to coordinate an ethics-distant and ethics-near approach in ways that I hope take us beyond the limits of each, drawing on multiple discourses in ethics, law, religion, political theory, and philosophy. Moving in the intermediate space between distant and near perspectives, I aim to develop a critical idiom that is connected to the lived world of pediatric care, drawing on and refining convictions of which care providers are (sometimes unconsciously) aware.

That said, I should note an idiomatic oddity of which I am aware: The language of "alliance" as it appears throughout this book has political resonances, somewhat foreign to biomedical ethics and to the moral culture of pediatric care. Yet in my view, we can draw valuable insights from political theory when thinking about the social and institutional worlds of children, ethics, and modern medicine. Thus I will draw on political philosophy in ways that are atypical for medical ethics. John Rawls and Michael Sandel inform my treatment of social responsibility, rights, liberty, and equality in medical contexts; Hanna Pitkin provides the parameters of my account of representation and proxy consent; Dennis F. Thompson and Amy Gutmann instruct my views of democratic deliberation in institutional settings. The ideas of Charles Taylor and Michael Walzer, though less pronounced, cast light on how to consider respective problems of recognition and intervention when treating children and families. What should emerge from this mix is a moral poetics that is political—or, stated differently, a politically informed approach to the moral culture of pediatric care. Drawing on political theory in this way, I hope to provide terms for liberal social criticism about biomedicine and social responsibility toward persons who are young and sick.

A penultimate word of introduction: The idea of moving in the intermediate space between an ethics-near and an ethics-distant approach seems to suggest that this book will draw on partial, contextual thinking, often associated with an "ethics of care," in dialectical relation with impartial, detached thinking, typically associated with an "ethics of justice." But I will resist the parallels between contextuality and care, on the one hand, and impartiality and justice, on the other.[20] That is because care should be seen in more robust, theoretical ways. In Chapter 2, I will thus argue that there is a general duty to care, a duty that presupposes but goes beyond justice, and that this duty must be understood apart from contextual, embedded formulations of care.

———

Drawing on local and general knowledge and on small and grand ethnographic epiphanies does not permit a crisp methodological formula for bioethical writing. It rather involves procedures that are more artistic than scientific, more interpretive than formulaic. I will begin the next chapter with a few remarks about the importance of that idea for biomedical ethics, developing what I call a moral poetics as a necessary ingredient in the healer's art.

Another goal in the next chapter is to address the existential challenge of dealing with sick children, focusing on how illness assaults not only the body, but also identity and personal relationships. In the care of infirm children, those assaults invite not only a philosophical analysis of rights and responsibilities, but a religious analysis of love, loss, and human vulnerability. Even in the best of family circumstances, pediatric care is a cause of anguish, dread, and grief. Those features of a patient's or family's experience of illness are frequently omitted in medical ethics, whatever its methodology might be, and it is my wish to begin this book by considering them.

Part I

MORAL
CONTOURS

ONE

Parental Responsibility in Fear and Trembling

MORAL POETICS AND THE HEALER'S ART

When Adrienne St. Jacques left her home in Lucian Heights one clear, cold January morning, the easier part of her day was over. She had dressed and fed two of her children and sent them off to school. Her husband, Michael, was out the door and heading for work, not to return until after dinner. Adrienne's thoughts about a job for herself would have to be put aside, at least for the time being. She would inquire about the listing for a nurse's aide later in the month. For now, it was time to go to see her infant son, Jean, a patient in the intensive care unit (ICU) at Baylin Pediatric Medical Center. She checked her purse for her small Bible, found a subway token, and headed downtown.

Jean lay atop a small metal stand, tiny, frail, and asleep, surrounded by a coterie of nurses, respiratory therapists, residents, fellows, and an attending physician, all of whom were monitoring his medications, feedings, metabolism, blood flow, and ventilation. When he was born in September, Jean was two months premature and weighed less than two pounds. After staying for eight weeks in a neonatal ICU, Jean went home for twenty-eight days before his pulmonary system was attacked by a virus, sending him to Baylin's ICU in January with respiratory problems. He was soon placed on extracorporeal membrane oxygenation (ECMO) that extracted his blood and sent it through an oxygenating filter before returning it to his body. For more than two weeks, Jean was unconscious, heavily sedated, and connected to ECMO, an IV, and numerous monitors. His first X-rays showed diminished lung fields, a condition that slowly (and unexpectedly) improved. After eighteen days, Jean's hose-size tubes became infected with fungus, and he developed a clot in his inferior vena cava. Worried that the ECMO was allowing the fungus to grow, house staff switched Jean to a high-rate oscillating ventilator to keep his weak lungs open. He quickly began to show signs of improvement. Within a week, he was placed on a conventional ventilator, his feedings were increased, and he was briefly taken off antibiotics.

"I come here every day," Adrienne says slowly and methodically in her thick French-Haitian accent. "You cannot not come. Definitely you have to come. But you don't know who you are anymore. You cannot say anything. You lose your faith. You are not conscious. I just come and face the situation. I open the Bible to whatever passage is there. It gives me hope and I can see Jean is getting better. I want God to give me my son back. To listen to me, to answer me. The doctors and nurses are doing a very great job. Jean is in their hands. I ask them to give me my son back. My hope for Jean, I would like to have him back. Back home sleeping with him, feeding him, playing with him. I want him back the same way as before."[1]

Throughout his stay in the ICU, Jean's condition remained precarious. His nutritional situation left his bones so brittle that his hip and shoulder were fractured on separate occasions during routine examinations. Moreover, house staff feared that removing ventilation support would require him to burn up much-needed calories in his attempt to breathe, thereby diminishing his low body weight. Adrienne and Michael were routinely confronted with bad news: Jean did not do well on ECMO; his bowel appeared to be necrotizing at one juncture; his blood oxygen levels dropped during the early stages of conventional ventilation; he spiked a temperature immediately after coming off antibiotics, suggesting an underlying immune deficiency, a nagging infection, or both; and, it was (wrongly) suspected, he contracted renal tubular acidosis, a condition in which the kidneys are unable to excrete the normal amount of the body's acid, leading to an excess level of acid in the bloodstream. It would be months and perhaps years before anyone would know whether or how much Jean had been neurologically compromised by his ECMO treatment.

Adrienne was not a blind optimist about her son's circumstances or about those working on his behalf. Early in Jean's admission, house staff implicated her in his situation. "In the first week, they asked me to take the HIV test. That made me very, very angry. I was insulted. I have never been with any man but my husband. You know, no other man. We meet in Haiti. I had to tell him, they ask me the test. They think Jean maybe has HIV from me. So I sleep on it and say okay. The test, it turn up negative. I say to you, you are never ready. You cannot prepare yourself for this. I had two other children premature. One left the hospital at four pounds, the other five pounds. Before, I thought I was a mother. But I did not become a mother until I had Jean. I was not a mother until now.

"In my country," she added, "it is bad luck if you have a dream about marriage when a family member is sick. When Jean came here [to Baylin], I had a dream of getting married, and the man goes to another church. I grabbed him and go to that other church, too. [After the dream:] Then, the next day, I know I'm going to lose my baby. I put everything away. I called the Salvation Army to give away my crib. Then I talk to the priest. He say God is going to give Jean back, that my dream means something different [here] than in my country. He say that God is creator. He [God] build his home for him [Jean]. Now I have more hope. Jean has been different since then."

Adrienne's remarks emphasize the importance of diagnosing and coordinating a child's care within the interstices of parental anguish, cultural and ethnic heritage, and religious tradition. Health care providers must not only treat a patient's disease, but also attend to personal and social context as these bear on the patient's medical condition. In this respect, pediatric contexts can be demanding, for they require health care providers to work with children and with those who are responsible for making medical decisions in their child's basic interests.

That is to say, proper medical care of children is guided not only by moral norms and the skill to connect them to experience. Equally important, medicine requires the healer's art, the ability to understand how illness assaults a patient's and family's identity, affecting their rhythms, hopes, self-understandings, and interpersonal relationships.[2] For pediatric care providers, the healer's art includes skills of discerning how well a patient is coping with the challenge of illness, and how family members are shouldering the weight of decision-making responsibilities regarding their child's well-being. Those decisions often take place in the context of disappointment, self-blame, cultural and ethnic pluralism, and indeterminacy about future outcomes.

The healer's art, among other things, is a diagnostic talent, an excellence of discernment and discriminating judgment. It is a metavirtue, a "virtue of virtues," on which sound professional practice relies. The art of caring for others is a nonformalized skill, not easily distilled into principles or recipes for action. Accordingly, it is shaped less by well-wrought procedures than by symbols and images that illumine how health care providers ought to care for patients and families as persons. Images and symbols inform professionals' perceptions of clients and contexts; they enable practitioners to interpret a patient's overall condition, thereby assisting in diagnosis and treatment.

I want to devote this chapter to thinking in symbolic and imagistic terms, recognizing that such an approach stands somewhat apart from the more straightforward philosophical arguments that will follow in this book. I will do that out of the conviction that medical ethics must aim not only to provide guidelines for policy and action, but also to articulate the healer's art. That is to say, there are matters of *seeing* moral reality in a certain way that are important for ethical action and reflection. Medical ethics thus requires a moral poetics—the art of configuring experience so as to highlight its morally relevant features, existential challenges, cultural variables, and, when relevant, its religious dimensions. The healer's art is informed by the ethicist's moral art and the need to inform the imagination.

The symbols and images to which I will turn come from a religious tale, the story of Abraham and Isaac, aspects of which I want to discuss here with an eye to the moral poetics of pediatric care. Widely known outside the Jewish and Christian communities in which it is regularly narrated, this controversial story seems wildly irrelevant to issues that are associated with medical care in general and pediatric medicine in particular. I will address those reservations in passing as we proceed in this chapter. For now, I want to focus on a feature of that narrative that provides an important backdrop for imagining the ordeals that parents such as Adrienne often face when confronted by their child's infirmity. Indeed, these challenges are so important and profound that they invite religious interpretation. Norms and paradigms for pediatric medical ethics I subsequently develop in this book are framed by the poetics of parental responsibility that is exercised in fear and trembling.

As told in Genesis 22, the story of Abraham and Isaac is as follows:

God tested Abraham. He said to him, "Abraham!" And he said, "Here I am." He said, "Take your son, your only son Isaac, whom you love, and go to the land of Moriah, and offer him there as a burnt offering on one of the mountains that I shall show you." So Abraham rose early in the morning, saddled his donkey, and took two of his young men with him, and his son Isaac; he cut the wood for the burnt offering, and set out and went to the place in the distance that God had shown him. On the third day Abraham looked up and saw the place far away. Then Abraham said to his young men, "Stay here with the donkey; the boy and I will go over there; we will worship, and then we will come back to you." Abraham took the wood of the burnt offering and laid it on his son Isaac, and he himself carried the fire and the knife. So the two of them walked on together. Isaac said to his father Abraham, "Father!" And he said, "Here I am, my son." He said, "The fire and the wood are here, but where is the lamb for a burnt offering?" Abraham said, "God himself will provide the lamb for a burnt offering, my son." So the two of them walked on together. When they came to the place that God had shown him, Abraham built an altar there and laid the wood in order. He bound his son Isaac, and laid him on the altar, on top of the wood. Then Abraham reached out his hand and took the knife to kill his son. But the angel of the LORD called to him from heaven, and said, "Abraham, Abraham!" And he said, "Here I am." He said, "Do not lay your hand on the boy or do anything to him; for now I know that you fear God, since you have not withheld your son, your only son, from me." And Abraham looked up and saw a ram, caught in a thicket by its horns. Abraham went and took the ram and offered it up as a burnt offering instead of his son. So Abraham called that place "The LORD will provide"; as it is said to this day, "On the mount of the LORD it shall be provided." (Gen. 22:1–14, NRSV).

The story of Abraham and Isaac is not instructive to the healer's art because pediatricians routinely encounter families who believe that God has commanded them to sacrifice their children. There is no parallel between parents who believe they have been divinely authorized to kill their child and parents who respond with care to their child's infirmity. Nor do I want to valorize an image of divine and human relations as patriarchal, hierarchical, and arbitrary; endorse a divine command morality that is morally offensive; or impute such beliefs to parents such as Adrienne. As Søren Kierkegaard reminds us in his classic midrash of this tale, *Fear and Trembling,* the trial of Abraham should not be interpreted literally.[3] Exactly how it ought to be interpreted to illumine situations such as Adrienne's involves several steps and disclaimers.

In Kierkegaard's mind, the story of Abraham and Isaac is a story about the trials of faith and commitment—about trusting powers and purposes that lie beyond human understanding. In large part, the story is about how God tests Abraham's faith. In addition, it raises issues of adult responsibility and care: What are Abraham's obligations toward Isaac? How is he properly to care for him as his father? How can he exercise the virtues and duties entrusted to him as Isaac's parent? To whom does Isaac finally belong, and where does Abraham fit in Isaac's life?

In response to God's command, Abraham acts "on the strength of the absurd,"[4] without calculating benefits and burdens to himself or to Isaac, and without doubting that God would not take Isaac from him. For Kierkegaard, Abraham represents the rare "knight of faith," a person who courageously hurls himself trustingly into a void of unknown and unconditional commitment, thereby expressing an "absolute commitment to the absolute." Abraham expresses a double movement: He is willing to give up Isaac in obedience to God, but he remains confident that he will not lose Isaac as his son. Kierkegaard contrasts Abraham's faith with that of other individuals, whom he calls "knights of infinite resignation"—persons who are willing to give up worldly inclinations and attachments, but who cannot believe that all things are possible, that our expectations are constrained by our own finitude, that it is possible to get Isaac back.[5]

Kierkegaard emphasizes Abraham's capacity for acting on unconditional terms, focusing on the religious psychology of commitment and trust. If taken literally, *Fear and Trembling* seems to encourage belief in miraculous intervention and supernaturalism (which is neither Kierkegaard's intention nor Adrienne's expectation). Later in this book, I will indicate why such a belief can run contrary to basic features of pediatric medical ethics and how it can lead to unwarranted decisions. Using Kierkegaard's language, we might say that sometimes it is necessary for pediatric care providers to enable knights of faith to become (only) knights of infinite resignation about their child's prospects. That fact points to other features of Abraham's (and Adrienne's) trial that I want to highlight here. Rather than enjoining trust in divine intervention or asking us to consider the ethics of child sacrifice, the story of Abraham and Isaac points to the tasks of parenthood and the existential gravity of making decisions, sometimes about life and death, on children's behalf.

To see this point, it is important to focus not on miraculous possibilities but on the fact that relinquishing one's child to another's powers, or recognizing that the child is beyond the reach of curative powers, enters parents and families into a void of indeterminacy and potential culpability in wrongdoing. At the very least, Abraham learns that his authority over Isaac is limited; Isaac's life is not for Abraham to dispose of as he wishes, for he would never have chosen to sacrifice him. But the limits on Abraham's authority are marked by his confrontation with an incomprehensible and hostile power. A medical midrash of Abraham and Isaac must attend to the fact that his parental responsibilities must confront powers of destruction that seem so arbitrary and absurd as to shatter any sense that the universe is benignly ordered. Both Abraham and Adrienne are forced to reckon with the basic question of theodicy: Is a world that allows the suffering of innocent children truly just? How is a parent to act in a universe that seems uncaring—indeed, malevolent? Abraham's duties to Isaac, like Adrienne's to Jean, are suddenly overpowered by contingencies whose magnitude is immeasurable. Except for the most routine pediatric examinations, any discussion of moral norms and practical reasoning in pediatric medicine must be framed by Abraham's challenge. When a child's welfare is seriously at risk, responsible parents such as Adrienne face decisions of Abrahamic proportions. And in the direst of situations, they must reckon with the unfathomable horror of losing a child.[6]

I realize that parental decision making about pediatric care often involves much more than acting or omitting action in life-and-death situations. Less dramatic, more quotidian examples than Abraham's or Adrienne's abound, especially in the context of primary care medicine. Decisions of Abrahamic proportions might describe the tragedies or triumphs of tertiary care medicine, but they obscure the more frequent though less controversial interactions between care providers and families in settings of lower intensity.

But if we focus narrowly or exclusively on the potentially sacrificial aspects of our biblical legend, we miss some of its broader (and more generalizable) features. The story of Abraham and Isaac is instructive to the healer's art not because Isaac's life is in imminent danger, but because the summons to Abraham is *alarming, particularizing, depersonalizing, and capricious* (perhaps macabre). Abraham's ordeal bears not only on his son's interests, but also on his own *identity.* His attachments are exposed as fragile and vulnerable to contingency. His encumbrances, crucial to his self-interpretation, are at risk. Let us consider these ideas.

MEDICAL MIDRASH

Noteworthy is the fact that the biblical tale begins with an alarming summons from without. Before God makes specific demands of Abraham, he alerts him and bids him to make his presence known. The challenge to Abraham comes as a surprise; he is unprepared. Among other things, God requires Abraham immediately to account for himself. He must surrender to God's demands and quickly modify his activity. The trial to which he will soon be subjected is entirely other; it has an alien agency that demands a response. Abraham is not in control of events or circumstances; he finds himself having to adjust his actions according to (prior) forces that act on him and Isaac.[7]

In addition to its alarming strangeness, the summons has a particularizing aspect. Both Abraham and his son are particularized, for they both are named. Abraham cannot remain one among others and, recognizing that fact, announces himself: "Here am I." Likewise, the boy is immediately specified as "your son, your only son Isaac." Neither Abraham nor Isaac is an anonymous figure. Their particularity is demarcated, their profiles delineated, by the summons from without.

Yet when we consider the ties between God, Abraham, and Isaac, this particularity has a paradoxical quality. God wants Abraham to sacrifice his firstborn son, a generic category into which Isaac happens to fall. Isaac's importance turns on being classified in this way. The strangeness of the summons and command penetrates a particular relationship, imposing terms that recast that relationship along general lines. God's command derives from cultic requirements that bind all within his care. In contrast, Abraham and Isaac address each other in terms of their specific kinship ties, as "my father" and "my son," implying a shared set of expectations that touch on them and them alone. Preference and partiality are expressed by the possessive. An asymmetry is palpable: To Abraham, Isaac is a son whom he loves, his only offspring; to God, Isaac is a firstborn son, like other firstborn sons offered up by other families in keeping with cultic duties.

This alarming and particularizing-yet-depersonalizing trial is also capricious: Abraham is selected for no apparent reason. He must experience the summons as arbitrary and inexplicable. Indeed, God's summons and subsequent command seem absurd. Before Genesis 22, we are told that Abraham and Sarah tried for years to conceive. Begetting and bearing Isaac occurred late in their lives and involved divine assistance. That God would now request Isaac's life cannot but seem manipulative and fickle.

Abraham's treatment of Isaac during his trial involves either blind faith that is subsequently vindicated or a paternalistic lie. When Isaac asks his father where the sacrificial lamb is, Abraham replies that God will provide the animal, thereby averting Isaac's attention from the ominous circumstances that surround them both. In either case—as a lie or an expression of faith—Abraham's reply is shaped by a beneficent commitment not to alarm Isaac. If Abraham is speaking a falsehood intending to deceive Isaac, he is acting so as not to harm his son. If Abraham is speaking out of faithful confidence that God will not take Isaac—the source of Kierkegaard's emphasis—then he is convinced that God will not require him to perform a harmful deed. In either case, Abraham's response to Isaac seems premised on a tacit understanding of Isaac's vulnerability and basic needs.

Finally, Abraham's identity and his experience of family are implicated in the trial. If Isaac is indeed to be sacrificed, then the family unit and Abraham's paternal role must change. Before the trial begins, Abraham is the father of Isaac in a family unit with Sarah. If he loses his son, his role as father in that unit will cease. Part of the story's force lies in the (final) divine decree not to place Abraham in such an unconsoling wilderness, a decree that may say less about the bountiful goodness of God than about God's realistic reckoning with the limits of human endurance.

Seen in this way, Abraham's trial provides a suggestive set of symbols to illumine the dramatic and quotidian contexts of pediatric medical care. The illness of a child is a dramatic summons to parents from without. They are called to respond to the alien and alarming agency of illness, which isolates them and their child; they are singled out from others and enter a journey of risk and sacrifice. Often they must leave home and rely on friends and families. Subsequently, even those allies might be left behind; other relationships may materialize. Parents experience the depersonalizing effects of illness, seeing an offspring's sickness plotted against medical data precisely when parents are challenged to become deeper and more attentive to their child's special needs. The capriciousness with which infirmity occurs—the fickleness of the social and genetic lottery—challenges any parent's sense of a benign cosmos. Parents' decisions must be informed first and foremost by a commitment to their child's basic interests. Whatever the outcome, the experience of the family itself, and the parents' identity within that family, are likely to undergo important transformations. Moreover, medical outcomes can seem ad hoc and capricious, requiring parents to arrange (and rearrange) their story and to ascertain its meaning in light of events that were unforeseeable at the outset.

Interpreted as a medical midrash, the story of Abraham and Isaac helps us understand the existential burdens that parents such as Adrienne face as they weigh treatment options for their children. Like Abraham, they are confronted by radical contingency and must respond to an emotionally vertiginous context of trust and uncertainty, hope and confusion. Adrienne and Abraham must ask themselves about the limits of the possible. How professional health care providers are to comport themselves in relation to such parents and families is a question that will dominate the rest of this book. As I shall emphasize throughout these pages, professional responsibility should protect the child's basic interest within the context of a therapeutic alliance with that child's family, constrained by considerations of fairness. Such responsibility must be exercised under the weight of a basic— and sometimes gigantic—human burden. Why there are countless Abrahams, Sarahs, and Isaacs in hospitals and clinics and is a question that I cannot answer. But that their history repeats itself in cases like Adrienne's and others is a fact with existential dimensions that we should not ignore.

Pediatric ethics and medical education that focus on proper procedures for producing therapeutic outcomes to the exclusion of parental trials is deficient. No less than Abraham, parents of sick children find themselves tested in ways that cut to the core of their identity. They are challenged to determine how best to care for persons who have had to trust them from the beginning. When a child is ill, parents are summoned not only to make the right decision on that child's behalf, but to endure a trial of faithfulness and trust while fighting anguish, uncertainty, and fatigue. Parental responsibilities to offspring seem infinite, their ordeals beyond description. The task of deciding about a child's fate rightly invites religious symbols not to generate hope in a God who is supernaturally present and who might intervene, or to solicit fear in a God who commands parental violence and abuse. Rather, those symbols illumine the fact that the challenge of exercising parental responsibility in the face of dark and mysterious forces, involving a love that has no measure or equivalent, cannot be easily fathomed according to conventional canons of philosophy or common morality. Parents of sick children, with their friends and loved ones, bear the weight of radical contingency. They remind all of us of our humanity, our vulnerability, and our limits.

Adrienne's remarks point to the emotional challenges of representing the interests of children, especially (but not only) when their prognoses change. She also reminds us about religious, ethnic, and cultural differences as they bear upon a parent's interactions with health care providers. In her case, cultural and racial differences led to a brief but deep personal injury, further complicating her trial in the ICU. Had she been an affluent white American parent instead of a black French-Haitian, it is unlikely that she would have been approached for an HIV test after the medical staff suspected that Jean had an immune deficiency. Parents' ordeals and the healer's art require medical professionals not only to ascertain the requirements of responsible decision making, but also to form a proper alliance with relevant parties in the context of cultural, ethnic, and religious differences.

Issues of religious and cultural pluralism are not illumined by our biblical tale, but they do not render it irrelevant. They expand and deepen the dimensions of a parent's ordeal. Such differences highlight the importance of identity and commitment in our everyday affairs, and they reveal how interactions with health care professionals touch on matters central to an individual's self-respect. In Adrienne's case, not only was her particularity as a black French-Haitian delineated in Jean's admission, it was briefly experienced as a liability. She was informed that she was not only Jean's mother, but a member of a (different) patient population.

As I have presented it, the challenge to Adrienne, like that to Abraham, bids us to concentrate on the demands of exercising parental responsibilities rather than on respecting children's rights. Reasons that are less religious than philosophical have led me to conclude that focusing on family and professional duties is the correct way to proceed when thinking about the ethics of pediatric care. Whatever rights a child may have correlate with the responsibilities of adults, but, as we shall see, some responsibilities of adults do not generate a specific set of children's rights. Focusing on parental and professional responsibilities draws a broader and more comprehensive outline for those who work with children and families. Exactly how we are to understand adults' duties toward children, and how those duties bear on the responsibilities of pediatric health care professionals, is the topic of the next chapter.

TWO

The Duty to Care

I strongly believe that at this end of life [children], there is far
less ambiguity about the appropriate place of medicine. That
makes me feel better about what I do. In most (but not all) cases
there's no debate about goals—to relieve children's suffering and
cure the child's disorder. If you can do that you don't know what
that kid will go on to do. That's really satisfying. When I was
with adults as a med student, they would say, "leave me alone." I
asked myself, what am I doing [with adults]? Medicine always
involves some discomfort to relieve suffering and attempt a cure.
You feel better about yourself at this end of life.
—*Dr. Michael DeVries, attending physician
in Baylin Pediatric Medical Center's Intensive Care Unit*[1]

I like to hug my patients. There's an extra level of care
that's possible with kids. You can't do that with adults.
—*Dr. Sarah Radford, a resident at Baylin*[2]

You can learn a lot about a culture by learning about
the people it marginalizes. Certainly children do not fare well
in America. . . . There's something in me that wants
to give children a shot at justice in the world. . . .
I'm committed to care of the family and of the vulnerable.
—*Rev. Charlene Dodson, head chaplain at Baylin*[3]

THE QUESTION OF CARE

Why should Abraham care for Isaac? Why should Adrienne care for Jean? Why should we care about the fates of these (and other) parents, or accept their claims to care for their dependent minors? In pediatrics, health care providers face similar questions: Why should medical professionals care about the welfare of families and children? Assuming that there is a basis for care, how should that care obligate parents who are presumably responsible for their children?

These queries about parental and professional obligation do not admit of obvious answers. Various religious traditions have approached such issues with reference to the command to love others, compassion for others, or role responsibility. Jews and Christians, for example, are admonished to love their neighbors as themselves, although each tradition exhibits considerable diversity about who counts as a neighbor, what it means to love oneself, how to rank and order love of different neighbors, what kinds of dispositions and actions count as loving, and whether it makes sense to speak of love as commanded.[4] However these issues are resolved, the love command implies the virtue of benevolence, a disposition to consider the well-being of others and to act on that disposition in appropriate circumstances. Buddhists hold up the ideal of compassion as a virtue that directs adherents to attend to the suffering of others and the general contingency of life.[5] Hindus regulate their lives according to the requirements of dharma, which involve duties within various social roles.[6] Muslims believe that adherents have duties to preserve, develop, and beautify God's creation, duties that include acting for others' welfare.[7] In all of these instances, emphasis falls on how religious believers are to attend to the needs of others, regardless of others' religious or cultural affiliations. Religions are often seen as encumbering their adherents with a sense of social responsibility, especially toward the vulnerable and needy.

For health care providers, professional practice is informed by the Hippocratic tradition, which appeals to patient welfare as a cardinal principle. The Hippocratic oath states, "I will apply dietetic measures for the benefit of the sick according to my ability and judgment; I will keep them from harm and injustice. . . . Whatever houses I may visit, I will come for the benefit of the sick, remaining free of all intentional injustice, of all mischief and in particular of sexual relations with both female and male persons, be they free or slaves."[8] Following the Hippocratic tradition, the Principles of Medical Ethics of the American Medical Association (1957) state, "The principal objective of the medical profession is to render service to humanity with full respect for the dignity of man. Physicians should merit the confidence of patients entrusted to their care, rendering to each a full measure of service and devotion."[9]

Venerable though these traditions are, they fail to indicate why persons who are not religious, who are not members of the medical profession, or who are not from mainstream religious backgrounds should care for others. That is, they do not provide a general basis for the duty to care. Often it is assumed that parents' and professionals' actions should be guided by the general requirement to care for others, but a rationale for that requirement is not obvious. Is there a duty to care? If so, how are we to care?

To clarify these matters, let us first consider the general obligation to care and then turn to specifications of that obligation for parents and pediatric health care providers. These considerations, although surely not exhausting pediatric medical ethics, provide broad parameters for understanding the challenges of adults' responsibility in pediatric contexts.[10] We will thus proceed, as Aristotle would say, "roughly and in outline" regarding the virtues and duties of care in parental and professional role morality.[11] With that general outline in place, we will turn to specific cases in the second section of this book.

CARE AS AN OBLIGATION

The responsibility to care for others, grounded in common morality rather than in religious teachings or professional oaths, derives from the Kantian rejection of indifference. To see this point, consider the opposite of care—namely, apathy toward others. Individuals who decline to care for others accept the value of indifference as a policy of action. In so doing, they deny themselves the care and beneficence of others, for it would be inconsistent to expect others to reject indifference while not rejecting it oneself. Herein lies the force of Kant's simple but profound principle of universalizability: A principle of action is unacceptable if I cannot will that it be a principle for all. Assuming that I will need assistance and care from others, I deny myself such resources by committing myself to indifference and neglect as a program of action. Only agents who are entirely invulnerable or self-sufficient can coherently embrace a life plan that neglects the needs of strangers; finite and vulnerable agents have no such license. Needy and incomplete, we depend on other persons and institutions for nurturance, support, and direction. Summarizing this line of argument, Onora O'Neill writes,

> No vulnerable agent can coherently accept that indifference and neglect should be universalized, for if they were nobody could rely on others' help; joint projects would tend to fail; vulnerable characters would be undermined; capacities and capabilities that need assistance and nurturing would not emerge; personal relationships would wither; education and cultural life would decline. . . . Those with limited and variable capacities and capabilities *must* plan to rely in various ways on one another's capacities and capabilities for action, so *must* (if committed to universalizable inclusive principles) be committed to doing at least something to sustain one another's capacities and capabilities, hence committed to rejecting inclusive principles of indifference and neglect.[12]

Given that nobody is self-sufficient, persons who are indifferent to others' needs act inconsistently. They make exceptions of themselves, imposing expectations on others that they refuse to adopt on others' behalf. Indifferent persons deny goods to others that they expect for themselves, given the conditions of finitude in which all action occurs. In this way, Kant provides a basis for making sense of our interdependence and for judging indifferent persons as selfish.

Conceived in these Kantian terms, the responsibility to care is premised on a version of the Golden Rule: Do unto others as you would have others do unto you. Assuming, as is reasonable, that I rely on the caring actions of others, it would be unfair to refuse to act toward others in caring ways, leaving them vulnerable to danger or harm while relying on deeds or institutions that enable me to avoid danger or harm. The duty to care, in short, is a function of justice, broadly conceived. Beneficent action is a requirement of fairness, encumbering me with the duty to care for others as I am cared for, and hope to be cared for, by others. If I fail to do unto others as others have done unto me, then I selfishly absent myself from patterns of reciprocity on which social life relies.

Thus, there is a general responsibility to care for others, premised on (1) the principle of universalizability and (2) the fact of vulnerability and dependence in all human agency. Still, this line of argument does not tell us for whom to care or what counts as caring activity. As such, it is what Kant calls an *imperfect duty,* for it fails to specify how and when it is to be deployed. An imperfect duty defines a norm of character, a general disposition toward others and the world. It refers to the virtue of benevolence, which requires further specification to determine proper acts and recipients of beneficence.

At the very least, however, this duty helps to address some of my opening questions about caring for those whose welfare is at risk and provides a critical norm for assessing our loyalties, loves, and dispositions. The absence of benevolent dispositions marks a weakness of moral character, an exceptionalist attitude, an inconsistent program of action of dependent and vulnerable agents. Those who fail to order their affections and attachments toward the good of others are morally diminished; they are unable to recognize the neediness that accompanies our common humanity. Conversely, persons with benevolent dispositions understand something that is basic to our nature: We rely on the kindness of each other in our various quests for growth and self-discovery. Love and care are not always acts of supererogation, but flow from the character of persons who recognize the ubiquity of human finitude.

Moreover, and equally important, this responsibility helps us understand how we have obligations that do not neatly correlate with others' rights. Obligations to others as matters of character do not entail a specific set of claims recipients. Determining exactly who is to benefit from our dispositions depends on additional moral and practical considerations.

Seeking to clarify these matters, O'Neill distinguishes between duties in terms of their *structure* and in terms of their *proper scope.* Following Kant, O'Neill draws the structural distinction between perfect and imperfect obligations. Perfect obligations hold between obligated parties and identifiable recipients. Imperfect obligations, as we have seen, impose duties on individuals without entailing identifiable recipients. Moreover, perfect and imperfect duties are to be distinguished in terms of their proper scope: There are universal duties, owed to all persons, and special duties, owed more narrowly to specific persons within domestic, professional, or other institutional arrangements. Bringing these categories together, we have four sets of obligations: perfect universal and special duties, and imperfect universal and special duties. Understanding these obligations enables us to proceed from the general duty to care to a more focused conception of parental and professional responsibilities toward children.

A perfect universal duty includes all persons within its range of identifiable recipients. For example, each owes to all the prima facie duty not to injure others. This duty obligates all persons in relation to everyone. A perfect special duty is also a duty that has identifiable recipients, but not everyone. Unlike a perfect universal duty, it can be discriminating, for it relies on background practices and corresponding expectations that connect specific agents to specific recipients. In such cases, specific recipients may rightly be said to be rights holders in the sense that they have justifiable claims on the actions of others. For example, the duty not to stigmatize gay and lesbian persons on the basis of sexual orientation includes identifiable persons as rights recipients and grows out of background practices and corresponding expectations that derive from the values of dignity and equality.

Imperfect duties, in contrast, are obligations that do not correlate to identifiable recipients. Such obligations, as I have said, pertain to dispositions of character and require individuals to be prepared to exercise such virtues in certain contexts. An imperfect universal duty refers to an obligation owed by each but not to all; its specific recipients remain unidentified. Such duties, as O'Neill points out, can best be understood as "required virtues," embodied in agents' characters.[13] An imperfect special duty likewise involves dispositions or character traits, but within role relationships. Thus, like perfect special duties, this duty can be discriminating, but it is less specific. Imperfect special duties are best understood as preferential loves: They generate caring dispositions regarding the needs and wants of specific persons within role or other institutional relationships. Warmth or affection in the family is an imperfect special duty. It defines a character trait within roles and relationships, but it does not specify how and in what circumstances an individual should act warmly or affectionately toward family members.

As I have characterized it, the responsibility to care is an imperfect universal duty. It is owed by each (thus it is universal) but not to anyone in particular (thus it is imperfect). A stranger on the street does not have a right to my beneficence, however much we all ought to be benevolently disposed. I would have a deficient character if I were not a benevolent person, but that does not mean that I must give of myself to everyone.

Parental duties to children, however, are more than an imperfect universal obligation; they involve perfect and imperfect special obligations. That is because, as we shall see more fully below, parents typically adopt roles according to social conventions in our culture that presuppose a special relationship between them and their children. Parents' perfect duties involve the responsibility to assure the welfare of their children, to satisfy an appropriate standard of care within the opportunities and constraints afforded by the natural and social lottery. Children have corresponding rights to protection and well-being that must be assured by their caretakers.[14] Further, parents have imperfect obligations that ought to inform family life. In liberal, Western culture, for example, parents who are unable to provide an affectionate, reliable, and trustworthy environment for their children may be able to satisfy some of their perfect obligations, but they lack the traits that caring individuals exhibit as matters of virtuous character.

CARE AS A SPECIAL DUTY

Given children's cognitive, psychological, and physical deficiencies and vulnerabilities, they cannot be presumed to care for themselves. Generally incapable of protecting their basic interests, they depend on others to guard their claims and needs, and that charge typically falls on parents, relatives, or guardians. The main idea is that family life generates special duties, both perfect and imperfect. Yet the rationale for that idea is not altogether obvious. How is it that some persons encumber themselves with special duties to care for children? What justifies us in imposing such moral expectations on parents or guardians?

In modern Western cultures, it is generally assumed that individuals take on parental responsibilities because they consent to do so. Individuals who beget children assign responsibilities to themselves by agreeing to adopt the role of caretaker. Persons who have conceived but who decide against parenting may either abort or place the child up for adoption. (I will not discuss the ethics of abortion here. I will assume its availability.) Biological parents of a child are not obligated to raise that child.

However, this liberty does not mean that duties to children are entirely a matter of parental whim, or that consent to rear a child is sufficient to ground the duty to rear a child. Parents who refuse to consent to rear a child nonetheless have a duty to make reasonable efforts to ensure that child's welfare. Parents who commit infanticide or who abandon their children commit a deep moral wrong. Moreover, that wrong must be understood as a breach of *parental* obligation. Appeals to consent alone do not capture the basis for parental responsibility or help us evaluate parents who beget but decline to raise their offspring. The critical question is how the commitment to raise children can be justified, and how we are to understand the implications of that justification for those individuals who beget children but decide not to raise them. In either case (raising or not raising), responsibilities require assessment at a second-order level. That assessment, in turn, enables us to understand why, morally speaking, some parents act rightly by encumbering themselves with special duties to their children, and why those who do not assume the role of caretakers nonetheless have other obligations that relate to the welfare of their offspring.

Duties of rearing can be rendered intelligible by turning to John Rawls's argument on behalf of paternalistic principles in *A Theory of Justice*. Those principles are situated within Rawls's more comprehensive project of producing principles of justice that presume neither a common vision of morality nor an antecedent order of being against which to measure particular institutions or social arrangements. Instead, for Rawls, principles of justice must be constructed by participants within a hypothetical situation in which they conceive of principles that will constrain the distribution of primary goods and shape the design of political and social institutions. Central to this theory is the aim of producing moral principles that do not privilege any particular class or group of persons, or valorize features of social life that are a function of the natural or social lottery. The goal, in brief, is to produce principles of fairness in the design of social institutions that do not favor hereditary advantages. The central device for the construction of such principles is the hypothetical "veil of ignorance," behind which persons are asked to conceive of principles of justice without knowing who they will be or how they will be situated once the veil is lifted and their "real" stations in society are revealed. They will not know their conception of the good, their race, gender, generation, or place in society. The imaginative place that is created by imposing this veil is what Rawls calls the "original position." That position requires impartiality of participants, thereby preventing them from crafting principles that would favor the positions they are to occupy, or advance their prejudices and hereditary advantages vis-à-vis others.

Within this account, Rawls delineates what he calls "principles of paternalism."[15] These principles are norms that would be derived by participants within the original position to direct the fair treatment of persons whose will or reason is compromised, and who need assistance from others. As with Kant and O'Neill, with Rawls considerations of vulnerability inform the construction of moral norms, however much Rawlsian liberalism might seem incapable of including considerations of finitude and dependence.[16] He writes,

The principles of paternalism are those that the parties would acknowledge in the original position to protect themselves against the weakness and infirmities of their reason and will in society. Others are authorized and sometimes required to act on our behalf and to do what we would do for ourselves if we were rational, this authorization coming into effect only when we cannot look after our own good. Paternalistic decisions are to be guided by the individual's own settled preferences and interests insofar as they are not irrational, or failing a knowledge of these, by the theory of primary goods. As we know less and less about a person, we act for him as we would act for ourselves from the standpoint of the original position. We try to get for him the things that he presumably wants whatever else he wants.[17]

With children, as we will see, the principles of paternalism imply the duty to provide primary goods, understood in terms of physical, intellectual, and emotional welfare; respect; and the right to an "open future."[18] For the moment, note that Rawls's argument functions to encumber those who beget children with obligations to act on the child's behalf. The core idea is as follows: If we are to construct principles of fairness without knowing our social position, age, or gender—behind the "veil of ignorance"—we would produce norms that would ensure that we were not abandoned if infirm or dependent once the veil has lifted and we learn about our actual position or condition in society. Those norms would guarantee that, as a matter of fairness, we would be treated in our actual circumstances according to principles that are rational and caring, aimed to protect our wishes, if possible, or our fundamental welfare. Behind the veil of ignorance, we would fashion principles that are intended to encumber others to care for the needs of the infirm or dependent.

We should note, however, that in order to produce principles of paternalism that are relevant to children, an important clarification to Rawls's theory is necessary. In Rawlsian liberalism, persons are owed just treatment according to principles derived behind the veil of ignorance only if they are moral persons, understood as persons with the capacity for a sense of justice and a capacity for developing a conception of the good as expressed in a rational plan of life.[19] For Rawls, participants in the original position do not know what their particular plan will be, but they *do* know that they will have one. Rawls's view of moral persons (or "moral personality") provides the baseline for his understanding of the equality of citizens. To be sure, this condition would nullify grounds for justly treating those who are severely retarded, as Donald VanDeVeer has trenchantly argued, for such persons obviously lack a capacity for a conception of the good as expressed in a rational plan of life.[20] But this idea would not undermine crafting principles that establish responsibilities to care for children and other needy persons with a capacity for a sense of justice and a conception of the good. Rawlsian liberalism is often viewed as applicable only to independent, autonomous subjects who have fully developed powers of self-determination. Such an interpretation overlooks Rawls's core agenda: to correct for the inequities that result from the accidents of the natural or social lottery—to protect persons who are disadvantaged by natural or social circumstances. Rawls goes to considerable length to say that civic equality relies on minimal capacities, which can include the case of infants and children. Moral personality refers to the *capacity* for a sense of justice and a conception of the good, but that capacity need not be realized in order for the duties of justice to apply.[21]

Situated behind a veil of ignorance (clarified in this way), participants would be motivated to construct principles of fairness that would ensure that those whose reason or will is underdeveloped owing to relative youth would not suffer from neglect as a result of their circumstances. Although Rawlsian liberalism is conceived largely with adults in mind, it can produce principles that can be more inclusive and egalitarian in their protective scope, including children whose capacities are undergoing development.

Clarified in this way, Rawls's principles of paternalism can encompass the case of young persons as needy and dependent. Children are owed duties of justice (and care) not in spite of, but *because* they are not independent, freestanding, and autonomous. As regards parents' duties to their offspring, my interest here is to note that the principles of paternalism and their corresponding responsibilities bear on groups who decide to raise their children as well as those who do not. Members of the former group are to provide children with goods that children need whatever else they would want. Members of the latter group are similarly obligated. Their decision not to raise their child does not free them from the responsibility to arrange for that child's well-being. At a minimum, parents are not free to perform infanticide or to abandon their children. They are morally required to seek a home or setting in which the children's needs can be provided for or protected. They are free not to raise their children, yet they are responsible for making reasonable efforts to ensure the subsequent welfare of their children. The principles of paternalism require that parents make reasonable efforts to provide either first-party or second-party care of their offspring.

It is sometimes thought that Rawls's theory of justice is premised on an account of what Michael Sandel calls "unencumbered selves," a view of persons who are free to choose their ends regardless of roles, received traditions, or relationships.[22] Rawls's account of the principles of paternalism, properly refined to cover the treatment of children, shows that this accusation can mislead. Parents encumber themselves with special duties to their children. They do so not as a matter of consent alone, but by virtue of principled constraints on choice to which reasonable persons behind the veil of ignorance would agree.[23]

Issues of parental custody and responsibility are often understood to be a function of consent rather than biology, because being a biological parent does not obligate an individual to raise a child. But if my account of Rawls is correct, it is only partially (and unhelpfully) true to say that individuals assign themselves duties of parenthood owing to consent rather than biology. It is more accurate to say that our understanding of parental responsibilities needs to be reframed in terms that avoid the consent/biology dichotomy. Individuals discharge duties to ensure the welfare of a child in one of two ways: by conceiving, bearing, and consenting to raise the child according to paternalistic principles; or by begetting and releasing their child to another's presumably reliable care. In either case, the principles of paternalism obligate those who beget children to arrange to meet the fundamental needs of their offspring. Taken alone, consent is not sufficient to ground the moral encumbrances of parenthood. Such consent can be fleeting and ad hoc, leaving the child vulnerable to the notorious vagaries of parental commitment. Adults' consent must be constrained by principles that reasonable people would agree to follow, principles that are produced in the design of fair institutions. What Rawls calls the principles of paternalism aim to enshrine such protective responsibilities, thereby providing a second-order justification of care as a special responsibility of parents to children.

What does this argument mean for couples who conceive a child unintentionally? What of instances in which couples conceive owing to faulty contraception, or cases of rape or incest from which conception results? In such cases, the generation of life is involuntary. Arguments that are premised on the idea that parents incur parental duties (only) voluntarily in a social contract are unable to require couples to discharge parental responsibilities to their unwanted offspring, for conception occurred contrary to the couple's will.[24] But Rawls's principles of paternalism function more rigorously than liberal social contract theory might suggest. Individuals or couples who bring a fetus to term obligate themselves to seek the infant's welfare, at least to the extent of finding a second party to care for that child. The child's well-being is not entirely a matter of parental volition; volition must be constrained by principles of fairness that are constructed to protect the interests of vulnerable persons.

PEDIATRIC ROLE MORALITY: JUSTICE AND MEDIATED BENEFICENCE

Thus far, I have argued that each person has a general obligation to care, understood as a universal imperfect duty. Parents have special duties that ought to constrain their decisions regarding their offspring. Later I will provide content to such duties in terms of the rights and virtues they generate.

For the moment, we should consider how these general responsibilities bear on the role morality of pediatric health care providers.

Like parental obligations, the duties of health care professionals are examples of special duties, and they divide into perfect and imperfect categories. They are special because they arise in specific social and institutional arrangements, generating a set of expectations from identifiable children and families. Perfect duties benefit identifiable recipients who have claims to an appropriate standard of treatment. Imperfect duties include the responsibility to produce an ethos of trust, comfort, and care, a commitment not only to heal the patient's infirmities, but to do so with grace and affection. In pediatric role morality, then, the general responsibility to care is specified in two ways: first, in acts of beneficent treatment toward children and families; and second, in virtues of character that convey trustworthiness and warmth. Patients and families who receive beneficent acts outside an ethos of benevolent care have been morally shortchanged.

However, the duties of health care providers relate to those of parents in complicated ways. At one level are the virtues and duties of justice, and these are of several kinds. Most fundamentally, there is the duty of commutative justice, the obligation to discharge goods and services according to contractual agreements between the family and the health care institution. This is an obvious point that I will not discuss further.

The second kind of justice is more amorphous and can be the source of moral conflict between care providers and families. By seeking to improve the health of children, medical professionals work to remove disadvantages owing to the social and natural lottery. Providing health care resources is, among other things, a fundamental feature of liberal justice. One aim is to treat the physical, emotional, intellectual, and psychiatric needs of infirm or disadvantaged children, needs that, left untreated, would produce inequalities that are arbitrary from a moral point of view. By treating children's physical or psychological infirmities, health care practitioners work to increase their access to a fair share of opportunities in society. The underlying idea is that leaving individuals to suffer the fate of social and natural circumstances is unjust, for it allows society to say that individuals' nature or inherited social context is their enduring misfortune. It seems intuitively unfair for individuals to be advantaged or disadvantaged owing to social or natural circumstances for which they are not responsible.[25] Although health care may not aim to transform individuals into new persons, it works in part to nullify what Rawls aptly calls "the accidents of natural endowment and the contingencies of social circumstances."[26]

In addition to duties of commutative and distributive justice, and perhaps better capturing the actual motivations of health care providers, is the commitment to care, enshrined in the virtue of benevolence and the norm of beneficence. These ideas inform professional oaths that are both venerable and modern, and set general priorities in what I have called the pediatric paradigm. Like the norm of justice, the norm of beneficence is a special perfect duty, arising in the interactions between professionals and identifiable persons who come to them for comfort and care. Here, too, health care providers' relationships with families can become complicated, for adhering to beneficence may put care providers at odds with families, who are primarily responsible for their children.

Stated differently, the role morality of pediatric health care providers includes the commitment to justice and patient benefit, but these commitments can put professionals at odds with a child's family. Herein lies one complicating feature in the professional life of pediatric health care practitioners and the first reason for amending the pediatric paradigm: Professionals' role morality can clash with the respect for parental authority and family privacy, about which I will say more momentarily. Parents or guardians, not professionals, are presumed to be principally responsible for children, and honoring the various customs and practices according to which children are raised is one of the hallmarks of a free society. Pediatric role morality is complicated in ways that professional morality in the adult context typically is not, for pediatric care providers must coordinate their work with children, their families, and their own professional and moral sensibilities. That coordination renders care providers accountable to patients and their caretakers, who are presumably entrusted to act in their children's basic interest. Professionals' responsibility in the care of a child is thus a matter of mediated beneficence, requiring them to triangulate their duty to care with patients and their families.

Disagreements about what counts as the child's basic interest can be a source of considerable tension. I will return to such tensions below when we consider nonideal circumstances in which professional responsibility is carried out. For the moment, it is necessary to clarify some fundamental presumptions and priorities. Given that parents or guardians are presumed to be the child's primary caretaker, a health care provider's duty to care for children is mediated by parental obligations. Medicine should aim to complement and, if necessary, supplement a family's special duties of beneficence. Presumptively, this means that the aim of pediatric care is to form *therapeutic alliances* with children and their primary caretakers. These alliances are therapeutic in the obvious sense that they aim to heal the patients or, when only palliative measures are appropriate, to ease patients' pain. They are alliances in the sense that health care providers are summoned first to discharge their responsibilities in concert with those of the family. As a result, it is necessary for medical professionals to heed, at least presumptively, the demands of parental autonomy and family privacy.

PARENTAL AUTONOMY AND FAMILY PRIVACY

To focus ideas about respect for parental autonomy[27] in pediatric care, consider first some features of autonomy in the adult context. In what I have called the adult paradigm, respect for autonomy generally works as a side constraint on the exercise of patient care.[28] That means that patients have a right to refuse treatment, that they have negative rights of noninterference. (It does not mean, as I will argue in Chapter 4, that patients have positive rights—for example, the right to demand treatment that is not in their medical interest.) Autonomy is justified philosophically by the principle of respect for persons and the equality of all human beings. Accordingly, professionals may not place patients in positions of subordination or dependence; they must treat patients as persons who are equal.[29] In practical terms, physicians, nurses, and house staff are to seek the patient's benefit according to the informed consent of patients when they are competent. Informed consent enshrines a commitment to treat patients out of respect for their (equal) humanity. When a competent patient provides valid consent to or dissent from treatment, health care professionals are presumptively obligated to heed the patient's wishes. Moreover, physicians are not to conclude that patients are incompetent because they do not consent to standard medical treatment. An adult Jehovah's Witness who refuses potentially lifesaving blood products makes a decision that doctors are legally and morally obligated to respect, however irrational that decision may seem from a medical point of view, unless that decision immediately puts another party (e.g., fetus at term) at risk. In adult contexts, respect for autonomy can mean, among other things, tolerating viewpoints that are medically unwise.

Whether and under what conditions a health care provider may override a patient's refusal in order to protect that patient's welfare is the topic of considerable debate among those who have sought to clarify how (for adults) respect for autonomy generally has priority to beneficence. James F. Childress argues, for example, that such acts are justified only when they promise clear benefit to a patient whose competence is compromised, in what is called "weak paternalism."[30] Others, such as Tom L. Beauchamp, argue that physicians can justifiably override the wishes of a fully competent patient if the issue is trivial—for example, elevating side bars alongside a postsurgical patient's bed, against that patient's competently stated wishes. For Childress, beneficence may override only compromised autonomy; for Beauchamp, beneficence may override uncompromised autonomy in trivial cases.[31]

However these specifics are resolved, debates in medical ethics about respecting adult autonomy are carried out on the prima facie assumption that autonomy constrains the professional's pursuit of beneficence. Overriding a patient's competent consent or dissent carries an enormous burden of proof. The effect has been to validate an ethos in medical care that is generally value-neutral and nondirective. Out of respect for patient autonomy, professionals are not to allow their religious or other comprehensive beliefs to intrude into their professional counseling of patients. To do so would compromise the decision-making authority of those who must bear the consequences of medical decisions.

Respecting parental autonomy and family privacy in pediatric care does not follow this pattern in its main contours, for these values should not be conceived on the model of treatment choice, respect for equality, and the presumptive requirement to tolerate medically irrational decisions. Rather, respect for parental autonomy and family privacy is a function of the prerogatives assigned to a social institution primarily responsible for the care of a child. As such, parental autonomy and family privacy are conditional in ways that adult autonomy is not. Parents may not make medically irrational decisions about the medical treatment of their children, for that would deny basic goods to offspring, contrary to the principles of paternalism and the special duties of care. The ethos of pediatric care should not be nondirective and value-neutral. Rather, the norm of patient benefit occupies a much larger role in pediatric than adult care, constraining the powers of parents and injecting into the professional ethos more expansive prerogatives in decision-making situations.

That is not to suggest, however, that parents' decisions are to be ignored or disrespected, that pediatricians should operate within an ethos of inequality and intolerance, or that medical professionals should disregard the requirements of informed consent. Rather, it means that the basis for respecting family privacy only vaguely resembles the adult model of respect for autonomy—that it is mistaken to conceive of pediatric role morality as the stepchild of the adult model of health care. In pediatrics, family privacy is to be heeded, at least presumptively, for five reasons, each of which reflects the demands involved in the special duties of parental care.

First is the intimacy reason. Given the increasingly impersonal, contractual, and institutional modes of interaction in social life, the family as an intimate association provides an important context in which individuals find meaning in their lives, experience affection, and transmit values across generations. As a source of love and unconditional care, the family is an important sphere of moral and psychological development. Moreover, families serve as foci for identification because family membership is premised on belonging rather than accomplishment; we typically relate positively to social arrangements that welcome us for who we are instead of what we have achieved. Because intimacy requires a good measure of privacy, professionals and other agents in society should be reluctant to attempt to control a family's decisions unless those decisions are clearly harmful to dependent minors. To intrude in the domestic sphere compromises the right to privacy, which is instrumental to protecting the conditions for young persons' growth, as well as their experience of care and protection. In this respect, family intimacy is necessary for children's well-being. Those who intervene must draw on those same reasons to justify their actions—childhood welfare—for they otherwise intrude in a realm in which they have no rightful authority.

Second is the epistemological reason: The family generally knows the child better than the health care professional and is in a better position to decide on the child's behalf. This knowledge includes more than information about the child's physical history or background; it includes aspects that derive from the intimacy reason. Parents and guardians know better than professionals about the values and priorities according to which the child is being raised. Intruding into a family's decision presumes a level of knowledge about the transmission of value that the health care provider usually cannot claim.

Third is the authenticity reason: The family is better off when its members are the principal decision makers. Taking decisions out of the hands of caretakers can be demeaning, for it suggests that medical experts are better than a child's primary caretakers at rendering good judgments. In general, parents care deeply about their children and know their needs better than strangers. Their knowledge and affection are legitimated, and potentially deepened, when they are assigned responsibility to decide on their children's behalf. When the family's commitments and affections are legitimated, in turn, the child's well-being is enhanced by the experience of family self-esteem. Heeding parental autonomy, in short, can contribute to a child's welfare.

Fourth is the fact that families play a central role in forming individual identity. We come to understand and interpret ourselves through the languages and thought-forms that are provided by a family and its cultural heritage. As a bearer of cultural or religious traditions, the family helps individuals develop their powers of reflection and choice against a background of meaningful options. Participation in family life helps to determine "the boundaries of the imaginable."[32] As persons develop, they adopt practices and forge self-understanding by drawing on family custom, value, and lore.[33]

A fifth reason turns on issues of freedom and responsibility. The family bears the financial and psychological burdens of making decisions on behalf of a child, and so should have considerable control of treatment choices. It would be unfair to encumber families with consequences of choices that they did not authorize or participate in making.

Seen in this way, there are good reasons for respecting parental autonomy and family privacy, reasons that produce a strong presumption against intervening in a family's decision-making process. Like the ethics of war, the ethics of children's medicine is constrained by a prima facie duty of nonintervention.[34] Families resemble sovereign states: They are presumptively free to define and order their domestic affairs. Decisions to intervene on behalf of a pediatric patient are not necessarily wrong, but they carry a heavy burden of proof.

Those who justify intervention should do so by remembering that the reasons for respecting family privacy are conditional: They presuppose the family as the unit principally responsible for the child's welfare. Simply stated, domestic privacy is to be respected insofar as it meets the criterion of protecting the basic interests of the child. The first four reasons presuppose this criterion directly, and the fifth does so indirectly. Intimacy, knowledge, authenticity, and the formation of identity are all valuable insofar as they protect and promote the child's basic interests. The fifth reason requires some qualification, and in the process likewise makes sense in light of the child's welfare. Because the child bears the immediate consequences of parental (or professional) choice, the child's interests should provide the criterion for allowing parents to shoulder the burdens of decision making. We justifiably allow parents the freedom to decide for their child on the assumption that allowing them to shoulder the financial and psychological burdens of decision-making would likely be done with the basic interests of that child in mind. Parents have to live with the child's condition, or the child's absence, as a consequence of their decision.

Respecting parental autonomy and family privacy in pediatric care, then, differs from respecting autonomy in adult contexts of medicine. Family privacy is instrumental and conditional, constrained by the criterion of childhood welfare. It is premised on understanding the family as a social institution with moral legitimacy and responsibility. In this respect it differs from adult autonomy, which is not measured by standards of medical welfare as a justifying criterion. When pediatric care providers heed the decisions of families, they are not respecting persons in the same sense that other medical professionals heed the decisions of adults. Rather than following freedom and its underlying values of equality and dignity, pediatricians act in alliance with individuals who must justify their actions as beneficial, or at least as unharmful. In such cases, health care professionals' commitment to patient welfare is mediated by the family's responsibility to the child. Such caring conduct on the part of parents or guardians divides into two categories.

SPECIAL DUTIES: PERFECT AND IMPERFECT

As I have explained, the principles of paternalism encumber biological parents to seek the welfare of their offspring either by discharging that duty directly or by making a reasonable attempt to place their offspring in the care of others who can discharge that duty. Caretakers who assume such responsibilities encumber themselves with two kinds of special obligations to children: perfect and imperfect responsibilities.

Duties of special perfect care, or beneficence, involve specific acts or omissions in relation to an identifiable child and generate legitimate moral expectations on the part of that child. Such expectations include dependency claims (primary goods of welfare and claims to respect) and claims to an "open future." Duties of special imperfect care, or the virtue of benevolence toward children, refer to the character of parents and the quality of the family's ethos, its internal culture. Duties of beneficence entail a set of rights; duties of benevolence entail a set of virtues. Let us consider each—rights and virtues—in turn.

Like all perfect duties, duties of special perfect beneficence correlate with identifiable recipients, namely, parents' or guardians' children. Children have justifiable claims to the beneficent action of their caretakers, and the denial of such claims violates a basic set of rights. This is not to say that children have a right to the maximal level of beneficent action that their caretakers can provide, for caretakers must accommodate their children's claims within a complex array of other duties. Parents must weigh duties to one child against duties to other family members when appropriate, and they must weigh duties to children against other family, civic, professional, economic, and social responsibilities. Moreover, parents have duties of fairness to themselves, and they may be unable to discharge their duties to others without appropriately attending to their own needs and commitments. As I noted earlier, modern liberal societies grant families tremendous leeway in deciding how to set intrafamilial priorities. As a matter of fairness to parents, other family members, and society at large, children do not have the right to maximal beneficence from their parents. Hence, it makes more sense to talk about children's *basic* interests, rather than best interests, when considering the special claims of beneficence.[35]

The rights that children possess can be specified in two ways: (1) as dependency rights, which include goods that are instrumental to their basic physical, intellectual, and emotional interests, including (when appropriate) the need to have their wishes respected, and (2) what Joel Feinberg calls "rights to an open future."[36] Together, these rights constitute a "thin theory" of the good for children, a set of what Rawls calls "primary goods."[37] Such goods are not the final or complete goods toward which a child's life is aimed. Primary goods are not teleological in the sense that they outline the contours of a child's identity or basic, self-defining commitments; they do not constitute the ends of human life. Rather, primary goods are instrumental to the pursuit of life's more comprehensive goods. They are goods that children need whatever else they might want now or later. As provisions that enable children to embark or continue on the process of self-discovery, self-determination, and self-fulfillment, primary goods aim to provide reasonably favorable circumstances for children as they develop. Rights to such goods enshrine claims to basic levels of protection and care. They are a function of the fact that children are dependent and vulnerable and, with care and good fortune, will develop into adults who have their own interests, at least some of which may be independent of their caretakers' interests.

Seen in this way, claims to primary goods are need-based, and they hark less to Kantian theories associated with Rawls than to the ideas of Aristotle and concerns about our natural needs for nurture and development. I shall not pursue those differences of philosophical pedigree here. My core point is as follows: As a result of physical, psychological, and cognitive vulnerabilities, children have rights to beneficent treatment by those who are encumbered with their protection and well-being. A child's helplessness generates what Feinberg calls "claims against the world," to which relevant caretakers are obligated to respond.[38] Needs-based rights, as Jeffrey Blustein observes, authorize caretakers "to control those aspects of their children's lives that are relevant to protecting their physical, emotional, and psychological development."[39] In keeping with the argument I have developed, a child's needs generate claims to care. Primary goods aim to satisfy those claims at a minimal level and thus correspond to the positive rights of protection, supervision, and nurturance.

Rights to physical, intellectual, and psychological welfare include goods that are instrumental to a child's basic well-being both now and later, including medical care, education, proper diet, shelter, recreational opportunities, social sources of self-esteem, a safe and healthy environment, and opportunities to participate in society and culture. Childhood dependence imposes on caretakers the responsibility to seek these goods for children as specifications of the principles of paternalism.[40]

In addition, children possess rights to have their wants respected. Duties of respect are obligations to heed the wishes of children when those wishes are not potentially harmful to themselves or others, when they are not overly difficult to honor, and when they do not disregard other weighty and legitimate family interests. When such conditions can be met, caretakers are to respect the wants of children because children have the need to be themselves and to enter into the process of identity formation and self-definition.[41] Without the right of noninterference, children would lack the freedom necessary to participate in the process of self-discovery. The right of noninterference is designed to enable children to learn from the consequences of their purposive actions. As future adults who will be expected to act reflectively and purposively, children must be able to enjoy the freedom requisite for, and appropriate to, their agency in development. The rights of respect, then, are central to fostering the process of self-discovery and the exercise of responsible freedom.

When needs-based rights conflict, the first set must usually take priority over the second because they are more basic to a child's well-being. If physical goods are subordinated to children's free wishes, then children can place themselves in considerable jeopardy. To be sure, exercising freedom and expressing desire are central to the formation of one's identity. But to use that freedom at the expense of other primary goods can significantly if not unalterably compromise a child's long-term prospects and the possibility of expressing wishes in the future.

In addition to the primary goods of welfare and respect, children possess a claim to what Feinberg calls an "open future." These rights function in part to protect children from making choices now that will compromise their powers of choice and self-discovery later. The right to an open future is also a primary good in that it is something that children need whatever else they may want. It captures a unique right, one that understands children as protoadults. The right to an open future refers to rights that are saved for children until they are adults, but which can be violated prematurely, before children are able to claim or use them. Feinberg writes: "The violating conduct guarantees *now* that when a child is an autonomous adult, certain key options will be already closed to him. His right while he is still a child is to have these future options kept open until he is a fully formed self-determining adult capable of deciding upon them."[42] Such "rights-in-trust" are claims of a future self on the conduct of the child and the child's current caretakers. In this respect, rights-in-trust differ from the claims of autonomy that adults may seek to protect. With an adult, present autonomy takes precedence over one's later good, "even at the expense of the future self that he [or she] will one day become."[43] With children, matters are different. Respecting children's future autonomy and welfare can require denying their free choice now.

The right to an open future means that children's future selves can be protected from decisions by their current selves as well as from some decisions by their current caretakers. Rights-in-trust thus cut in two directions. They may restrict the authority of caretakers whose decisions may seriously handicap children's future options, or they may empower caretakers to exercise authority over children's conduct should those children make decisions that promise seriously to attenuate their opportunities as adults. In either case, the same general point holds: The future self has more moral weight in our treatment of children than it does with adults.[44]

Feinberg argues that a child's right to an open future is compatible with different theories of morality—that it can be grounded either in terms of the basic value of self-determination, the basic value of self-fulfillment, or a balancing of these two values.[45] Those who embrace the value of autonomy or those who embrace a substantive vision of the human good can both provide a basis for affirming rights-in-trust because such rights are instrumental either to the good of adult freedom or the good of adult self-fulfillment. We need not pursue that line of inquiry further. What is important to our purposes is to note how, in practical terms, children's right to an open future generates obligations on the part of caretakers. The right to an open future authorizes parents or guardians to ignore children's wishes should those wishes seem harmful to their future interests. In this respect, the right to an open future generates a possible source of tension for parents because it may mean ignoring the right to respect now in order to protect interests that children have now but cannot foresee. In this way, we can see one source of paternalism in family life: Parents might ignore or override children's wishes now in order to protect their later good. Moreover, such rights provide critical norms for assessing how parents make choices that bear on their children's future opportunities. Parents who rigidly enforce practice regimes on their child in hopes of grooming a future tennis professional might compromise that child's freedom to explore life's possibilities and to deliberate about which are best for him or her.

In addition to the perfect special duties of beneficence that children are owed, there are special imperfect duties. In family life, the imperfect duty of care, or the virtue of benevolence, involves the disposition to provide comfort, affection, and warmth, which are conducive to an ethos of trust and reliability. In this respect, the imperfect duty of care says more about the agent than the recipient, for it refers to character traits and inclinations that shape an individual's orientation to the world.

Consider again the example of Adrienne. When she came to visit Jean in Baylin's ICU, he was rarely conscious of her presence. Sedated and intubated, he slept long hours. When he was awake, his consciousness was often a function of discomfort or the effects of withdrawal from morphine. Seldom did he see or hear Adrienne, know that she was praying beside his bed, or realize that it was her touch that caressed him. It is tempting to think that Adrienne's daily visits were morally insignificant because Jean hardly seemed to benefit from his mother's presence. Adrienne's benevolence seems paradoxically nonbeneficent. But the idea of a special imperfect duty shows why it would be wrong to ignore Adrienne's conduct, for her actions testify to a strength of character that is noble and praiseworthy. The fact that, as she remarks, "you cannot not come" to the hospital is a function of a commitment to and solidarity with her suffering child. Her actions remind us that love is, in part at least, agent-referring. Each of Adrienne's daily visits was a deeply moral act.

In Baylin's ICU, nurses in particular registered their sense of a family's attention to their child's well-being and to his or her daily status. Each child's medical chart includes a place for nurses or residents to comment on the child's family. Although daily medical rounds rarely devoted much time to these "social" issues, they were seldom ignored altogether. (A separate "psychosocial team," composed of social workers, nurses, a speech therapist, a family therapist, and a chaplain met each week to address families' needs and anxieties. Strangely, this team never included a physician.) Parents' recurrent or long-term absences, although not always recorded, were noticed. When health care professionals worry about parents who do not seem appropriately affected by and attentive to their children's needs or changing health status, they rightly express moral intuitions that draw from an inchoate commitment to the importance of special, imperfect duties.

Of course, to distinguish between benevolence and beneficence is not to separate them. Benevolence includes, among other things, the disposition to act beneficently, thereby blurring virtues and duties, feelings and actions. Love's dimensions have internal relations that belie a scholar's quest for neatness. Moreover, benevolent dispositions directly affect a child's self-image—his or her confidence and self-regard. As I will argue in this book's Conclusion, parental love's salutary consequences are a primary good, one that families should protect and nurture. Thus it is not entirely correct to say that children have rights to beneficent but not benevolent action, because children have rights to primary goods that include sources of self-esteem. Distinguishing the dimensions of care may be easier to do conceptually than experientially.

The requirements of special, imperfect duties bear on the character and ethos of medical professionalism as well. Health care providers who assume that care and compassion is supererogatory—an "add-on" to their professional responsibilities—fail to recognize the imperative nature of benevolence: It is an obligatory disposition, not a virtue that may be adopted or put aside at a professional's whim. Parents and patients who object to perfunctory or officious treatment from medical professionals—an all-too-frequent complaint in medical settings today—rightly express moral indignation. Their frustrations express a clear sense of the requirements of benevolence as a virtue of professional life.

This expectation of professional performance, aspects of which I adumbrated earlier in this chapter, can cut different ways, however. If care as a virtue bears on how professionals ought to interact with families and children, then certain kinds of acts are appropriately expected of families and patients. Care is not a matter of benign tolerance; it includes responsible judgments about and responses to the conduct of others. Benevolence and beneficence have implications for the interpersonal dynamics between health care providers and families, implications that remind us once again of the limited and conditional place of family privacy in pediatric health care. Stated simply, the commitment to care as a virtue obligates health care providers not only to attend to the pain and suffering of patients and families, but also to transform their understanding of health and illness prevention when necessary. As I will argue more fully in Chapters 6 and 8, the duty to care in pediatrics is not nondirective and value-neutral.

William F. May has recurrently called attention to this and related ideas, though in my mind his views apply more directly to pediatric than to adult care. For May, viewing medicine in "transactional" terms differs crucially from a "transformational" understanding of the profession.[46] The former is contractual and value-neutral, contributing to the nondirective ethos of modern biomedicine. Although not without commitments and agreements, a transactional approach is confined to an exchange of information and the guarantee that practitioners will provide adequate goods and services to their clients. Transactions do not require doctors to instruct patients about how to decrease the likelihood of future illness or how to improve their health-related habits. Echoing recent critiques of professionalism, May argues that a transactional approach privatizes professional responsibility by reducing it to a commodity to be bought and sold in the marketplace.[47] A transformational approach, in contrast, requires physicians to get to the bottom of their patients' problems and envisions professional life as part of the larger commonweal. It opens the door to more directive and intersubjective communication between professionals and patients. A doctor confronted by an insomniac patient, for example, may be asked to provide the remedy of a sleeping pill. But in a transformational approach, a physician "may have to challenge the patient to transform the habits that led to the symptom of sleeplessness."[48] The aim is not to satisfy patients' preferences but to address patients' long-term problems with an eye to prevention and public health. In this way, May encourages an approach to professional relationships that borders on what I will call in the next chapter *moderate paternalism.*

A transformational approach to medical responsibility generates more robust moral expectations than those of transactional dealings. For May, medical responsibility acquires an expanded set of implications for health care practitioners given transformational dynamics: The demands of professional virtue are amplified; their range of application is broadened owing to background assumptions regarding the proper meaning of beneficent action. May's position illustrates how the virtue of benevolence affects our understanding of the duties of beneficence: The general commitment to care ought to translate into concrete acts that aim to improve the health-related practices of patients and families.

May's views may run into difficulty in adult contexts, where the value of patient autonomy enjoys considerably more strength as a limit on a physician's action. But in pediatric contexts, as I have indicated, the tension between autonomy and beneficence plays out differently. It may be entirely uncaring to assume that a child has the same level of autonomy as an adult patient. More to the point, in pediatrics, there are appropriate times to assume that a professional's prerogatives are not presumptively restricted by a patient's right to refuse treatment. In those instances, it is appropriate to care in ways that involve transformational dynamics.

PEDIATRIC MORAL COMPLEXITY

A child's right to primary goods helps us to clarify how certain persons ought to discharge the perfect special duty of care. A child's rights correlate with parents' and professionals' special perfect duties. Let me state again that honoring such rights-claims does not exhaust adults' responsibilities toward children, that adults also should also embody virtues of benevolence that generate dispositions of love and trustworthiness. For now, I want to focus on the primary goods that help to specify the special duties of care and how such goods can clash with each other and with the legitimate claims of others. One challenge to practical reasoning turns on how to weigh one set of claims against another. Tensions between special perfect duties to children and the duty to respect other persons generate the need for discernment and practical reasoning in families and the helping professions.

Such tensions are especially acute in the context of pediatric health care, for the professional stands one step removed from the primary care of children. As I have noted, a pediatric health care provider's responsibilities are mediated by parents' autonomy and their duties to the well-being of their child. That means, among other things, that health care providers must not only consider the child's claims, but parents' or guardians' claims to have their decisions respected. Complicating matters further, pediatric professionals must sometimes consider the health of existing children as well as public health and the health of future children. Such considerations are especially acute in research settings, in which experimental treatment is sometimes proposed with an eye to improving future health care. Taken together, these various obligations generate considerable moral complexity in the lives of families and medical professionals. Here we should note how various obligations can conflict, and how presumptively to weigh one set of claims against another.

1. *Tensions between a young person's right of physical well-being and right of respect.* Some children or adolescents may refuse treatment that is in their

immediate or long-term medical interest. When this interest is weighty and involves primary goods, such patients decide against their own welfare. If the patient is deemed incompetent to make decisions on his or her own behalf, it is justifiable to override treatment refusals. (I will discuss matters of competence and incompetence in the next chapter.) In many instances, it may be justifiable to override the young person's decision in order to prevent a harm or produce a good. Generally, children's interest in their freedom or self-determination is not an interest *as children* to make decisions for themselves, but an interest in developing the *ability to decide as self-governing adults*. Allowing young patients to refuse medical treatment out of a respect for their autonomy can result from misinterpreting and misapplying that value to matters of decision-making authority.

Yet to override patient autonomy is not to ignore it altogether. Rather, attempts should be made to persuade the patient to accept the treatment recommendation. That way, families and professionals combine the value of concern for the young person's medical needs with the value of respect for his or her identity and personal wishes. In such instances, health care providers seek the patient's assent, aspects of which I will address in the following chapter. When tensions cannot be resolved, however, physical needs outweigh wants, for those needs are more basic. As instrumental to the child or adolescent's physical, intellectual, and psychological development, primary goods and their proper ordering aim to ensure that the developing patient will have the resources necessary to self-discovery and eventual self-determination or self-fulfillment as an adult.

2. *Tensions between the young person's right of respect and right to an open future.* Some young patients may embark on a course of action now that jeopardizes their long-run chances for self-discovery and growth. Children who wish only to play street hockey each day, with no regard for their schoolwork, household or community responsibilities, friends who are not hockey players, or other recreational activities, make choices that, if left unchecked, could seriously limit their opportunities for work and recreation later. The general rationale for overriding decisions with an eye to a young person's open future, as I have noted, is that with children and adolescents considerations of the future self can outweigh respect for the present self. Helping young people explore a range of interests and activities enables them to make decisions against a background of meaningful choices. Care of this type aims to leave basic options open until the child is in a position to deliberate more reflectively about them.[49]

3. *Tensions between the right to physical well-being and respect for family privacy.* Some parents may make decisions that are not in the immediate or long-term medical interest of their offspring. The fact that a parent's authority over his or her child is constrained by the principles of paternalism limits the respect that a parent is owed. Parents or guardians who refuse

standard medical treatment for their children for religious or cultural reasons deny those children primary goods. Such decisions may be justifiably overridden in order to protect the children's therapeutic interests.

4. *Tensions between the young person's right to an open future and respect for family privacy.* Some parents or guardians may make decisions that restrict the freedom of the child later to reflect on and evaluate life's challenges. This tension, like the previous one, should presumptively be resolved in favor of the young person's basic interest. Principles of paternalism not only constrain a family privacy as it bears on a child's immediate welfare, but also on the child's long-term prospects of development and skills at reckoning with the demands of adulthood. Although it may be difficult to override decisions that are likely to foreclose basic options from a child-as-a-future-adult, the principles of paternalism imply that adults' decisions that unduly constrict a reasonable range of future opportunities do not require others' respect.

5. *Tensions between the young person's right to respect and respect for family privacy.* Resolving this tension between a young person's freedom and parental authority depends in part on the issues at stake and the age of the child. For reasons that I have mentioned, it is presumptively true that families best know the interests of their child, that family experience involves intimacies and priorities that are unique to each child's experience. It is also the case that parents must be allowed a considerable measure of freedom and discretion in order to arrange a family's internal life, and such arrangements may require children sometimes to sacrifice their interests for the good of the family unit. Parents are responsible not only for providing and protecting the basic interests of their children, but also for settling intrafamilial differences and needs. One child's right to physical well-being may justify parents requiring a sibling to assume some medical risks—say, to donate blood or bone marrow—despite that sibling's protestations. Children not only have rights vis-à-vis parents, but duties to obey their parents given the importance of cooperation for family life as a whole. The tension between individual rights and collective interests is a perennial one in philosophical and religious ethics; that tension finds its experiential roots in family life. When children's wishes contradict the family's and the family is deciding in the children's basic interest, then the family's wishes outweigh the children's. In other cases, the balance may shift in favor of heeding children's wishes out of respect for their budding self-discovery when those wishes do not override other weighty and legitimate intrafamilial interests or the rights of others.[50]

6. *Tensions between respecting the claims of the patient-child (with present and future interests) and the claims of other children to improved health care.* This tension, unlike any of the previous five, pits the claims of some children against those of others who are not siblings. Such cases arise when re-

searchers consider nontherapeutic treatment of young patients. In such instances, children become research subjects, relying on proxies to provide consent.

In part, this tension asks us how to specify the perfect duty of care. May medical researchers use some children in order to benefit others? Generally, this question should be answered restrictively, given the priority of negative over positive duties as well as the vulnerability of young patients to manipulation and coercion. That priority prohibits us from harming identified persons in order to benefit unidentified others. However, if the research involves "minimal risk" to children as research subjects, it seems plausible to permit such acts, as the National Commission for the Protection of Human Subjects of Biomedical and Behavioral Research recommends.[51] (I will provide an independent rationale for such research in Chapter 11). If a presumptively promising research protocol entails no grave risks to the patient-subject, then (with the research subject's consent and parental approval) nontherapeutic measures are acceptable.

These six tensions point to ways in which parents and professionals might consider ignoring the decisions of children in pediatric health care, or professionals might consider ignoring the decisions of families and children. My comments here about those tensions are deliberately sketchy. Several of these tensions raise the specter of medical paternalism, in which health care providers attempt to decide what is best for patients without their presumed or stated wishes, or without the wishes of their family proxies. In paternalistic action, individuals ignore a person's wishes in order to produce a good or remove a harm for that person. I have discussed why it is necessary to conceive of issues of autonomy and beneficence differently in pediatric than in adult settings. In order to clarify and deepen our understanding of paternalism in pediatric care, a more straightforward discussion is needed. To that subject the next chapter is devoted.

THREE

Pediatric Paternalism

> I remember walking into a room and seeing
> one of our nurses with her hand on a teenager's knee.
> That kind of touching is not unusual with young children.
> I told her that it was totally unacceptable with teenagers.
> But that is a danger in a children's setting: infantilizing patients,
> presuming that they are less mature than they are.
> —*Kathy Thompson, charge nurse in Baylin's Intensive Care Unit*[1]

About allowing adolescents with cystic fibrosis to refuse treatment, even if that meant they will die:

> CF kids have lived with their illness and the suffering it causes
> their entire lives. They know more about it and what it does to
> them than anyone else. Chronically ill children have been in
> and out of hospitals a lot, and know more about that than most
> adults. Why should we be telling them what they should decide?
> —*Sharon Johnston, director of the Office of Ethics,*
> *Baylin Pediatric Medical Center*[2]

MEDICAL COMPLICATIONS

I began the last chapter by focusing on the category of *responsibility* as providing the framework for understanding adults' duties and virtues and their connection to children's rights. In addition to defending children's basic rights, I argued that the idea of responsibility extends beyond those rights to acts and dispositions that define a broader basis for encumbering adults with the duty to care for children. I then sought to refine that idea by looking at adults' responsibilities in special relationships with children, especially family and professional relationships. There, I argued that professional responsibility in pediatrics should be guided by the norm of mediated beneficence, which requires medical professionals to triangulate their commitment to patient welfare with the opportunities and constraints provided by the child's needs and the family's desires and background. Therein lies a medical professional's challenge of forming a therapeutic alliance.

That triangulation makes for professional contexts that are typically more complex than those in adult care. In pediatric medicine, health care providers must situate their caring conduct within the contours of a family's wishes; there is a second party with whom to work. Parents or guardians are presumptively responsible for making decisions on behalf of their children, and parental autonomy, as I have argued, is an important value in decision making in pediatric medicine. That is not to say that family relations are irrelevant to contexts of adult care. But, as I will argue in the next chapter, family representatives in adult care are obligated to represent the patient's presumed or stated wishes and may turn to considerations of the patient's basic interest only when they lack sufficient information about those wishes. With adults, proxy representation typically presumes that the patient has undergone childhood development or, for various reasons, cannot develop beyond his or her current state. In contrast, in cases with children (especially young children with no history of informed decision making), family members typically have less information about the patient's wishes and must attend to the child's immediate welfare as well as considerations that bear on the child's development. In pediatrics, professionals must form an alliance with the patient's parents or guardians, whose responsibilities include protecting the child's present and future interests, as well as the family's own interests in sustaining its cultural, religious, and other commitments.

Yet as child neglect and abuse statistics regrettably indicate, parents cannot always be trusted to protect and promote their children's interests. Hence the second reason for revising the pediatric paradigm: Presuming a therapeutic alliance with a family can be naive, and in some cases dangerous, for a dependent minor. At times, interventions are necessary and justified. This revision qualifies our first revision of the pediatric paradigm, for it reminds us that the norm of parental autonomy is not absolute. As such, this second revision reminds us of core values that lie at the heart of the pediatric paradigm, in which beneficence has general priority to autonomy. Because the norm of beneficence is less qualified in pediatrics than in adult contexts, care providers may assume more prerogatives that derive from the substantive duty to care. Medical professionals may act with an eye to a child's interests with fewer restrictions on their decision-making authority than in cases involving adult patients.

In adult medicine, patients have rights that operate as side constraints on the conduct of health care professionals, rights that aim to protect patients' dignity, equality, and autonomy. Children's rights, as I outlined them in the previous chapter, derive from principles of paternalism that help to specify the duty to care. Such rights are aimed less at protecting well-developed autonomy than at protecting the basic medical interests of patients who are vulnerable, dependent, or "protoautonomous." Children are often presumed to be incompetent, or at least below the threshold of adult competence, and thus unable to make informed decisions about their present and long-term interests. Often there is room for parents, guardians, or medical professionals to discount a child's wishes or dissent in medical decision making. Thus, in the popular mind, it is a truism that pediatric health care is (and ought to be) more "paternalistic" than its adult counterpart. In this vein, Ruth Macklin states that "the undisputed paradigm of justifiable paternalism is the proper treatment of infants and very young children."[3] Similarly, Tom L. Beauchamp and James F. Childress write, "The paradigmatic form of justified paternalism starts with incompetent children in need of parental supervision and extends to other incompetents in need of treatment analogous to beneficent parental guidance."[4]

These statements, and the truism to which they point, are nonetheless misleading. If we consider the paradigmatic case of paternalism to be an act that ignores the stated wishes of a free, informed, and competent patient, then the example of treating or supervising children is not illuminating. Paternalism is controversial when some individuals assume sovereignty over the decisions of other free, informed, and competent persons. It is to treat them as things rather than as persons, as objects rather than as subjects, as instruments of one's own wishes or ideas of a good life rather than as self-determining agents. Insofar as children are inexperienced and dependent on others for care, ignoring their wishes is a matter of assuming decision-making authority for persons who lack the capacity to do so for themselves. Such actions are, at most, "weak paternalism," justified in part by the absence of factors that normally make paternalism controversial. Insofar as competence is one indicator of individual sovereignty, assuming sovereignty over the decisions of incompetent individuals poses fewer problems to patient dignity than similar actions involving competent persons.

Yet even this clarification has a misleading element. Although it is true that many children are presumptively incompetent, it is also true that children are usually not incompetent in ways that some adults are, and treating children and adult incompetents as members of the same class can oversimplify medical decision making in ways that fail to accommodate children's special needs and abilities. As a general rule, children below the threshold of competence are *precompetent,* whereas incompetent adults are temporarily or permanently incompetent, or were formerly competent. Moreover, children at a certain stage of development have wishes that ought to be respected. Such concerns have pushed pediatric care in the direction of seeking children's participation in medical decision making in some circumstances. Considerations of competence in pediatrics are a function of maturity, which varies considerably with age. Treating children as incompetent en masse on analogy with incompetent adults fails to honor children's needs and wants as developing persons. It discriminates against some children in ways that appear arbitrary.

Moreover, standard cases of paternalistic action involve one party ignoring the presumed or stated wishes of another in order to remove a harm or produce a good for that person. In pediatric care, however, a paternalistic action may involve a professional's decision to ignore parental wishes where a therapeutic alliance breaks down or has never existed. "Paternalism" in pediatrics may involve ignoring parental autonomy rather than patient autonomy; the "paternalistic" action is mediated by family relations.[5]

Complicating these matters even further are considerations of risk and benefit. Heeding a child's or family's refusal of treatment that has few risks and promises great benefit seems intuitively more difficult to justify than heeding the refusal of treatment that has many risks and promises low or uncertain benefit. Given the importance of beneficence in pediatric care, the merits of the family's or patient's decision may be complicated by the stakes involved.

Hence, we have numerous variables when triangulating decisions in pediatric health care: the age and relative maturity of the patient; the stakes involved in the medical decision; and the family's conditional legitimacy as decision maker. The truism in the popular mind—that pediatric health care is, or ought to be, more "paternalistic" than its adult counterpart—is considerably more complicated than it first appears.

I will devote this chapter to sorting through the issues of pediatric paternalism, hoping to shed light on the role responsibility of care providers who are making decisions with families and children in pediatric contexts. My aim here is to provide important terms for moral judgment and practical reasoning. I will argue that it is possible to treat some children paternalistically and that some of that treatment is unjustified. I will also consider when to override parental authority, focusing on actions that resemble paternalism in its main outline. That discussion will rely on the distinction between first-party and second-party paternalism. Along the way, we will need to consider assumptions that ground considerations of paternalism, and the related notions of pediatric consent and assent.

THE NATURE AND TYPES OF PATERNALISM

Typically, paternalism is viewed as occurring when an individual ignores the presumed or stated wishes of a competent person in order to prevent a harm to or to produce a good for that person. But that understanding of paternalism is too broad, for it would include someone who denies a match to a stranger who wants to light a cigarette, or a doctor who refuses to prescribe antibiotics to a patient with a viral infection who requests such a prescription. In those cases, it is counterintuitive to think that a stranger has a claim on another's behavior to cooperate with his or her unhealthy habits, or that a patient has a right to nonbeneficial treatment from a physician. No person has a positive right to demand that another assist in untoward conduct. Ignoring such requests is not a paternalistic act; it is rather a refusal to *cooperate* with another's harmful or undesirable behavior.

It is more accurate to say that paternalism occurs when an individual ignores the presumed or stated wishes of a competent person in order to prevent a harm to or to produce a good for that person, when those wishes express *negative rights*—that is, the right not to be interfered with or violated in word or deed. A paternalistic act occurs when an individual ignores another's negative rights in order to produce a good or prevent a harm to that person. (Neither the stranger nor the patient described above has negative rights that are ignored by a refusal to heed their wishes.) Two clear examples of paternalism, then, would be (1) failure to heed a patient's refusal of a blood transfusion in order to save that patient's life, or (2) failure to provide a truthful answer to a patient's question in order to reduce that patient's anxiety. In those instances, negative rights (not to be touched, not to be deceived) would be violated in order to enhance patient welfare. When I discuss paternalism below, it will be framed in terms of the conflict between the norm of beneficence and negative rights that express respect for persons as self-determining agents.

With these qualifiers in mind, an individual who acts without the informed, valid consent of the beneficiary assigns greater weight to the value of beneficence than to (negative) rights that connect up with the value of autonomy. Paternalistic acts often, but not always, involve contrariness and a zero-sum situation: They can run against the grain of what individuals wish for themselves, requiring compromises of liberty. In interpersonal or professional settings, paternalism can involve an agonizing clash of wills.

In addition to this volitional factor, paternalism has cognitive and psychological dimensions. Paternalists express epistemological superiority— the belief that they "know better" than the beneficiary. The recipient of paternalistic treatment is deemed deficient on cognitive grounds, and this appraisal can have damaging psychological results. If identity and self-esteem are partially a function of having one's own decisions and judgments respected, then paternalists can inflict harm on those whose ideas or plans are judged to be wrong. This fact is important in the treatment of children. Our identity is partly shaped by recognition or nonrecognition, and a person can suffer damage if authority figures convey the impression that he or she is unworthy of respect.[6] In seeking to do well for an individual, paternalists can actually do harm. A paternalist might not only compromise autonomy; he or she might also (paradoxically) compromise beneficence.

Paternalism is thus morally controversial, touching on matters of free-dom, care, identity, and the potential for harm. Inquiring into various general features of human action can generate a useful taxonomy of paternalistic conduct that has relevance for adult and pediatric settings alike. I want to develop that taxonomy in this section, calling attention to some familiar distinctions along with some new categories. My preliminary aim is to sift through some of the complexities of paternalism as a first step toward considering justifications for paternalistic behavior in the treatment of children and families. Consider the following eleven distinctions.

First, as Joel Feinberg has argued, is the difference between *strong* and *weak* paternalism.[7] Strong paternalism ignores the presumed or stated wishes of an autonomous person in order to prevent harm or produce a good for that person. Laws that require adults to use seat belts seem strongly paternalistic to competent adults who do not wish to use them. In medical contexts, strong paternalism involves a medical action intended to benefit a person despite the fact that the person's decision or action (including refusal of treatment) is informed, voluntary, and autonomous.[8] A strong paternalist acts beneficently at the expense of a competent person's autonomous wishes, choices, or actions. In weak paternalism, an individual seeks to protect another against substantially nonvoluntary actions—for example, when consent is not adequately informed, severe depression occludes rational deliberation, or addiction prevents free choice.[9] Weak paternalism occurs when beneficent actions are performed on individuals whose autonomy is attenuated or underdeveloped.

Second are differences between *hard, moderate,* and *soft* paternalism. These categories are meant to capture the relationship between the goods that a paternalist imposes and the beneficiary's own commitments and values.[10] In hard paternalism, I impose alien values on the beneficiary; in soft paternalism, I impose values that accord with the beneficiary's presumed or stated wishes, but without the beneficiary's valid consent; in moderate paternalism, I appeal to one set of the beneficiary's values to ignore another set. Hard paternalism is imperialistic and involves a clash of wills. Soft paternalism involves deciding for another on the basis of what that person would presumably want given what is known about his or her prior statements, commitments, or practices. In soft paternalism, the paternalist may infer what the beneficiary wants based on that individual's personal history when that person is unable to communicate his or her wishes. Such acts are paternalistic insofar as they proceed without the recipient's explicit consent. Moderate paternalism recognizes that the beneficiary has various values, and appeals to one set, ignoring that individual's possible preference for another set. A spouse who enrolls her husband in an antismoking program, against her husband's stated desire to continue smoking, commits hard paternalism. A parent who enrolls his budding soccer player in a summer soccer camp, without that child's explicit consent, commits soft paternalism. A professor who advises her junior colleague to use his pretenure fellowship year to produce a manuscript for tenure rather than to broaden himself intellectually tends toward moderate paternalism. In the last case, the paternalist regards one set of the beneficiary's values (job security) as superior to another (intellectual enrichment).

A third distinction calls attention to a beneficiary's *present* and *future* interests. Present interests would be those that a beneficiary would immediately enjoy as an effect of a paternalist's activity. Future interests are those that the beneficiary might not see or enjoy, but that the paternalist seeks to protect by ignoring the beneficiary's wishes now. A friend who turns off my computer so that I end a long workweek and embark on a hike through spring wildflowers acts to protect my present interests. A parent who tells his daughter that one day she will thank him for requiring her to take piano lessons acts with an eye to future interests.

Fourth, consider the distinction between *objective* and *subjective* interests and their connection to a paternalist's activity. Objective interests would pertain to primary goods—goods that individuals need, whatever else they might want. Subjective interests pertain to what individuals want as part of a clearly wrought set of preferences and wishes. Now consider two examples that combine this distinction with the previous one. First, a paternalist could ignore a person's present subjective interests in order to protect his or her immediate objective interests. Such a description seems to capture what most theorists have in mind when they discuss paternalism—for example, a physician who transfuses a comatose patient, ignoring that patient's written refusal of blood products. Second, a paternalist could ignore a person's present subjective interests in order to protect his or her interest in having a future that is open to making a wide range of choices later. This latter example, although scarcely unique to children, helps us to understand the weight that future interests can have when assessing the interests of those who are young. In this latter instance, a paternalist would ignore the wishes of a person now in order to protect access to important opportunities later. Requiring children to participate in a broad range of recreational and creative activities, often against their stated wishes, aims to keep their horizons open so that they may make future decisions against the backdrop of known activities and experience. Their subjective interests are curtailed now in order to protect both objective and subjective interests later. In this way, a child's right to an open future may lead to some forms of paternalism.

Fifth is the distinction is between *passive* and *active* paternalism, which is meant to indicate whether the philanthropic act is one of omission or commission.[11] Passive paternalism involves omissions that prevent harm or promote a good for the recipient. In passive paternalism, individuals refuse to acquiesce in another person's presumed or stated wishes, or they deny that person vital information when discussing matters bearing on that person's concerns. Active paternalism is more explicitly coercive and interventionist in ignoring an individual's stated or presumed wishes for beneficent reasons. Withholding information from competent patients in order to prevent them from becoming overly anxious is an instance of passive paternalism. Taking throat cultures from patients while examining their tonsils, without their informed consent, is an example of active paternalism.

Sixth, consider the distinction between *direct* and *indirect* paternalism. Direct paternalism omits or commits action against a person's presumed or stated wishes for that person's benefit. Indirect paternalism restricts the activity of some individuals in order to prevent harm to or promote the good of *others* who cooperate with or participate in a harmful act. Requiring motorcyclists to wear helmets is a form of direct paternalism. Banning the production of marijuana is an example of indirect paternalism. In this latter instance, one is restricting the liberty of one group in order to protect others.[12]

A seventh distinction obtains between *first-party* and *second-party* paternalism. Admittedly, this distinction is not unlike the previous one. Once again, we are invited to examine whose liberty is affected by the beneficent act, but in this instance, each form of paternalism has a direct effect. First-party paternalism directly ignores the presumed or stated wishes of another for that person's benefit. Second-party paternalism directly ignores the wishes of a second party who presumably represents the first party's interests. In second-party paternalism, the judgment of a patient's proxy is deemed deficient and thus without authority. Decisions are thus left to others whose authority is a function of the extent to which they represent the patient's basic interest. Many controversial cases in pediatrics involve second-party paternalism: Parents' judgments are ignored, or at least modified, in order to prevent a harm to or promote a good for their child.

An eighth form of paternalism focuses not on the relative autonomy of the patient (strong or weak), the paternalistic act in relation to the recipient's wishes (hard, moderate, or soft), the act's temporal orientation (present, future), the beneficiary's interest (objective, subjective), the structure of the act (passive or active), the restriction on potentially harmful behavior (direct or indirect), or whose judgments are ignored or liberties compromised (first or second party). It focuses instead on how the beneficial action is authorized, giving rise to the distinction between *unreflexive* and *reflexive* paternalism. In unreflexive paternalism, one agent acts on behalf of another without regard for the other's presumed or stated wishes. It is unreflexive not because the paternalist is unaware of his or her actions, but because the paternalist is assuming decision-making authority without the patient's consent. In reflexive paternalism, the paternalist acts on the basis of the potential beneficiary's prior, voluntary decision to waive his or her rights of autonomy in order to authorize a second party to act in the beneficiary's interests without further, specific consent. The beneficiary has reflexively transferred decision-making authority to the paternalist, who acts on that authority. The decision involves a paradox: An individual freely decides to leave some matters to chance, outside his or her direct control. The case is paternalistic insofar as specific acts occur or decisions are made that do not have the beneficiary's express consent. Many agreements and hospital consent forms are of this variety: They assign broad powers to medical professionals to act on a patient's behalf, without securing consent for specific procedures that may become necessary in the course of treatment.[13] They are paternalistic because they assign responsibilities to health care providers to make specific decisions for the patients' good, but those specific decisions lack the patients' express consent.

Ninth is the distinction between *personal* (or local) and *impersonal* (or general) paternalism. Here the key element is the form in which the paternalistic treatment is expressed. Personal paternalism refers to an act that ignores an individual's presumed or stated wishes to prevent harm or promote a good for that particular individual. Impersonal paternalism occurs in institutional policies or legislation and is neutral to interpersonal details in its application. Parents who forbid their adult offspring to smoke during holiday visits but who allow others to smoke during cocktail parties at their home commit personal paternalism when their prohibitions derive from beneficent principles. Laws that require motorcycle riders to wear helmets are impersonally paternalistic insofar as they do not presume knowledge of or familiarity with the putative beneficiaries; they are applied outside the context of interpersonal relationships.

A tenth class of paternalistic actions distinguishes between *pure* and *impure* paternalism.[14] Pure paternalism ignores individuals' presumed or stated wishes in order to prevent harm to them or to promote their good, whereas impure paternalism mixes paternalistic and nonpaternalistic motives. Parents who forbid their adult offspring to smoke during holiday visits commit impure paternalism when their rationale combines a concern for their offspring's good with their own desire to be free of the toxic effects of second-hand smoke.

Finally, consider the distinction between *presumptive* and *actual* paternalism. Presumptive paternalism refers to the *disposition* to treat individuals or groups according to the norm of beneficence without presuming to heed their wishes. Presumptive paternalism can also refer to the ethos in which such dispositions are fostered. In either case, the presumption is premised on the idea that some persons are generally unable to exercise sufficient autonomy when important decisions need to be made. Teacher–student relationships in many elementary schools and day care centers are shaped by an ethos of presumptive paternalism. Actual paternalism, in contrast, refers not to a disposition or an ethos but to acts that are paternalistic.

In summary:

Types:	Based on:
1. Strong or weak paternalism	Relative autonomy of beneficiary
2. Hard, moderate, or soft paternalism	Degree to which paternalistic act accords with beneficiary's presumed or stated wishes
3. Present or future interests	Temporal interests on which the paternalist focuses
4. Objective or subjective interests	Whether focus is on primary goods or beneficiary's wishes
5. Active or passive paternalism	Commission or omission
6. Direct or indirect paternalism	How another's liberty is restricted by paternalistic act
7. First- or second-party paternalism	Whose judgments are ignored by paternalistic act
8. Unreflexive or reflexive paternalism	Whether beneficiary's express consent is ignored or voluntarily waived
9. Personal or impersonal paternalism	Whether act is directed toward known or unknown parties
10. Pure or impure paternalism	Whether beneficent act includes some self-interest
11. Presumptive or active paternalism	Whether paternalism is a disposition or act

Three of these distinctions are arguable, and I want to address doubts about them here.

First, the category of weak paternalism seems to extend concerns about paternalism into a class of uncontroversial cases—namely, those that ignore the wishes of individuals whose autonomy is compromised or underdeveloped. Overriding the wishes of such persons is not acting disrespectfully, because the ground of an individual's wish and the proper object of respect—that individual's autonomy—does not count as a competing value in the overall moral equation. Weak paternalism is a confusing way of describing acts that are more accurately seen as (only) philanthropic. To justify weak paternalism is thus to settle a nonproblem, for the beneficiary is not being protected from a genuinely self-induced harm.[15] Stated simply, justifying weak paternalism is merely a way of authorizing some uncontroversial actions—namely, beneficent ones.

The concern is legitimate, and it is complicated by another consideration: Terms denoting *relative differences* (strong, weak) are used to separate individuals into *two distinct classes*: those whose autonomy suffices as a norm that rivals beneficence, and those whose diminished or underdeveloped autonomy does not. The problem, in short, is that a distinction of degree is used to produce a distinction of kind. If, as Beauchamp and Childress write, strong paternalism ignores "*substantially* autonomous" choices,[16] how "substantial" must autonomy be for a paternalistic act to be classified as strong rather than weak?

The answer is difficult to state in a philosophical formula that can be applied mechanically to specific cases. General criteria for measuring factors relevant to autonomy in potentially paternalistic actions will be discussed below. For the moment, we should note that the problem of relative differences enables us to understand why it makes sense to retain the language of weak versus strong paternalism in some cases. So long as we understand weak paternalism as referring to beneficent actions that ignore the express or presumed wishes of those whose autonomy is diminished or compromised, then the fact that it is presumptively problematic can be better understood. That is to say, so long as we do not view weak paternalism as referring to a class of *nonautonomous* patients, then the category does important work. Although it functions to distinguish between two classes of patients, those in one class should not be viewed as having "null and void" autonomy as opposed to those whose autonomy is sufficiently robust to render paternalism controversial. In other words, what becomes a difference in kind must not be "read back" into patient populations to obscure differences of degree.

Children, at least those in early adolescence, are a case in point: As protoautonomous persons, their capacities for self-determination are budding. Although not in full bloom, their autonomy is incipient and in need of support. That fact has two implications. First, it should remind us that self-discovery and self-determination are not all-or-nothing affairs, but matters of ever-increasing competence. Second, childhood development involves learning from and interacting with authorities, whose judgments are vital to the experience of recognition and self-respect. Viewing paternalistic action in relation to children as "weak" should not obscure the fact that paternalism can be experienced as a lack of respect, and thus can damage a child's self-image and self-regard. Weak paternalism is not uncontroversial, and one class of individuals to which it is relevant presents genuine moral challenges to health care providers (and others).

For these reasons, it can be confusing to consider children as members of the same class as adults whose autonomy is diminished by, say, drugs or depression. Normal children are not afflicted and should not be classified with adults who are. Ignoring children's developing autonomy is arguably more controversial because the paternalistic act is an affront to their identity, not a corrective to autonomy that has been diminished by a malady. *The language of weak paternalism, properly conceived, points to controversies sur-rounding beneficent actions that ignore the wishes of patients whose autonomy is developing.*

The distinction between first- and second-party paternalism is also problematic. That distinction extends the notion of paternalistic behavior beyond the specific beneficiary to representatives and family members, and that extension is confusing. A paternalistic act seeks to remove a harm or promote a good in violation of a beneficiary's rights. Because parents or representatives are not the obvious beneficiaries of a putatively beneficent act in second-party paternalism, it is odd to call restrictions on their decisions for others' well-being "paternalistic." It would seem wiser to begin by asking whether the parents' decisions or judgments are potentially harmful to their child. If the answer is yes, then one can tackle the problem by appealing to the idea that liberties may be restricted when they threaten to harm others. The language of second-party paternalism only confuses matters by suggesting that representatives, and not children, have their liberty restricted *and* are putative beneficiaries of others' decisions. Restrictions on their liberty are best understood as deriving from acts that aim to protect the child. Accordingly, such restrictions are nonpaternalistic.

Although this correction is doubtless true about nonfamilial settings in which the liberty of one party is restrained in order to protect another party, it is phenomenologically misleading in the treatment of sick children and their families. When parents' or guardians' authority is ignored, they are told that others are in a better position to serve "parentally." Parents or guardians are informed that they are treating their wards according to harmful principles; they are also disqualified as agents who are responsible for exercising the special duty to care.[17] Second-party paternalism is meant to capture the judgment that putatively beneficent decisions by parents or guardians are wrong and that the family would benefit from the decisions of outside authorities. Families are told that "the doctor knows best"—an idea that lies at the heart of the problem of paternalism, against which the patients' rights movement first directed itself.[18] In such instances, the issue is not only that parents' decisions are harmful *simpliciter*; it is also that their claim to represent the child's interests is illegitimate. In other words, not only their autonomy, but also their role responsibilities to act on duties of care are ignored. Parents are told that they are better off leaving matters of their child's care to others. *Second-party paternalism is meant to distinguish between counterfeit and real claims to beneficence for those who have role responsibility to care for others. It provides a language that captures not the challenge of dealing with harmful people, abstracted from their roles, but the challenge of dealing with individuals acting within the role of parenthood or guardianship.*

The distinction between direct and indirect paternalism suffers from the same problem that appeared to afflict the distinction between first- and second-party paternalism: The party whose decisions are restricted does not appear to benefit from the action. In the example above, the indirect effects of a paternalistic ban on marijuana do not benefit marijuana growers. In that case, a second party is affected but not benefited.

Once again, that point is true in nonfamilial settings when the liberty of second parties is compromised by the attempt to protect others. But matters are different in the context of family relations. As with second-party paternalism, the aim of indirect paternalism is to correct the problem of counterfeit care as it touches on parental roles and the identities that such roles presuppose. The (hypothetical) case of a Jehovah's Witness who refuses a potentially life-saving blood transfusion for his child provides an example. Should legal authorities or relevant medical professionals override that decision, the family would be treated paternalistically insofar as the intervention informs family members that they are better off leaving matters of care to others. The action does more than protect the child's interests, for the child and the parents are presumed to benefit from the intervention. Such parents are told that they are disqualified as medical decision makers because they embrace beliefs that are contrary to their family member's good. The effect of that judgment is to restrict the role that parental beliefs may play in medical decisions for children because such beliefs are considered to be counterfeit beneficence, contrary to the special duty to care. Parents are informed that they are better off leaving matters of care to others, that the family as a whole will benefit from the judgments and actions of outsiders.

For this reason, it seems wise to apply the distinction between direct and indirect paternalism to situations in which second parties have special role responsibilities to protect the interests of the putative beneficiary. *Accordingly, role relations and expectations provide background conditions for applying the distinction between direct and indirect paternalism.* It is incorrect to say that banning the production of marijuana is a paternalistic restriction on the liberty of marijuana producers,[19] but families with certain religious or cultural beliefs can be a different matter insofar as they are presumed to benefit from the paternalistic action.

COMPETENCE AND INCOMPETENCE

Underlying concerns about paternalism, and informing them in important ways, are considerations about competence and incompetence in decision making. According to the Report of the President's Commission for the Study of Ethical Problems in Medicine and Biomedical and Behavioral Research, *Deciding to Forego Life-Sustaining Treatment,* patients are judged competent when they have "sufficiently stable and developed personal values and goals, an ability to communicate and understand information adequately, and an ability to reason and deliberate sufficiently well about choices."[20] Competence is one of three components in the provision of informed consent—the other two being the patient's *understanding* of relevant diagnostic information and a decision's probable consequences, and the patient's *freedom* to choose in an uncoerced way.

Patients' competence is a vital matter when considering whether to heed their wishes. As we have seen with weak paternalism, an act is less paternalistic, and less controversial, when it seeks to benefit persons of diminished or underdeveloped ability. Insofar as informed consent requires patients to understand their diagnoses, the nature and consequences of proposed treatment, the availability of alternative treatment, and the implications of refusing treatment, then a vital component is missing when care providers seek informed consent from individuals who are unable to comprehend relevant information. As a result of their diminished capabilities, some patients need others to represent their interests or wishes.

Determining competence is a basic feature of assigning decision-making authority in medical contexts, and age plays an important role in assumptions surrounding patients' decision-making prerogatives. In the United States, the age of majority sets a basic set of presumptions in law and medical practice, presuming individuals at or above the age of eighteen years to be competent unless proven otherwise. In the presumptively antipaternalistic ethos of adult care, the burden of establishing incompetence rests on medical professionals. Below that age, individuals are presumed to be incompetent and thus in need of a proxy. In the presumptively paternalistic ethos of pediatric care, in contrast, the burden of establishing competence, and the right to acquire responsibility for medical decisions, rests on the patients.

Accordingly, there is some room for persons below the age of eighteen years to establish their competence. Three classes of minors who may be considered competent are widely recognized. Emancipated minors are those under the age of eighteen years who need not seek the permission of an adult in medical decision making. This category includes individuals who are married, parents, in the military, self-supporting, or declared emancipated by the court. Having assumed the risks of adulthood, they have effectively freed themselves from parental authority. Second, many states assign decision-making authority to minors who are not emancipated but who are otherwise deemed competent ("mature minors"), those who are near the age of majority and who are able to understand the nature and consequences of medical treatment. Third, states assign permission to minors to seek health care or counseling without parental consent if seeking consent might compromise or deter the quest for treatment—for example, treatment for sexually transmitted diseases or drug abuse.[21] Yet as legal scholar Walter J. Wadlington observes, states have created these classes out of expedience rather than out of a desire to protect children's rights or prerogatives. Little clarity exists about the presumption of incompetence from which specific laws depart.[22]

A standard for competence in medical decision making can be conceived in two ways: the basic threshold approach, and the sliding scale approach. Both focus attention on competence as a *process* of deliberation rather than as a skill in *reasoning correctly*. Competence in medical decision making is not a matter of producing the correct decision about what is in one's medical interest. It is rather a matter of integrating information, weighing and judging its implications in light of one's values and commitments, and communicating one's reasons to relevant health care professionals. One may competently decline a professional's recommendation of medical treatment. The idea of competence presupposes contexts in which care providers and patients may disagree, and health care providers must sometimes tolerate such disagreements. At a minimum, disagreements require health care providers to consider how patients' decisions fit into an overall picture of life that makes sense to those patients, if to no one else. Such differences do not mean that patients are unable to deliberate about what is in their interest, only that their deliberations involve values and commitments that professionals may not share.

The first approach to competence defines a standard in terms of a minimal ability or range of abilities—the skills of understanding information, forming a judgment that is consistent with one's values, and communicating that decision coherently. This standard of competence presumes a fixed, minimal set of deliberative traits. The second approach conceives of a standard of competence as variable, relative to the complexity and risks that accompany the decision at hand.

Advocating the first approach, Beauchamp and Childress understand competence to mean "the capacity to understand . . . material information, to make a judgment about the information in light of their values, to intend a certain outcome, and to freely communicate their wishes to care givers or investigators."[23] On that view, competence is determined by whether a person has the capacity to decide autonomously, not by whether a person's best interests are protected. Arguing against the view that a person's competence is contingent on the decision's importance or on some harm that might follow from that decision, they note that "a person's competence to decide whether to participate in cancer research does not depend upon the decision's consequences."[24] The standard of competence that Beauchamp and Childress embrace protects the value of self-determination.

The second approach, advocated by Allen Buchanan and Dan Brock, argues that any reasonable standard of competence joins the value of self-

determination with the value of promoting individual well-being or protecting against harm. If patients' preferences were allowed to suffice as a
measure of competence, then many individuals would be free to make decisions that jeopardize their welfare. Standards of competence should seek to
safeguard the value of individual well-being by requiring a higher threshold
than statements of subjective preference alone. Yet if a competent decision
is one that must produce medical welfare, then some patients would be denied the right to refuse care for reasons of religious or other cultural commitments. A "patient welfare" standard of competence could produce a
criterion that would fail to honor the value of self-determination. The best
standard, they argue, would roughly balance these two moral values.

In addition to coordinating the values of self-determination and individual well-being, standards of competence must account for the fact that
competence is a decision-relative matter. I am more competent to balance
my checkbook than to solve differential equations, better able to interpret
Aquinas than theorems of nuclear physics, more skilled at driving a car than
flying an airplane. On this account, competence cannot be conceived along
the lines of a minimal threshold, for that conception oversimplifies the different ways in which our capabilities are challenged.

According to Buchanan and Brock, a reasonable standard of competence—one that balances self-determination and medical interest—should
be measured along a sliding scale, taking into account the complexity and
risks of a medical decision. The higher a medical procedure's risk or complexity, the higher the level of ability that a patient must demonstrate to
establish competence. Conversely, the lower the complexity or risk of a
procedure, the lower the level of ability that a patient must demonstrate to
establish competence.

Standards of competence can thus be calibrated in ways that honor the
values at stake in medical decision making. That means, among other
things, that consents and refusals may need different assessments. Even if a
patient is deemed competent to consent to a treatment,

> it does *not* follow that the patient is competent to refuse it and vice versa.
> For example, consent to a low-risk lifesaving procedure by an otherwise
> healthy individual should require only a minimal level of competence, but
> refusal of that same procedure by such an individual should require the
> highest level of competence.[25]

Competence surrounding a consent or a refusal should take into account
whether patients' decisions expose them to significant risks. Calibrating
competence to complexity and risk is meant to ensure that the value of self-
determination is not to be held hostage to the value of patient well-being,
and vice versa.

In order to prevent paternalistic applications of this sliding scale formula, Buchanan and Brock add that an account of patients' well-being must accord with their values and beliefs. They adopt a "corrected preference account" that grounds "individual well-being more squarely in the underlying and enduring aims and values of the persons in question."[26] Practically speaking, attention to patients' underlying and enduring aims and values limits how a care provider may interrogate those patients' decisions. Regarding patients' high-risk decisions, medical professionals are not to inquire on the basis of what they believe the correct decision to be, but on the basis of what the patients themselves ought consistently to decide. (Whether this account of patient well-being is sufficiently distinct from the value of self-determination is doubtful. Let us put aside that difficulty for the moment.) Physicians are not to ask patients who are making high-risk decisions, "Are you sure that's what you want to do?", thus implying that the patient is wrong. Rather, in the words of Buchanan and Brock, the physician is to say, "Help me try to understand and make sense of your choice. Help me to see whether your choice is reasonable, not in the sense that it is what I or most people would choose, but that it is reasonable for you in light of your underlying and enduring aims and values."[27] A decision that seems medically unwise should trigger greater inquiry into the coherence of patients' deliberations in light of their underlying and enduring commitments. For Buchanan and Brock, high-risk decisions provide contexts in which health care providers may scrutinize the internal consistency of patients' decisions.

The problem with this argument is both theoretical and practical, at least when the argument is applied to adults. At the theoretical level, Buchanan and Brock's attempt to introduce the value of patient interest into considerations of competence is confused and, on its most charitable reading, untenable. At the practical level, they confuse ideas about the *burdens of competence* with criteria for the *standard of competence*. As a result, they confuse who is responsible for providing information in exchanges between health care providers and patients considering high-risk decisions.

Consider the theoretical problem first. According to Buchanan and Brock, two values inform the standard of competence: self-determination and patient welfare. Self-determination refers to the ability to direct one's life and to reflect critically on one's choices and commitments. Honoring the value of patient welfare, they say, means enabling patients to decide what is in their interest according to their own stable commitments, heeding patients' "underlying and enduring aims and values."[28] Patient welfare is not equivalent to what is medically wise, viewed from the medical professionals' therapeutic standpoint. For that reason, inquiries into patients' deliberations may not impose alien values onto those patients; professionals must seek to ascertain what is reasonable for the patients in light of their stable and sincere commitments.[29] Brock and Buchanan's views approximate the idea of moderate paternalism, as I have defined it above. That point aside, the problem here is that they fail to indicate why we should distinguish between the values of self-determination and patient welfare. The latter is conceived as a species of the former. The theoretical problem, in short, is one of redundancy.

Buchanan and Brock might rejoin that individual well-being functions as a value independently of a patient's underlying aims and commitments insofar as objective medical interests can justifiably *trigger* an inquiry into patients' capabilities when they make high-risk decisions.[30] The health care provider can be informed by but not bound to considerations of patient welfare. Patient welfare can operate as a norm that swings wide of the patients' own values and justifies medical professionals in imposing stricter standards for ascertaining the competence of patients who are weighing high-risk decisions. Judgments of patient welfare provide the background conditions that raise the investigative bar when evaluating patients who make high-risk decisions, but they do not justify ignoring patients' decisions if the physician disagrees with them.

The problem with this rejoinder is that it fails to avoid the problem of paternalism in the care of adults. It means that adult patients must demonstrate higher deliberative capacities when making high-risk decisions. In effect, those patients have shifted regimes from presumptive antipaternalism to presumptive paternalism. In matters of high-risk decision making, patients' competence has to be proven; it is not presumed. Not only is that shift vulnerable to abuse, it confuses the presumptions that ought to shape interactions between physicians and adult patients who are considering high-risk decisions.

Various practical problems follow from the shift to presumptive paternalism. One difficulty surrounds the matter of *calibrating competence with complexity* in decision making. Although it is true that one can be less competent to make decisions that involve complex procedures and facts, that does not mean that the *burdens* of competence thus increase for the *patient*. Rather, it means that health care providers have greater responsibilities to simplify explanations so that lay individuals can understand them. In complex decisions, patients may be "less competent" only because they are not properly informed, not because they are deliberatively unskilled. Allowing health care providers to presume individuals to be incompetent because they cannot understand complex medical information increases the incentive to complicate medical explanations in order to secure medical professionals' decision-making authority. Surely that is wrong. Given the highly compressed, technical, jargon-laden, and "in-house" mode of communication that characterizes many medical settings, it is incumbent on medical professionals to learn how to translate their language into something that patients can understand and deliberate about. Brock and Buchanan's way of calibrating competence with complexity removes incentives for health care professionals to provide such translations. If patients must bear the onus of proving competence in situations of medical complexity, they are placed at a considerable disadvantage in power relations with medical providers.

A second practical problem turns on *calibrating competence with risk* in decision making. Here, too, Brock and Buchanan err, but for different reasons. If complexity requires professionals to work harder to provide information that will enable patients to make informed decisions, risk requires patients to provide a more explicit account of their decisions when providing informed consent. That is not to say that patients are incompetent or "less competent" because they are weighing risky medical procedures. No (paternalistic) presumption of incompetence is warranted when seeking consent from such patients. Rather, patients' willingness to assume a high level of risk warrants an inquiry into their reasons; physicians who easily accede in patients' high-risk decisions fail to exercise their responsibilities to care. Here, again, Brock and Buchanan confuse the *standard of competence* with the *burdens of competence.* Requiring patients to shoulder burdens of competence in risky decisions is not to raise the standard of competence according to a sliding scale, but to ensure that the standard in place has been reasonably met.

Given these problems, it seems wise to adhere to a minimal threshold as the standard of competence. Following Beauchamp and Childress, let us say that competence refers to patients' "capacity to understand . . . material information, to make a judgment about the information in light of their values, to intend a certain outcome, and to freely communicate their wishes to care givers or investigators."[31] Brock and Buchanan are correct to point to important variables in decision making, but these variables are relevant to the burdens of competence. Those burdens are shouldered either by the professionals or the patients, depending on whether the decision is characterized by complexity or risk.

The distinction between the standard of competence and the burdens of competence is likewise relevant in the treatment of children. Having endorsed Beauchamp and Childress's standard of competence, let us consider the matter of burdens once again as it applies to situations in which children or their proxies are to satisfy that standard.

In pediatric care, as I have noted, considerations of patient welfare are less constrained by considerations of patient autonomy. In the care of children, we may justifiably view the burdens of competence as balancing the value of individual well-being, understood from the care providers' therapeutic standpoint, with the value of individual self-determination. In pediatric health care, one key motive for determining competence is the need to protect patients against decisions that are contrary to their medical interests.

Given the presumptive paternalism that characterizes much of pediatric care, it is often fair to integrate considerations of patient welfare into the moral equation when determining proper burdens of patient competence. That is not to say that the standard itself should be subject to a sliding scale, but that the burdens of competence must be calibrated given the complexity and risks of treatment, objectively understood.

For practical purposes, that means that pediatric care providers may have to work harder to inform pediatric patients about complex medical procedures. If the burdens of adult competence increase as complexity increases, then those burdens are even greater in the care of many children. Rather than relieving care providers of the responsibility to inform patients, the norm of mediated beneficence increases their responsibilities when they are dealing with children and families. Similarly, the burdens of competence increase in high-risk decisions, and these burdens bear on the kinds of reasons that families or children must give when considering such decisions. That means that care providers may inquire directly into a child's or proxy's reasons when decisions are risky or medically unwise. Rather than asking patients, "Help me to see whether your choice is reasonable, not in the sense that it is what I or most people would choose, but that it is reasonable for you in light of your underlying and enduring aims and values,"[32] it is warranted for care providers to ask patients (or proxies) a question that presumes a medically correct answer, when appropriate. If patients or representatives refuse to undergo a lumbar puncture to draw fluid for a meningitis test, it may be entirely fitting for caregivers to respond with the statement, "That decision would increase your risks because alternative diagnoses are more time consuming, and time is of the essence here to reduce the risk of life-threatening or serious illness." A decision that seems medically unwise should not only trigger inquiry into the depth and consistency of a patient's deliberations, it should also allow care providers to make explicit recommendations, when appropriate, that run contrary to patients' or families' express wishes. The kind of indirect speech that Brock and Buchanan suggest for interactions between professionals and adults has less to recommend it in pediatric settings guided by the norm of mediated beneficence.

Children or families who reject medically recommended treatment of certain benefit do not necessarily decide "incompetently." Once again, it is important to distinguish criteria for determining the standard of competence with criteria for determining whether a recommendation is therapeutically "correct." Pediatric health care providers who consider patients' or proxies' decisions that are contrary to that patients' basic interest may at times justifiably ignore those decisions not on the grounds that they are incompetent, but on the grounds that they are contrary to the patients' medical welfare.

AGE

I have not yet touched on the obvious issue of age in evaluating children's competence. The age of majority provides a rough division, separating individuals into the regimes of presumptive antipaternalism and presumptive paternalism in law and in medical practice. I have already noted that the latter regime is subject to further gradations, depending on age, maturity, occupational or marital background, and other "maturing" events. It is no great insight to say that the presumption of paternalism about those under the age of eighteen years should not be uniform or monolithic. Hence the third reason for revising the pediatric paradigm: Children have an interest not only in medical well-being, but also in assuming ever-expanding freedom and responsibility for themselves. That fact reminds us of the value of autonomy and how it demands greater recognition and respect as children grow.

Studies of children indicate that self-determination should be taken into account earlier than the age of majority, and that decision-making authority can be appropriately assigned to minors in many cases. In a widely cited survey of developmental studies of children's competence, Thomas Grisso and Linda Vierling claim that psychological grounds exist for assigning competence to minors who are fifteen years of age and older.[33] Subsequent studies have more or less confirmed Grisso and Vierling's findings and, with strong caveats, can provide guidelines for modifying the presumption of incompetence for some minors.

Grisso and Vierling frame their survey by citing three legal criteria for establishing competence: knowledge, intelligence, and voluntariness. They note that data from parallel categories in developmental psychology can inform our understanding of children's capacities to consent to medical treatment.[34]

As a psychological category relevant to consent situations, *knowledge* refers to "understanding the semantic content of the information that is provided by the professional."[35] It can be measured by matching "the information given to the patient and the patient's own paraphrase of that of which he/she has been informed."[36] When it comes to evidence from developmental psychologists about thresholds at which children are progressively capable of knowing the meaning of terms that are likely to be used in medical circumstances, "we have practically no systematic information regarding children's understanding."[37] That is, we have no reliable information about how children conceptualize the treatments that are proposed to them, and little understanding of how children conceive of relevant legal and moral categories like patients' rights, consent, or confidentiality. About the criterion of knowledge, Grisso and Vierling add, professionals lack clear guidelines or expectations for satisfying patients' right to be informed, for it is not obvious how we are to measure children's knowledge of the information presented to them. In specific cases, health care providers might plausibly depend on whether minors can adequately paraphrase the information they have received. But such judgments are isolated and ad hoc. Grisso and Vierling remark, "Clearly there is a need for research regarding minors' understanding of basic terms and concepts related to treatment and consent."[38]

About intelligence and voluntariness, more data are available. *Intelligence* refers to the cognitive ability to assimilate and use information when arriving at a decision about proposed treatment. Relevant skills include "attention to the task, ability to delay response in the process of reflecting on the issues, ability to think in a sufficiently differentiated manner (cognitive complexity) to weigh more than one treatment alternative and set of risks simultaneously, ability to abstract or hypothesize as yet nonexistent risks and alternatives, and ability to employ inductive and deductive forms of reasoning."[39] "Response latency" enables children to reflect on information, use available cognitive resources, ask questions, and employ inductive reasoning more efficiently. On this score, however, "it is difficult to infer . . . at what age response latency and reflection are sufficient for consent or other decision situations."[40]

Information about a related developmental phenomenon can shed light on considerations of intelligence and consent in children: "locus of control," that is, the belief "that the consequences of situations are a matter of fate dependent upon external influences or are controlled by one's own decisions."[41] Development of this self-concept is connected to individuals' attentiveness and awareness of a situation's details, as well as the time that they are able to spend reflecting on problems. In short, whether or not one expects to be able to exercise control over one's circumstances "might mobilize or inhibit one's use of cognitive resources to deal with a consent situation." According to Grisso and Vierling's survey, developmental studies indicate that children at or above the ages of twelve to thirteen years are more prone to perceive themselves, and not external factors, as the locus of control.[42] As a child ages beyond this point, they add, one can expect increases in adaptive capacities in consent situations.

Another feature of intelligence is the ability to consider alternative treatments. In order to weigh several possibilities, individuals must be able to entertain both their own views and relevant alternatives. Grisso and Vierling state that such a capacity involves role-taking skills—the ability to comprehend the roles, intentions, and responsibilities of another person, to consider a position from another point of view. Developmental studies indicate that the basic elements of role taking are not attained until middle childhood or early adolescence: "The age range of about 8–11 years is a period of distinctive development, and by the ages of 12–14, many children are surprisingly adept at role-taking skills across a wide range of tasks and problems."[43]

Intelligence also involves inductive and deductive logic and abstract reasoning, employing capacities that Piaget associates with formal operations in cognitive development. Those skills include the ability to bring general, abstract ideas to bear on problems and to think flexibly and hypothetically. This stage also appears in early adolescence. Researchers have generally cited the age range of eleven to thirteen years as the period in which formal cognitive operations emerge. Summarizing these findings about development and intelligence, Grisso and Vierling state that younger minors do not possess many of the cognitive skills that are associated with "intelligent" consent. However, they argue that denying minors over the age of twelve the right to consent to or veto treatment decisions cannot be justified on the basis of uninformed judgments about minors' intellectual incapacity.[44]

The final variable is *voluntariness,* that is, the ability to "provide consent that is not merely an acquiescent or deferent response to authority."[45] The key consideration is whether minors' decisions derive from tendencies to conform to authority. Evidence from various studies points to a greater tendency toward conformity in early adolescence than at any other stage of childhood. Indeed, data indicate that children aged eleven to thirteen are more conforming in their conduct than children aged seven to nine. Such "deferent response tendencies" are a function of the desire to avoid negative consequences and are especially acute among young teenagers. Data strongly suggest that early adolescents generally exhibit an increased concern about social perceptions and expectations. Grisso and Vierling conclude, "Such observations suggest that the risk of deferent responses to requests for consent might generally be great until the ages of 15–17."[46] Below those ages, "there is reason to question whether minors in general can satisfy the voluntary element of competent consent."[47]

This last consideration leads Grisso and Vierling to raise the bar to the age of fifteen years and above to define the cohort of minors that can plausibly provide competent consent. Although data about the development of intelligence might suggest lowering that bar, Grisso and Vierling rightly note that matters of intelligence are not sufficient when weighing the validity of informed consent. Individuals must be relatively free from internal or external pressures that would compromise their abilities to weigh the merits of treatment options. Grisso and Vierling hasten to add, however, that some exceptions might be possible. The period from eleven to fourteen years is an important transition. Cognitive development during this time is such that "there may be some circumstances that would justify the sanction of independent consent . . . for limited purposes, especially when competence can be demonstrated in individual cases."[48]

Subsequent research points to developmental data about children's skills below the threshold of fifteen years. In a study of competence and developmental differences at four age levels (nine, fourteen, eighteen, and twenty-one years), Lois A. Weithorn and Susan B. Campbell conclude that four-teen-year-old adolescents do not differ from adults and that nine-year-old children are less competent in providing reasons for their decisions but not less prone to making reasonable choices when compared with adults. This latter fact leads Weithorn and Campbell to argue that "children as young as 9 appear able to participate meaningfully in personal health care decision-making."[49]

In their research, Weithorn and Campbell gave each group of twenty-four research subjects a set of hypothetical dilemmas, two from medicine and two from psychiatry, and measured their responses in light of four cri-teria: the ability to make a choice, produce a reasonable outcome, provide reasons for the decision, and understand the implications of the decision. The second criterion was based on judgments of "reasonableness" made by a panel of twenty experts in relevant fields of specialization.[50] This criterion introduced a standard that was arguably more stringent than those used in the studies surveyed by Grisso and Vierling insofar as it measured not only the capacity to deliberate about medical information, but also the ability to provide what medical and psychiatric specialists consider the objectively correct response. Adolescents were found to demonstrate competence on this scale comparable to adults. (However, Weithorn and Campbell did not assess developmental impediments to voluntariness among early adoles-cents.) Children who were nine and younger appeared less competent in giving reasons and understanding implications, but they succeeded in ex-pressing their preferences and arriving at reasonable outcomes. About this group of minors, Campbell and Weithorn conclude, "Their focus upon sensible and important reasons suggests that they are capable of meaningful involvement in personal health care decision-making, even if their develop-ing competencies are not sufficiently matured to justify autonomous deci-sion-making."[51]

Drawing on these and related studies, the Committee of Bioethics of the American Academy of Pediatrics recommends seeking informed con-sent from minors in most instances of the following: performing a pelvic ex-amination on a sixteen-year-old; diagnostic evaluation of recurrent head-ache in an eighteen-year-old; long-term oral antibiotics for severe acne in a fifteen-year-old; surgical intervention for a bone tumor in a nineteen-year-old. More important than these specifics is the Committee's general recom-mendation about informed consent and adolescents. In the Committee's judgment, "adolescents, especially those age 14 and older, may have as well developed decisional skills as adults for making informed health care decisions."[52]

Yet this trend toward lowering the threshold for seeking informed consent from patients below the age of majority is subject to several qualifications. Although I do not claim expertise as a social scientist to provide contrary evidence, I want to identify limits to the findings on which policy and practice have relied. My reservations are based on the fact that children vary widely in developmental competencies. Moreover, data about them are sparse, produced in highly artificial environments, and fraught with biases regarding class, race, and gender.

First, although it may be true that one stage invariably follows another as a child matures from infancy to adulthood, it is also true that wide developmental variations exist among children of the same age group. For this reason, relying on ages as fixed categories is insensitive to the particulars of each child's personality. Medical policy regarding consent that relies on age differences below majority should be complemented by discernment and discretion about each child's personality and capabilities.

Second is the absence of significant data regarding children and competence. Grisso and Vierling's survey has functioned more or less canonically for those in law and ethics who have written on the subject of children's competence, but that survey was published in the late 1970s.[53] Moreover, it is limited insofar as it produces information about only two of the three categories pertaining to informed consent; it acknowledges the lack of data about children's capacity to understand relevant factual and moral categories that pertain to medical or psychiatric decisions. Weithorn and Campbell's findings rely on data provided by ninety-six research subjects, divided into four age categories with twenty-four persons in each group. On that basis they make general statements about the capacities of minors who are nine and fourteen years old. But policy and practice that rely on findings from forty-eight children rest on a slim reed of information.

Third is the issue of research contexts. Grisso and Vierling and Weithorn and Campbell admit that their information presupposes artificial environments, and that none of the subjects was asked to make a decision that was influenced by their own physical illness or psychological disorders, or by factors that accompany such conditions (e.g., anxiety, familiarity with disease in chronic cases, or emotional regression). Weithorn and Campbell readily note, "Further research must examine developmental differences in competency to make treatment decisions in naturalistic settings."[54]

Moreover, and finally, the research is flawed by biases regarding class, race, and gender. Weithorn and Campbell concede that their research's generalizability is compromised by the fact that their subjects "were 'normal,' white, healthy individuals of high intelligence and middle-class background."[55] Thus, their findings represent the decision making of only one race and class of children—hardly a model of broad-based research on which to base policy that will affect children of minority races, the poor, or those who have limited education.

Grisso and Vierling's biases are smuggled not into their research pool but into their criteria for evaluating decision making. Their survey presupposes an understanding of voluntariness that privileges independent and nonconformist decision making. That model of development has been seriously questioned by the well-known research of Carol Gilligan, who calls attention to the more contextual and cooperative modes of decision making among girls. Correcting that bias might lead to lowering the bar of competence for girls if cooperative decision making is not considered "conformism" or an impediment to voluntariness.[56]

For these reasons, families and care providers are wise to be cautious about imposing expectations of competence on minors without also acquiring information from each child that fills out his or her family background, cultural heritage, and individual capabilities. As I will indicate below, the data to which I have referred furnish broad parameters for thinking about first-party and second-party paternalism in pediatric practice. But broad parameters are no substitute for thoughtful and sensitive interactions between professionals and patients. There is the problem, in short, of expecting too little of minors or of expecting too much. Broad guidelines will not eliminate the danger that "we burden some minors with decisions that they cannot make intelligently (sometimes to their detriment) or inadvertently deny to some the opportunity to make decisions of which they are fully capable."[57]

PEDIATRIC ASSENT

Weithorn and Campbell's research points toward an important concern in the treatment of incompetent children—namely, empowering them to participate in medical deliberations about their own treatment. That is one aim of soliciting pediatric *assent*. In contrast to acquiring consent or establishing competence, acquiring assent does not presume that the patient will be the final authority in medical decision making. Of particular importance is the absence of patient veto power; families or physicians may ignore a child's assent or dissent in order to prevent a harm or produce a good for that child. But children's lack of veto power should not eliminate them from medical discussions in professional settings, for that lack of authority need not preclude other modes of involvement. Physicians are now frequently urged to integrate children into discussions of treatment options, consequences, and alternatives, in an ersatz version of informed consent. The Committee on Bioethics of the American Academy of Pediatrics states, "Patients should participate in decision-making commensurate with their development; they should provide assent to care whenever reasonable."[58]

It is tempting to envision considerations of pediatric assent on the model of informed consent as that pertains to adults or competent children. My view is that such an analogy is profoundly mistaken and reflects the hegemony of adult medical ethics in the care of children. Pediatric assent, properly understood, differs significantly from informed consent and relies on values that are considerably more qualified in adult settings.[59]

In the care of competent patients, an (admittedly ideal) informed consent situation occurs when the physician clearly explains the treatment along with its risks and benefits, describes relevant alternative treatments and their consequences, and discusses the implications of refusing treatment. That conversation occurs within an ethos of antipaternalism in which the patient's rights operate as side constraints on the care provider's conduct. When patients make medically unwise decisions, the physician may seek to persuade them to choose otherwise, but more forceful methods to impose medical treatment carry an enormous burden of proof and may implicate the care provider in a legal tort.

In cases of pediatric assent, the norm of mediated beneficence should be operative. Accordingly, assent should be guided by considerations of pedagogy with an eye to promoting patient welfare. That is to say, the care provider should instruct (incompetent) patients about self-care and cultivate a sense of health care responsibility. The Committee on Bioethics of the American Academy of Pediatrics articulates this point when it states: "As children develop, they should gradually become the primary guardians of personal health and the primary partners in medical decision-making, assuming responsibility from their parents."[60] In interactions between physicians and competent adults, the patient is dependent on the care provider's knowledge and expertise but is (or ought to be) free from the care provider's authoritative claims. In children's interactions with health care professionals, in contrast, patients are dependent on care providers' knowledge, expertise, and authority. Accordingly, the goal is not to liberate children from the hierarchical arrangements that presuppose professional authority, but to nurture a sense of "freedom for." With adults and some older adolescents, consent situations operate within an ethos of presumptive antipaternalism. Assent situations, in contrast, operate within an ethos of pedagogy and presumptive paternalism, guided by the norm of mediated beneficence.

Conceived as a spin-off of adult health care ethics, pediatric assent appears to impose weaker expectations on health care practitioners than the standard account of informed consent. The idea is that children are less competent and thus have a lesser claim on medical information than adults. Although perhaps true in a legalistic sense for most pediatric interactions, such an inference crowds out other morally relevant aspects of pediatric assent. If we conceive of pediatric assent along the lines of a pedagogical model as opposed to an antipaternalistic one, then we can see that pediatric assent imposes significant expectations on health care providers. Viewed in this way, securing pediatric assent *augments* rather than diminishes health care providers' social responsibility.

Sanford Leiken captures this point. The aim of securing pediatric assent, he writes, is "ethical, humanistic, and therapeutic."[61] Discussions with minors should "determine how they view illness, how it has changed bodily functions, and what personal significance it has to that individual."[62] This latter point bears not simply on the changes caused by illness in motor or other physical functions, but also on the meaning of such changes for the child-patient. Playing with friends, attending school, playing sports, participating in cultural or artistic activities, and other childhood activities are all relevant. Moreover, Leiken observes, "since young children frequently view illness as a form of punishment, an attempt should be made to detect and correct, when possible, any fears of self-blame, thus permitting a reduction in anxiety."[63]

Complicating matters further is the fact that some treatments produce unpleasant side effects that can be difficult for a child to understand, given the promise that he or she will improve as a result of medical care. Pediatric assent viewed on the model of pedagogy aims to teach children about infirmity in ways that are appropriate to their age, maturity, and familiarity with illness. Children's participation in conversations with professionals and family members should aim to empower them as they progressively assume ownership of their lives. Leiken recognizes the challenges that such responsibilities impose on care providers. He writes: "Although there has been some attempt to explain illness and its management in language and concepts appropriate to a child's level of development, much needs to be done to improve the communication skills of the pediatric health professional."[64]

Nancy King and Alan Cross identify several ways to empower children as they develop relationships with pediatric care providers. Children two or three years old might be allowed to decide such things as whether the examination occurs on the table or in the parent's lap. Pediatricians might try to obtain medical information and authorization for minor medical treatments from patients as young as four or five. For six- to eight-year-old patients, King and Cross write, health care professionals should direct their initial explanations to the child rather than the parent or guardian. For children who are eight to ten, some portion of the office visit might be set aside to allow privacy between the professional and the child. As the child gets older, more and more of his or her office visits might exclude the parent.[65] One goal of these procedures is not merely to secure authorization from the child, but progressively to impart a sense of responsibility as the child develops from infancy through adolescence. For primary care providers who expect to see patients over the course of their childhood, pediatric assent occurs against the backdrop of a patient–professional relationship that can deepen over time. In such contexts, securing pediatric assent aims to empower children so that they experience their freedom less as a burden than as an expression of their authenticity and personal responsibility.

CAN CHILDREN BE TREATED PATERNALISTICALLY?

Given the caveats and cautions about generalizing from data on childhood development, what can we say about pediatric paternalism? Three classes of children emerge from the data above, each of which poses distinct issues for the role morality of pediatric care providers. Here we are concerned with first-party pediatric paternalism—acting to benefit minors without their valid consent.

First is the class of emancipated minors, mature minors, and adolescents who are at least fifteen years old.[66] Individuals in these categories are presumably competent and thus ought to be treated as if they were adults. That means, among other things, that individuals in this group exist in the regime of presumptive antipaternalism. Within that regime, it is the care providers' responsibility to determine patient incompetence, not the patients' responsibility to establish their competence. Accordingly, the burden of proof shifts from standard pediatric interactions, in which the regime of presumptive paternalism (and presumed incompetence) holds sway.

Interactions between care providers and patients in this group can be paternalistic in one of three ways. First, and most obviously, an act is paternalistic if it aims to help the patient but ignores that patient's valid consent. Such an act would be an instance of *strong* paternalism, given the assumption that individuals in this group possess substantial autonomy. Although paternalistic acts may be justified, especially if they involve trivial interests, they shoulder a heavy burden of proof.

Patients in this category who demonstrate less than adequate competence but who express strong wishes can be treated paternalistically by those who fail to heed or respect those wishes in order to prevent a harm or produce a good for such patients. In those cases, the act is an instance of *weak* paternalism, in which the paternalist acts against the patient's desires in order to help him or her. Such acts can be justified when they seek to protect an adolescent's primary goods, are likely to produce beneficent outcomes, and use the least coercive methods. Although such acts shoulder a lesser burden of proof than acts of strong paternalism, it should be noted that ignoring the wishes of an adolescent is an expression of disrespect, and that such expressions can affect a teenager's budding self-image and sense of self-worth. Acts of weak or strong paternalism must weigh the good that is sought against the potential harm to adolescents' self-image that may occur when their claims are ignored.

Third, care providers can treat patients in this group paternalistically by presuming that they are not competent. This kind of paternalism has less to do with actions or omissions than with the *disposition* to treat patients in an infantalizing way. As Feinberg observes, paternalism in the care of children means treating a child at a given stage as if he or she were at some earlier, less developed stage.[67] Kathy Thompson, a charge nurse in Baylin's intensive care unit, provides a provocative example, one that I noted at the outset of this chapter: "I remember walking into a room and seeing one of our nurses with her hand on a teenager's knee. That kind of touching is not unusual with young children. I told her that it was totally unacceptable with teenagers. But that is a danger in a children's setting: infantalizing patients, presuming that they are less mature than they are."

The second class of children is between eleven and fourteen years old. Drawing on the data from Grisso and Vierling, we can say that children in this group are presumably incompetent. That presumption may be rebutted in specific cases of mature children, but the burden of proof lies with the patient rather than with the health care provider. Relaxing the burdens of competence in appropriate cases respects and nourishes the patient's budding identity without jeopardizing his or her interests in well-being.

With children in this age group, paternalism can occur in two of the three ways that we saw with the first group. An act of *strong* paternalism can occur when a person fails to heed the wishes of a child who establishes competence and provides valid consent. In those more frequent cases in which children do not establish competence, ignoring their wishes would be an exercise of *weak* paternalism. As with older children, such acts are justified when they are likely to protect primary goods in the least coercive way, for the interest in providing primary goods outweighs the interest in respecting incipient autonomy. Once again, however, it is important to recall the importance of recognition of and respect for the patient's psychological well-being. Health care providers who act paternalistically should also lessen the harms involved by providing reasons to the patient for their actions.

Members of this class of patients are distinguished from the first class insofar as they cannot be treated paternalistically by an individual who presumes their incompetence. As such, they are not infantilized by care providers who do not initially assign decision-making authority to them (although they might be infantilized in other ways). Because the patient should shoulder the burden of proof for determining competence, the health care provider may properly act with dispositions that presume the regime of paternalism until competence is established.

Finally, there is the class of patients under the age of eleven years. For this group, it is safe to assume that the presumption of incompetence cannot be rebutted. In such cases, care providers do not infantilize patients by presuming limited decision-making capabilities. Ignoring the wishes of patients in this category are instances of *weak* paternalism. As before, protecting primary goods with the least coercive methods provides a sufficient justification; moreover, considerations of the child's self-regard should not be ignored.

Within each of these three groups, health care professionals will encounter incompetent patients at different levels of development. Incompetence is one barrier to providing valid consent. Yet as I have noted, considerations of assent must be introduced when consent cannot be secured. Obviously the pedagogy that surrounds assent must be calibrated to the needs and development of children in each group; assent from an incompetent thirteen-year-old is considerably different from that of a five-year-old. In all instances, however, the main aim should be to impart or empower a sense of medical responsibility and self-care.

Seen in this way, one challenge in pediatric health care turns on matters of judging competence and calibrating care accordingly. Children's care providers must operate within one of two regimes: that of presumptive paternalism or, with a special population of children, that of presumptive antipaternalism. One task for the professional is to determine what kind of care provider to be—a child's or an adult's. Depending on the patients' development and maturity, different presumptions and pitfalls accompany the challenge of respecting their wishes while seeking to produce therapeutic results. For a pediatric health care provider, it is important to know how to treat patients as children, and when not to do so.

FAMILIES AND SECOND-PARTY PATERNALISM

If one of the challenges of pediatric health care turns on calibrating decision-making authority to patients' level of development, another turns on whether to ignore the decision-making authority of those who purport to guard or represent the interests of patients who are judged to be incompetent. In *second-party paternalism,* a third party ignores the directives of the person who has assumed the role of proxy for a patient's interest. This form of paternalism is especially important in pediatrics, given the frequency with which incompetence is presumed and children are in need of a proxy. Whether a child's interests are adequately protected is a vital matter of professional judgment.

Justification for second-party paternalism bears on general issues of representation, the conceptual features of which have political parallels that I will explore in the next chapter. It also presupposes more general views about the limits of family privacy in liberal societies, ideas I will develop in this book's conclusion. For the moment I want to remain focused on the ethics of paternalism, and what I have argued thus far provides grounds for drawing a line between justified and unjustified second-party paternalism.

Paternalism would be justified when a child's parents or guardians refuse treatment that, on balance, is of certain benefit to the child. Second-party paternalism is not justified when treatment is, on balance, of uncertain or no benefit to the patient. In such cases, third parties cannot plausibly claim to protect a child's interests better than the child's parents or guardians. Third parties thus have no grounds for assuming legitimacy by virtue of the principles of paternalism, for they cannot point to primary goods that will be placed at risk without outside intervention. Accordingly, when treatment promises uncertain or no benefit, the role morality of pediatric professionals impels them to heed the family's refusal of treatment. As we have seen in the last chapter, families can exercise discretion with an eye to their own interests when those interests do not clearly violate the basic interests of the child.

Moreover, cultural and social factors that are relevant to second-party paternalism cannot be overlooked. Lessons from American law are instructive. As Hillary Rodham Clinton observes, when states have few standards to guide the exercise of judicial discretion, "the legal system will not only be likely to treat individuals capriciously, but will also subject members of social minorities to the prejudices and beliefs of the dominant sector of the community."[68] Benevolent intrusion is easier "in cases involving poor, nonwhite, and unconventional families."[69] As we shall see more directly in Chapter 8 with the case of Lia Lee, families that are relatively powerless for economic or cultural reasons may be especially vulnerable to state intrusion when a child's interests appear to be at risk. In medical and legal contexts, it is important not to allow the virtues and duties of care to become an excuse for intolerance or an expression of cultural prejudice. A searching investigation of a pediatric patient's basic interests should function as a baseline norm.

Whether second-party paternalism is justified turns in large part on whether medical professionals or legal authorities can demonstrate that they can better provide for a child's basic interests when those interests are, on balance, seriously at risk. In cases of children, adults who assume special relations with those children are required by the duty to care to defend their "claims against the world"—to "represent" their interests. Up to this point I have been referring to *representation* rather loosely, assuming that its meaning is obvious. However, what I have argued in this and the previous chapter suggests that understanding the need to represent children's basic interests is complicated by their development from infancy to early adulthood, and such developments imply changing expectations and role responsibilities for those who are attached to those children. To a more fine-grained understanding of mediated beneficence, pediatric role morality, and the challenge of representing young patients' basic interests we must now turn.

FOUR

Representing Patients

INTRODUCTION

Thus far, I have argued that the category of responsibility generates a more comprehensive framework for thinking about the morality of pediatric care than the idea of children's rights. Without wishing to weaken a commitment to children's rights, I have focused on the virtues and duties of professionals and families who form a therapeutic alliance on behalf of a child in need. A central feature of medical care understood in this way is the idea of representing a child's basic interests. The core idea is that care for a child should be mediated by those who are responsible for representing that child's basic interests when he or she is incapable of doing so. Although that idea should be a truism in pediatric medical ethics, what is meant by *representation* is hardly obvious.

In this chapter, I will attempt to clarify the idea of representation given what we have learned about responsibilities, rights, paternalism, and the fact that children are developing persons. I will do so by broadening my focus somewhat, drawing on categories in political philosophy to indicate what it means for one person to represent another. By way of introduction, I should note two points toward which my discussion will move.

First, because most children develop competence over time, those who act as their spokespersons must calibrate their actions accordingly. We have seen how this idea about childhood development provides the third revision of the pediatric paradigm. Responsible adults must act to guard children's basic medical interests early their lives, but such responsibilities must be adjusted appropriately as children gain greater powers of self-discovery and self-determination during late childhood and early adolescence. In a child's infancy and early childhood, responsible adults must guard his or her basic medical interests and modify that role in order to convey express or presumed wishes as that child matures.

Such adjustments are a function of the changing dynamics between patient benefit and patient freedom in pediatric care, dynamics that are conditioned by natural processes of human development. Care for a pediatric patient must be mediated by the laws of nature, understood as having physiological as well as psychological aspects. Changes in a child's powers of self-determination, and adults' appropriate responses to such changes, focus our attention on two fundamental norms in medical ethics, beneficence and autonomy, and prepare us for the second point toward which my analysis will proceed: The role responsibilities of a child's proxy are normed differently, depending on the age, maturity, and capacities of the patient. Expecting young infants to be represented according to the model of competent, autonomous adults is (wrongly) to impose a model that envisions children as "little adults" who have made decisions against the background of settled values and commitments. On the other hand, representing adolescents as if they are no different from young children offends their developing powers of self-discovery and self-determination, and this offense is both wrong and preventable. Spokespersons who are called on to represent children should find themselves prioritizing different norms—beneficence or autonomy—depending on the age, maturity, and capabilities of the patient in question.

Understanding these two points will be helped if we examine several court cases—*In re: Quinlan, Superintendent of Belchertown State School v. Joseph Saikewicz,* and *In the Matter of Eichner*—in which the norms of autonomy and patient benefit have been deployed to settle disputes about the proper care of patients with diminished autonomy. Although those cases involve incompetent adult patients, they invite renewed attention given their relevance to the care of children, many of whom are presumptively incompetent. We will then be in a position to examine *In the Matter of Martin Seiferth, Jr.,* and *Custody of a Minor,* in which disputes about the medical treatment of young persons have been litigated. Taken together, these five cases will help us sharpen the difference between the norms of autonomy and beneficence in medical care as well as clarify differences in the representation of incompetent adults and children. Let us turn, first, to general considerations of representation, drawing insights from political theory, as a step toward focusing on specific issues about representing voiceless persons' wishes and interests in medical contexts.

ELIGIBILITY, CONSTITUENCY, AND GOALS

What does it mean for one person to represent another? Why should anyone need representation? What does one *do* in the act of representation? These questions enjoy a long history of discussion in political philosophy, various aspects of which are directly pertinent to medical ethics and pediatric care. In her study *The Concept of Representation,* Hanna F. Pitkin argues that representing as a substantive activity means acting *for* others, making the represented individual or individuals present in the conduct of the actor.[1] Traditionally, political representation has often been seen as a "second-best" alternative to direct democracy when individuals are unable to participate immediately in the decisions of a polity. The representative *re-presents* what is not literally present—namely, the interests or wishes of others. That fact points to a paradox in representation: Representatives are both attached to and detached from the principals they represent, raising questions about the extent to which representatives may act independently of the presumed or stated wishes of their constituencies. I will return to that point momentarily.

Moreover, and equally important, persons who are represented must have certain competencies. Pitkin writes, "The represented must himself be capable of action, have a will and judgment of his own; otherwise the idea of representation as a substantive activity is not applicable."[2] Those who lack such capabilities have interests that can be *guarded* by others, but such interests cannot be *represented.* An interest that cannot be made present in an individual's action, will, or judgment is ipso facto incapable of being *re-presented* in the actions of another. Persons who are helpless or totally incompetent are ineligible to have representatives; they are protected by stewards, trustees, or guardians of their interests.[3] In Pitkin's mind, being *cared for* is different from being represented.

A representative, then, acts for others who are capable of action, will, or judgment in order to protect or advance their wishes or interests. The critical question turns on how we are to understand such interests, especially if they clash with the represented's wishes, and how we are to understand the representative's responsibilities toward such interests and wishes. Two extremes are to be avoided.

On the one hand, Pitkin observes, persons who act entirely independently of their principals' wishes can hardly claim to be their representatives. They rather presume to decide *in behalf* of their constituencies but not *on behalf* of them. Such a model of "representation" understands interests as detached from the persons they are aimed to protect. On this model, those who claim to be representatives are not obligated to be responsive to their constituencies' wishes, only to guard what they perceive to be the objective interests of the represented individuals or groups. According to Pitkin, persons are representatives "in name only" if they habitually do the opposite of what their constituents would do.[4]

On the other hand, a person is not a representative if he or she is nothing but a "mechanical reflection or delivery of the wishes of the constituents."[5] Such an individual is a mere instrument or megaphone of a constituency's wishes, "a servant, a delegate, a subordinate substitute for those who sent him."[6] This account of representation is deficient for two reasons.

First, representation as a substantive human *activity* must include a measure of autonomy, "of animation." Without some level of detachment, a representative lacks what is necessary to act as a *person* engaged in representative activity. Second, there are times when it is impossible to know a constituency's wishes. Pitkin observes, "Leadership, emergency action, action on issues of which the people know nothing are among the important realities of representative government."[7] In such circumstances, representatives are required to act according to their best judgment and discretion.

Representing thus involves a complex dialectic of attachment and detachment, mirroring the paradox that shapes the concept of representation as a whole: It is a making present of something that was present but is now absent. Noting that fact, Pitkin argues that there is an inescapable tension in the act of representing another person or group. Stated simply, representatives can neither entirely ignore a constituency's wishes nor be slaves to those wishes. They must be responsive without being denied a proper measure of autonomy when judging the merits of those wishes in light of the constituency's interests. Summarizing a broad norm of representation, Pitkin writes,

> representing . . . means acting in the interest of the represented, in a manner responsive to them. The representative must act independently; his action must involve discretion and judgment; he must be the one who acts. . . . Conflict must not normally take place. The representative must act in such a way that there is no conflict, or if it occurs an explanation is called for. He must not be found persistently at odds with the wishes of the represented without good reason in terms of their interest, without a good explanation of why their wishes are not in accord with their interest.[8]

Assuming that acting on behalf of a constituency's wishes generally coheres with their interests, departures from a constituency's presumed or stated wishes must be justified. We normally presume that what persons want is in their interest, and that any discrepancy between wants and interests cries out for explanation. It is difficult to imagine an interest that cannot be ascribed to actual persons, one that does not accord with their preferences, wishes, or individual longings. John Stuart Mill writes, "The . . . proposition . . . that each is the only safe guardian of his own rights and interests . . . is one of those elementary maxims of prudence, which every person capable of conducting his own affairs implicitly acts upon."[9] According to Pitkin, that fact should inform the representative's task, even when wishes and interests do not cohere. For her, the representative's duty "is to the constituent's interest, but the constituent's wishes are relevant to that interest. Consequently, the representative also has an obligation to be responsive to those wishes. He need not always obey them, but he must consider them, particularly when they conflict with what he sees as the constituent's interest, because a reason for that discrepancy must be found."[10]

Pitkin's broad norm attempts to pave a middle way between two accounts in Western political philosophy, an "independence" theory and a "mandate" theory of representation.[11] The first is exemplified in the writings of Edmund Burke, the second in the coauthored work of Hilaire Belloc and Cecil Chesterton. It is worth pausing to notice the characteristics of each account, for these authors assign different weight to interests and wishes when they conflict, and such differences illumine how we can consider representation in medical contexts.

For Burke, political representation means serving as a trustee of interests as objective, impersonal, and unattached realities. On his account, representatives may presume to act independently of their principals' presumed or express wishes; they act on behalf of collective, unifying interests rather than on behalf of individuals or local groups. Individuals or groups may participate in an interest, as in an agricultural interest, understood "as an objective reality . . . apart from any individuals it might affect."[12] Because everyday persons can be mistaken about what is in their rationally discernible interests, representatives must act independently of their principals' wishes when their wishes are clearly contrary to their welfare. Considerations of welfare, moreover, must be cast in national rather than regional terms. That is, the political representative is bound by the interests of the nation as a whole, not the specific opinions of local constituencies within that nation. Burke writes,

> To deliver an opinion is the right of all men; that of constituents is a weighty and respectable opinion, which a representative ought always to rejoice to hear, and which he ought always most seriously to consider. But *authoritative* instructions, *mandates* issued, which a member is bound blindly and implicitly to obey, to vote, to argue for, thought contrary to the clearest conviction of his judgment and conscience; these are things utterly unknown to the laws of this land, and which arise from a fundamental mistake of the whole order and tenor of our constitution.
>
> Parliament is not a *congress* of ambassadors from different and hostile interests, which interests each must maintain, as an agent or advocate, against other agents and advocates; but Parliament is a *deliberative* assembly of *one* nation, with *one* interest, that of the whole—where not local purposes, not local prejudices, ought to guide, but the general good, resulting from the general reason of the whole.[13]

A representative may originate from Bristol, but he or she should make decisions that redound to the good of the national community. The test of representation, then, is not whether representatives voice the opinions of their principals, but whether they have deliberated about the good of the nation according to the best possible reasons. Burke remarks, "If a part of the kingdom is being well governed, its interest secured, then it is represented whether or not it has the franchise."[14] Indeed, representatives need not be chosen by those in whose name they act. What is important is not the representatives' point of local origin or local constituency, but how well they advance the objective interests of the nation as a whole.

On Burke's account, it is possible to speak of detached interests in descriptive but not normative terms. A person or group may be detached from certain interests as a matter of fact, but that detachment is undesirable. Local groups can elevate their own interests above that of the general welfare; one task of a representative is to realign the local constituency's perception of its welfare in light of more comprehensive, long-term goods.

Burkean representatives should thus acquire a broader perspective than their constituencies'. One mark of good representatives is their intellectual superiority, their ability to put reason above interest or passion. They act on the presumption that they know better than the populace what is in the nation's best long-term interest. For that reason, Burke conceived of representatives as constituting a natural aristocracy.[15] Everyday persons are governed by opinion and feeling rather than reason, and cannot be trusted to conceive of general interests. Burke writes,

> The most poor, illiterate, and uninformed creatures are judges of a *practical* oppression. . . . But for *the real cause*, or *the appropriate remedy*, they ought never to be called into council about the one or the other. They ought to be totally shut out; because their reason is weak; because, when once roused, their passions are ungoverned; because they want information; because the smallness of the property which individually they possess renders them less attentive to the consequence of the measures they adopt in the affairs of the moment.[16]

On this account, citizens are incompetent to deliberate appropriately about civic affairs.

For Burke, then, representatives may operate completely independently of their constituencies' wishes. That view contrasts sharply with Belloc and Chesterton's, whose ideas can be stated more succinctly. For Belloc and Chesterton, a representative is not a trustee of objective, collective interests, but a deputy through whom the people exercise control over their government. As someone whose authority is deputized, moreover, representatives must be selected by those in whose name they act. Representatives are to advance their constituencies' attached interests, or wishes—not abstract, detached interests that presume knowledge of the collective welfare. That is because representation is the second-best alternative to "pure" democracy, according to which each citizen can advocate his or her position directly to others. But direct democracy is possible only in small communities; it is rendered impossible today given "the size of modern communities and the complexity of modern political and economic problems."[17] Representative democracy is to secure by indirect methods what pure democracy is able to accomplish in small social groups. Belloc and Chesterton write,

> Either the representative must vote as his constituents would vote if consulted, or he must vote in the opposite sense. In the latter case, he is not a representative at all, but merely an oligarch; for it is surely ridiculous to say that a man represents Bethnal Green if he is in the habit of saying 'Aye' when the people of Bethnal Green say 'No.'[18]

For these authors, a representative "is merely the mouthpiece of his constituents and derives his authority from them. And this is the only democratic theory of representation."[19] On this account, representatives are *agents* of their constituencies, accountable to them and no one (or nothing) else.

Pitkin claims that Burke and Belloc and Chesterton tend toward extremes that must be avoided: Burke tends toward the model of representatives "in name only," who are always free to act apart from their constituents' wishes; Belloc and Chesterton tend toward the model of representative as tool or megaphone of those wishes, lacking "animation" and discretion. As extreme positions, these accounts have different views of human capabilities in political affairs. Burke's tendency toward an "independence" theory assumes that people are generally incapable of seeing their own broader interests; Belloc and Chesterton's tendency toward a "mandate" theory suggests that we should not worry about whether people are capable of seeing their interests. Mandate theorists (along with others, such as Mill) allege that people know what is in their basic interests or that it makes no sense to speak of interests that people do not sincerely want.[20]

This last point is important when thinking about representation in medical contexts for, as I have noted, in health care, our assumptions about human capabilities must change depending on the patient in question. When a patient's competently expressed wishes cannot be divined or a patient cannot competently express them, "representation" must look to that person's objective interests. When, in contrast, a patient has competently expressed his or her wishes explicitly or implicitly, "representing" those wishes is presumptively required as an expression of respect and recognition. As models of representation in medical contexts, Burke's and Belloc and Chesterton's ideas provide less of a set of extremes than a trajectory along which considerations of representation must travel as patients grow and mature. Parents and proxies must shift from "independence" to "mandate" models of patient "representation." That fact complicates how we are to understand the role responsibilities of proxies in pediatric settings. To see this point, let us first examine representation in adult contexts, especially as its duties have been understood in landmark legal decisions, before turning to pediatric cases.[21]

REPRESENTING INCOMPETENT ADULTS

In medical contexts, the need to represent adult patients arises when they are unable competently to express their wishes about commencing or continuing treatment; they are unable to provide informed consent. Hence, the need exists for a mechanism to represent their consent, a mechanism that is borne by the patient's proxy. Patients in need of proxies are incompetent in one of three ways: they are temporarily incompetent; they have irretrievably lost competence; or they have never been competent.

The first two groups comprise individuals who were formerly competent and whose capacities now are diminished. Contrary to Pitkin's suggestion, they are not ineligible for representation because they are incompetent; their wishes have been stated or implied and can be re-presented by another agent. Depending on how clearly such patients have expressed their wishes, representatives have two options at their disposal: representing the patient's *express* or *inferred* wishes. In the former case, the proxy can rely on statements that the patient has made before becoming incompetent and perhaps in anticipation of such a contingency. In the latter case, verbal evidence of the patient's wishes is lacking. Here the proxy is expected to make a decision that is compatible with what he or she knows of the patient's life and personality; the decision is constructed from the materials of the patient's customs, beliefs, and commitments.

Persons in the third group, never-competent patients, pose a different challenge. They have provided no evidence of their wishes, no evidence that reflects *competent* judgment. In their case, matters turn less on "representation" than on guardianship.

How we have come to understand the precise demands of proxy consent for these populations owes no small debt to landmark court cases—specifically *In re: Quinlan, Superintendent of Belchertown State School v. Joseph Saikewicz*, and *In the Matter of Eichner*. Although these cases pertain to adults, I want to discuss each of them because they provide a complicated but instructive legacy for considering the challenges of proxy consent in pediatric care.

In re: Quinlan (1976)

On the night of April 15, 1975, twenty-one-year-old Karen Ann Quinlan stopped breathing for at least two fifteen-minute periods after friends brought her home in a state of wooziness from a birthday party at a bar.[22] Two attempts were made to resuscitate her, the second of which restored her breathing. Nonetheless, she remained profoundly inaccessible. Although the exact cause of her unconsciousness remains unclear, it appears that she consumed a mixture of drugs and alcohol. At admission to Newton Memorial Hospital, her initial blood and urine tests indicated the presence of quinine, aspirin, and barbiturates in the normal range, and therapeutic traces of Valium and Librium. Her pupils were unreactive and she was unresponsive to deep pain, and she had a temperature of 100°F. Karen was subsequently diagnosed as comatose with evidence of decortication, a condition relating to the derangement of the brain's cortex, and was put on a respirator to assist her breathing. Her initial neurological examination concluded that her condition was abetted by anoxia, a prolonged lack of oxygen in the bloodstream that starves the brain of its essential fuel. She was then transferred to Saint Claire's Hospital, which had a neurological staff to follow her condition. Dr. Robert Morse diagnosed Karen's coma as a sleep-like unresponsiveness that later changed into "sleep–wake" cycles, in which she blinked and cried out but otherwise showed no awareness of her surroundings. Her overall diagnosis was that of "chronic persistent vegetative state," in which the brain regulates body temperature, breathing, blood pressure, digestion, and heart rate, but has no higher cognitive function.

After several agonizing months, Karen remained in a coma and showed no signs of improvement or recovery. She required around-the-clock intensive nursing care, antibiotics, a respirator, a catheter, and a feeding tube. Karen lay in the fetal position, lost considerable weight, and showed increasing rigidity and emaciation. Controversy surrounding her treatment turned on whether her adoptive father, Joseph Quinlan, could assume judicial authority to arrange for physicians to withdraw her from the respirator and allow her to die. In November 1975, his request was successfully opposed by her doctors, the hospital, the Morris County prosecutor, the State of New Jersey, and Karen's guardian *ad litem*. Five months later, the Supreme Court of New Jersey reversed that decision, thereby allowing Mr. Quinlan to decide on Karen's behalf to discontinue the use of her artificial respirator. On May 20, 1976, she was completely removed from her respirator and a few weeks later was transferred to Morris View Nursing Home, where she lived in a persistent vegetative state for ten years. Karen died on June 11, 1985, at the age of 31.

Doubtless "the most celebrated of all medical cases,"[23] *Quinlan* provides a gnarled and ambivalent precedent for the ethics of representation in medical contexts, aspects of which spin out in two directions. One direction, as we will see in *Eichner* (1980), emphasizes patient autonomy as the basis of representation, focusing on the incompetent patient's (previous) express or implied wishes. The other direction, as we will see in *Saikewicz*

(1977), attempts to squeeze a concern for the patient's objective medical interests into the mold provided by the norm of patient autonomy in cases involving patients who are permanently incompetent. *Quinlan* provides a complicated precedent because its account of representation conflates two norms—patient autonomy and patient welfare—in its decision to allow Karen's father to assume complete control over her interests. It does so, moreover, because *Quinlan* echoes the mandate theory of representation, which subsequent courts attempt to extend. That extension can lead to serious mistakes in the care of other incompetent adults, and we do well to note that error before considering issues of a proxy's responsibilities in the care of children.

The core of *Quinlan* turns on its interpretation of the right to privacy —the court's vernacular for autonomy—as a value to be measured against the state's interest in the preservation of life. According to *Quinlan,* the state's interest diminishes and the individual's right increases in proportion to the degree of medical invasion and prognosis for medical recovery.[24] Writing for the court, Chief Justice Hughes argues that "it is for that reason that we believe Karen's choice, if she were competent to make it, would be vindicated by law."[25] According to Hughes, "If a putative decision by Karen to permit this noncognitive, vegetative existence to terminate by natural forces is regarded as a valuable incident of her right of privacy, as we believe it to be, then it should not be discarded solely on the basis that her condition prevents her conscious exercise of that choice."[26] The proper way to protect her right to privacy "is to permit the guardian and family of Karen to render their best judgment, subject to the qualifications hereinafter stated [regarding consultation with attending physicians and a hospital ethics committee], as to whether she would exercise it in these circumstances."[27]

Also relevant is the fact that the Quinlans argued, following Catholic teaching and supported by an *amicus curiae* by the New Jersey Catholic Conference, that certain medical means are extraordinary and thus not obligatory. Viewed as extraordinary means, Karen's ventilator may be discontinued. That distinction between ordinary and extraordinary means is premised on objective considerations about the relative benefits and burdens of treatment for a particular patient. As described by Gerald Kelly,

> *ordinary* means of preserving life are all medicines, treatments, and operations, which offer a reasonable hope of benefit for the patient and which can be obtained and used without excessive expense, pain, or other inconvenience. . . .
>
> In contradistinction to ordinary are *extraordinary* means of preserving life. By these we mean all medicines, treatments, and operations, which cannot be obtained or used without excessive expense, pain, or other inconvenience, or which, if used, would not offer a reasonable hope of benefit.[28]

Extraordinary means are those whose burdens are disproportionate to the patient's prospective welfare. At the heart of the controversy was Joseph Quinlan's request for judicial authority to arrange for the removal of means that were insufficiently beneficial to Karen, however customary the use of such technological devices may have become in intensive care settings.

In the wake of *Quinlan,* it has been widely assumed that representatives are authorized to make decisions that the patients would make if they could do so. Known as the doctrine of "substituted judgment," the idea is that, absent any clear directive from the patient, the representative may (or must) divine the patient's wishes from what he or she knows about the patient's lifestyle, values, commitments, and everyday practices. Richard W. Momeyer writes, for example, that the New Jersey Supreme Court

> relied upon designating a guardian who would best know and most respect her wishes. . . . A guardian so situated as Mr. Quinlan could be expected to know the character, convictions, and personality of the now comatose Karen; such a person would know what the religious or moral dogmas, if any, subscribed to by the patient prescribe; such a guardian would be presumed to know what, in the total context of the life and life-style of his charge, she would choose even if she had never explicitly given any expression of desire before. A guardian so situated, the court implied, could be trusted to discern and abide by a treatment decision compatible with what the patient herself would choose.[29]

In Momeyer's judgment, *Quinlan* sought to protect patient autonomy and provided "as plausible a means of doing so as we could hope to find."[30]

Contrary to this interpretation, however, *Quinlan* qualifies its claims about protecting patient autonomy by appealing to the norm of patient welfare. Indeed, the Hughes court entirely dismisses the strongest form of evidence regarding Karen's autonomy—namely, explicit statements she had made regarding the use of extraordinary means of medical care. Moreover, Hughes uses the phrase "substituted judgment" only once in *Quinlan,* and he does so with reference to the courts' role in overriding physicians' professional recommendations, not with reference to parents or guardians divining the wishes of incompetent patients.[31] But even if we grant that the court sought to craft a standard of substituted judgment as a mechanism for protecting a patient's right to privacy, the following question is of critical importance: What is meant by the claim that Karen's willingness "to permit this non-cognitive, vegetative existence to terminate by natural forces is . . . a valuable incident of her right of privacy"?[32] What is a "valuable incident" of a right of privacy? Is it "valuable" insofar as it expresses what she would have *genuinely wished*? Or is it "valuable" because it is *reasonable,* in keeping with an objective understanding of her welfare?

As Roger Dworkin has remarked, the phrase "valuable incident" is not a legal term of art.[33] Does it mean expressing a subjective wish or objective interest? Although the court is woefully vague on this important point, its comments support the latter interpretation and explicitly discount the former. In keeping with the trial court's finding of fact, Hughes acknowledges that Karen "firmly evinced her wish, in like circumstances, not to have her life prolonged by the otherwise futile use of extraordinary means."[34] When she was competent, Karen expressed "her distaste for continuance of life by extraordinary medical procedures, under circumstances not unlike those of the present case."[35] Such statements, the Supreme Court nonetheless held, "lacked significant probative weight," because they "were remote and impersonal."[36] Indeed, the Hughes court explicitly assigns to Karen a right to privacy *despite* the "testimony of her previous conversations with friends" indicating what she would choose for herself.[37]

What is more decisive, in the court's judgment, is the fact that we can infer what Karen would decide according to an objective standard of reasonableness. "We have no doubt, in these unhappy circumstances, that if Karen were herself miraculously lucid for an interval (not altering the existing prognosis of the condition to which she would soon return) and perceptive of her irreversible condition, she could effectively decide upon discontinuance of the life-support apparatus, even if it meant the prospect of natural death."[38] Such an inference about Karen's putative decision is not extracted from Karen's lifestyle. Indeed, we read *Quinlan* in vain if we hope to find a basis for understanding substituted judgment that is premised on inferred wishes. Rather, Hughes argues, the decision to withdraw the ventilator from Karen is a reasonable judgment. The court notes that accepted medical standards would argue on behalf of keeping her on the ventilator, and adds that such standards are irrational: "The question is whether there is such internal consistency and rationality in the application of such standards as should warrant their constituting an ineluctable bar to the effectuation of substantive relief for plaintiff at the hands of the court. We have concluded not."[39] In other words, there is no objective medical reason to support state action that would stand in the way of Joseph Quinlan assuming judicial authority over Karen's interests and arranging for the discontinuation of the respirator. The decision to cease artificial respiration is a reasonable judgment with which most people would agree. Upon assigning the right to Karen's parents to consider the discontinuation of treatment, the court writes, "If their conclusion is in the affirmative this decision should be accepted by a society the overwhelming majority of whose members would, we think, in similar circumstances, exercise such a choice in the same way for themselves or for those closest to them. It is for this reason that we determine that Karen's right of privacy may be asserted in her behalf, in this respect, by her guardian or family under the particular circumstances presented by this record."[40]

Does *Quinlan* straddle the fence between the values of patient autonomy and patient benefit? Does it confuse privacy rights with welfare interests? The answer requires us to step back from particulars of *Quinlan* and consider matters of representation in more general terms. If we recur to general ideas about representation, perhaps we can see that my way of posing these questions about *Quinlan* is overly stark. The court could respond by invoking Mill's assumption that bifurcating wishes and interests is, in general, wrong: Most people wish for what is in their welfare. Given that assumption, it seems plausible to infer the converse: What is in one's objective interest is also what one generally wants. This connection between interest and wish, moreover, can structure how Karen's rights to privacy can be understood. Assuming that what is reasonable for her is what she would actually want, it is fair to assign representative status to those who would act to protect her rights to privacy in this reasonable way and discontinue treatment. As I have noted, Hughes argues that the decision to withdraw treatment is one that most people would make for themselves or for others close to them. It passes a "reasonable person" standard. There is no basis, in short, to ask whether Karen's putative decision to refuse further treatment as a "valuable incident" of her rights should be understood in subjective or objective terms. The court may thus plausibly discount Karen's express wishes and nonetheless hold that someone expressing what she would reasonably decide for herself is representing her "right to privacy."

It is not always true, however, that what persons wish for is in their interest, or that what we consider to be in their basic interest is in fact what they perceive as good for them. Nor is it the case that all persons have been competent at some point in their lives. However much Mill's dictum seems generally correct, it does not capture cases in which there might be a wedge between a patient's competent wishes and his or her welfare.

That wedge can be a function of different factors. On the one hand, a barrier can be a function of a patient's prior voluntary decisions. Some patients have principles that they have chosen or acted on but that are not in their basic medical interest. Proxies for such patients should represent them on the basis of those individuals' competently expressed wishes, when possible, and when such wishes don't jeopardize others' reasonable interests. Representation in these cases turns on respecting adult patients' formerly expressed wishes, which in turn derives from a respect for those patients' autonomy and personhood. In order for individuals to discover meaning *for themselves,* they need an appropriate range of discretion and freedom to make and test choices. Respecting persons in this way, we allow them to discover their own authenticity, to place their unique stamp on their lives and relationships.

On the other hand, barriers may not be a function of a patient's freely chosen principles or wishes, but rather a function of involuntary forces—for example, developmental delay or retardation. To handle these cases, another standard is necessary. Here the relevant factors are a function of the genetic lottery, which pose an obstacle to the competent expression of any sort of wish. In such cases, another mechanism for protecting patients is needed, raising the specter of discriminating against different kinds of incompetent individuals. Whether and to what extent such worries are justified are issues to which we will turn our attention shortly.

For the moment, let me note that subsequent court decisions regarding incompetent patients and their proxies apply the *Quinlan* precedent to both sets of cases: previously competent patients whose express wishes about possible treatment interventions *are* sufficiently clear before their incompetence, and patients who are permanently incompetent and who have never had competently expressed wishes to be represented. Let us turn to cases concerning each, proceeding in chronological order, focusing first on the case of a permanently incompetent patient.

Superintendent of Belchertown State School v. Joseph Saikewicz (1977)

For permanently incompetent patients, spokespersons are obviously unable to rely on competently expressed wishes. In such instances, the model of Burkean "representation" should direct us, for we are shifting from cases in which a patient's competence—albeit former competence—can serve as a guide to one in which no such guide is possible. Consider the case of Joseph Saikewicz.[41]

Saikewicz was a sixty-seven-year-old man with an IQ of ten and a mental age of less than three years when he was diagnosed as having acute myeloblastic monocytic leukemia (AMML) in 1976. An incurable disease in adults, AMML can be treated with chemotherapy to produce temporary remission in 30 to 50 percent of cases and extend the patient's life two to thirteen months. The treatment increases the chance of infection and kills the patient's bone marrow; frequent blood transfusions are needed to counteract some of the treatment's toxic effects. It was believed that Saikewicz would suffer pain and confusion during treatment procedures, that he would need to be physically restrained during the administration of chemotherapy, and that he would not understand his treatment. William E. Jones, the superintendent of Belchertown State School in Massachusetts where Saikewicz had been a long-term resident, and Paul Rogers, the staff attorney at the school, filed for an immediate appointment of a guardian *ad litem,* with authority to make decisions concerning Saikewicz's care and treatment. In May 1976, the court appointed Patrick Melnik guardian *ad litem* with authority to decide the proper course of treatment—chemother-

apy and transfusions, or palliative care—as Saikewicz was able to communicate only with grunts and gestures. Melnick argued that Saikewicz's illness
was incurable, that chemotherapy had strong adverse side effects, and that
Saikewicz would not understand his treatment or pain. Melnick claimed
that palliative care would be in the patient's best interest. The Massachusetts Supreme Court upheld that view on July 9, 1976,[42] and Saikewicz
died two months later.

Writing for the court, Judge Liacos argues (1) that privacy rights, drawing from *Quinlan,* may be extended to Saikewicz and (2) the distinction between ordinary and extraordinary means allows for withholding extraordinary treatment, and that Saikewicz's treatment would be extraordinary.
The first line of argument lies at the core of Liacos's position and is seriously flawed. The second is more muted but contains a moral insight that the
Saikewicz decision should have developed. Let us consider each.

Regarding the first point, Liacos wrongly adhered to a mandate model
of representation in its account of how an incompetent's interests are to be
protected. In the court's view, there is a general right to refuse treatment,
and this right "must extend to the case of an incompetent, as well as a competent, patient because the value of human dignity extends to both."[43] A
patient's proxy must make every effort

> to ascertain the incompetent person's actual interests and preferences. . . .
> The decision . . . should be that which would be made by the incompetent
> person if that person were competent, but taking into account the present
> and future incompetence of the individual as one of the factors which
> would necessarily enter into the picture of the competent person.[44]

On this account, a permanently incompetent person's proxy is to render a
judgment premised on what the ward, if competent, would decide about
treatment as a never competent individual.

The court's argument begins with the principle that human life is intrinsically valuable, and it proceeds on the conviction that this principle
must be applied in a nondiscriminatory way to competent and incompetent patients alike. Incompetent persons are not to be assigned fewer protections than other persons, as if some lives are worth less than others.
Hence the need for a mechanism that is neutral to differences between
competent and incompetent persons, one that does not sneak in quality-of-
life prejudices.

The crucial question is whether the *procedure* for protecting all classes
of incompetent patients ought to be the same: Assuming that a mechanism
for protecting formerly competent persons is now in place as a result of
Quinlan, the question put to the *Saikewicz* court was whether equality of
dignity entails an identical procedure for protecting that dignity for differ-

ent kinds of incompetent persons. Liacos answered that question in the affirmative, and in this respect he erred. According to *Saikewicz,* we are to assure equal protection by extending the procedure of representing formerly competent patients to representing permanently incompetent patients. Citing *Quinlan* as explicitly defending the doctrine of "substituted judgment," the court states, "The primary test is subjective in nature—that is, the goal is to determine with as much accuracy as possible the wants and needs of the individual involved."[45] However difficult it may be to achieve that goal with a profoundly retarded individual, "the effort to bring the substituted judgment in step with the values and desires of the affected individual must not, and need not, be abandoned."[46] The underlying concern is that using a different procedure may be less protective and thus discriminatory, that it would open the door to "quality-of-life" judgments and thus introduce a standard for measuring relative degrees of human worth and assign fewer protections to some persons than others.[47]

What evidence exists that Saikewicz would not want chemotherapy? Herein lies the crux of the court's argument. Recognizing the importance of this matter for their application of the norm of substituted judgment, Liacos distinguishes among six relevant considerations, the fifth of which points to Saikewicz's inability to cooperate with the treatment. That factor

> introduces those considerations that are unique to this individual and which therefore are essential to the proper exercise of substituted judgment. The judge heard testimony that Saikewicz would have no comprehension of the reasons for the severe disruption of his formerly secure and stable environment caused by chemotherapy. He therefore would experience fear without the understanding from which other patients draw strength. The inability to anticipate and prepare for the severe side effects of the drugs leaves room only for confusion and disorientation. The possibility that such a naturally uncooperative patient would have to be physically restrained to allow the slow intravenous administration of drugs could only compound his pain and fear, as well as possibly jeopardize the ability of his body to withstand the toxic effects of drugs.[48]

The problem here is obvious: The court relies on factors "that are unique to this individual" that do not draw from *competent* expressions of that individuality. To use language from the previous chapter, the court conflates matters of *assent* with matters of *consent*. Saikewicz's anticipated conduct turns on a failure to assent to treatment, but that refusal is not the same as failing to provide informed consent. Only the latter presupposes instances in which patients are competent. Indeed, the court's argument is entirely convoluted, drawing on factors that pertain to Saikewicz's incompetence—his inability to understand treatment, and his likely confusion and disorientation—as reasons for applying the standard of substituted judgment, which "commends itself simply because of its straightforward respect for the integrity and autonomy of the individual."[49] In short, Liacos invokes data about a patient of considerably diminished autonomy in order to protect his autonomy rights.

The *Saikewicz* court fails to discern the relevant circumstances that surround different kinds of incompetence. In the case of a formerly competent patient, a proxy is to infer a patient's wishes from prior competent statements or competent behavior. In the case of permanently incompetent patients, however, such evidence is unavailable. Ironically, the court's logic imposes ableist assumptions on the second class of patients. Permanently incompetent patients have never crossed a threshold that grants their wishes moral weight in the calculus of medical decision making. The court's attempt to find a neutral, nondiscriminatory mechanism for protecting competent and incompetent patients presumes that no distinctions are plausible within the latter group. As a result, *Saikewicz* imposes an assumption about the prior abilities of one group of incompetent persons onto another incompetent group, abilities that the latter group clearly lacks. Herein lies a paradox: The attempt to produce a value-neutral, nondiscriminatory judgment nonetheless draws on assumptions that are obviously value-laden and prejudicial.

An additional, more muted, line of argument in *Saikewicz* refers to the distinction between ordinary and extraordinary means of medical care and contains a core of moral insight that the court unfortunately failed to develop. Without providing a definition of either means of treatment, Liacos referred to discussions in medical ethics according to which physicians may withhold extraordinary means and allow a patient to die: "The current state of medical ethics . . . is expressed by one commentator who states that: 'we should not use *extraordinary* means of prolonging life or its semblance when, after careful consideration, consultation and the application of the most well conceived therapy it becomes apparent that there is not hope for recovery of the patient.' "[50]

It is not clear why the court felt it had to claim that "our decision in this case is consistent with current medical ethos in this area" (of withholding treatment), given its concentration on privacy rights and the appropriateness of employing the standard of substituted judgment. Indeed, the *Saikewicz* court went to great lengths to discount the idea that *Quinlan* requires consideration of a reasonable person standard or an objective interests test in cases like Saikewicz's: "Evidence that most people choose to accept the rigors of chemotherapy has no direct bearing on the likely choice that Joseph Saikewicz would have made."[51] When discussing the sanctity of human life and the state's interest in preserving that life, Liacos speaks in expansive terms about the value of self-determination: "The constitutional right to privacy . . . is an expression of the sanctity of individual free choice and self-determination as fundamental constituents of life. The value of life as so perceived is lessened not by a decision to refuse treatment, but by the failure to allow a competent human being the right of choice."[52] Hence the court's reliance on a subjective test for the doctrine of substituted judgment.

That test, and the value of autonomy that it seeks to enshrine, does more work than the distinction between ordinary and extraordinary means. Practically speaking, it establishes greater negative liberties than the idea that extraordinary means may be permissibly withheld. Indeed, the distinction between ordinary and extraordinary means rests on an entirely different foundation and stands in tension with the assumptions that lie behind the doctrine of substituted judgment applied according to a subjective test.

As I have noted, the distinction between ordinary and extraordinary means is premised on objective considerations about the relative benefits and burdens of treatment for a particular patient. Extraordinary means are those whose burdens are disproportionate to patient welfare. Informed consent and substituted judgment, however, are premised in *Saikewicz* on subjective criteria, namely the patient's presumed or stated wishes. Indeed, if treatment may be withheld from a patient on the basis of substituted judgment that relies on divining the patient's wishes, then it is unnecessary to consider the relative merits of the treatment, for that patient may presumably express the wish to withhold any kind of treatment—ordinary or extraordinary.

It is easy to misunderstand this point and to run together considerations of informed consent and considerations of ordinary and extraordinary means. That confusion is, I believe, a function of two facts. First, it is probably true that most people who use living wills do so to express the wish not to have extraordinary means of treatment deployed in the event that they become incompetent. Second, the doctrine of informed consent and the category of extraordinary means function similarly: Both impose limits on a physician's conduct. But these two points, especially the latter, should be considered with care.

The first point draws a connection between the two ideas in ways that are contingent but not necessary. To suppose that informed consent *ought* to be guided by the distinction between ordinary and extraordinary means fails to recognize the full range of negative liberties that respect for patient autonomy allows in medical decision making. Those liberties permit patients to refuse treatment for many reasons, apart from whether its means are extraordinary. (For example, a patient may refuse ordinary means for religious reasons.) The second point needs to be nuanced in light of the limits it places on conduct. Extraordinary means refer to means that are *not medically required.* Physicians may withhold such means given that, on balance, they are not therapeutically necessary. Patients may not demand the use of extraordinary means, or, if they do, that demand may be denied. The idea of extraordinary means, premised on objective burdens and benefits, limits the demands that *either* the physician or the patient may make on the other. Reference to autonomy and substituted judgment, in contrast, may place limits on the deployment of medical treatment that *may be medically "required."* In that case, other values (autonomy) override the value of medical benefit.

I will return to this point and elaborate its more general features in the next chapter. Note for the moment that we are circling around a fundamental difference between the norm of autonomy and the norm of beneficence as barriers to action in treatment decisions. We see that difference here in the distinction between seeking substituted judgment regarding proxy consent, on the one hand, and considering the relative burdens and benefits of treatment, on the other. The former, as interpreted and applied by *Saikewicz,* rests on subjective criteria and seeks to protect autonomy. The latter rests on objective criteria and derives from estimations of a treatment's likely beneficial effects. If the court thought that Saikewicz's fate could be permissibly determined by the doctrine of substituted judgment—however flawed that reasoning happens to be—it did not need to rest part of its case on the fact that the treatment imposed burdens that were disproportionate to Saikewicz's benefit.

Given the obvious problems that surround the doctrine of substituted judgment in the representation of permanently incompetent patients, I am suggesting that Liacos would have done better to adhere to, and amplify, the idea of extraordinary means and to eschew the doctrine of substituted judgment altogether. That would imply more than one doctrine to protect human dignity when dealing with incompetents, but that fact would not leave some patients less protected than others. Rather, it would calibrate the mechanism of protection to the circumstances that surround their brand of incompetence. That is to say, the court's reasoning would have been less convoluted had it recognized that Saikewicz needed not a representative, strictly speaking, but a guardian. The latter's role, Pitkin reminds us, is distinct from the task of re-presenting what was present but is now absent. Instead, the guardian's role is to protect the objective interests of his or her ward, regardless of whether they are attached to or detached from the principal's wishes. The language of competence wrongly implies the ableist idea that, in cases of permanently incompetent patients, conditions of autonomy have been met and that the value of autonomy in such cases calls out for others' respect.

In the Matter of Eichner (1980)

Quinlan and *Saikewicz* establish an unclear legacy regarding the representation of incompetent patients. In *Quinlan*'s case, the court ruled that a formerly competent patient's express statements about nontreatment could be discounted, and argued on behalf of representing her medical interests on the assumption that interests connect with other presumed wishes. In *Saikewicz*, the court ruled that an incompetent patient's spokesperson can represent the autonomy rights of a patient who has never exhibited competency. Taken together, both cases suggest the paradoxical idea that permanently incompetent patients can have greater autonomy rights than formerly competent patients. How we are to represent the different cases of formerly incompetent patients and permanently incompetent patients required further thought and refinement, to which the court in *Eichner* addressed itself.[53]

That case focused on the plight of eighty-three-year-old Brother Joseph Fox, a devout Roman Catholic who resided with the community of Marianists at Chaminate High School in New York. Fox enjoyed a long-term relationship with the president of the school, Philip Eichner, a Catholic priest and superior of the Marianist community that lived on the school's premises. Eichner had known Fox since 1953, when Fox was prefect of novices during Eichner's novitiate. They had had occasional contact until 1970, when Fox asked to join, and was accepted into, the Chaminate community. While gardening on the school grounds one day in 1979, Brother Fox sustained an inguinal hernia trying to move large tubs of flowers. Fox arranged for corrective surgery and scheduled his operation for October. Near the conclusion of what was expected to be a routine procedure, Fox suffered a cardiac arrest. Emergency measures restored his heartbeat, but he experienced substantial brain damage as a result of the interruption of the flow of oxygen to his brain. Fox was moved to the intensive care unit of the hospital and placed on a respirator to assist his breathing. He then withdrew into a coma from which he was never to emerge.

When he learned of Fox's condition, Father Eichner approached hospital administrators and asked that he be removed from the ventilator. Those officials declined his request without direction from the court. Eichner, supported by Fox's surviving relatives and members of the religious community, then petitioned the court to be appointed the proxy for Fox and be permitted to authorize the cessation of the life-support system. An attending physician and examining neurosurgeon supported Eichner's petition. Controversy turned on the district attorney's opposition to the petition, requiring a special hearing and testimony about Fox's condition and his opinions about the use of extraordinary means.

In his affidavit, Eichner called attention to several statements that Fox had made regarding the use of extraordinary means of treatment, and these statements figured prominently in the court's decision to permit Eichner to assume judicial authority in conformity with those statements. Fox "had expressed the wish that if he ever entered into a state where his brain was rendered permanently incapable of sapient or rational thought 'the use of extraordinary life support systems' should be discontinued and 'nature allowed to take its course.' "[54] In 1976, when the *Quinlan* case was topical, the Chaminate community held discussions in which Fox actively participated, agreeing with Catholic teaching that allows for the cessation of extraordinary means. Eichner recalled one incident when Fox expressly stated that he "would not want any of this 'extraordinary business' "[55] done for him. Others testified that about two months before the hearing that Fox had said, "Well, why don't they just let us go? I want to go."[56]

The court ruled in Eichner's favor, arguing that Fox's common law right of bodily self-determination and the constitutional right to privacy could be exercised for him "since his wishes had been made sufficiently clear."[57] No countervailing state interests—the preservation of life, the integrity of the medical profession, the protection of third parties, the ban against suicide—were relevant. The crux of the case turns on the proper mechanism for protecting such rights. Writing for the court, Judge P. J. Mollen argues that the ideal is to have sufficient evidence so that "all concerned may rest easy in the knowledge that they are merely carrying out the stated wishes of the patient."[58] In the court's judgment, Eichner succeeded in providing that evidence. Fox's statements were closely connected in time to his operation and directly pertained to his circumstances after that operation. Unlike Quinlan's statements, Fox's claims were "highly probative."[59] Mollen adds, "Common sense dictates that when an 83-year-old man undergoes surgery —even 'routine' surgery—he contemplates the possibility of death."[60]

The *Eichner* court allows for proxies to exercise the privacy rights of incompetent patients when sufficient evidence exists regarding that patient's prior competently expressed wishes. In such cases, third parties are exercising what Pitkin would call the "megaphone" model of representation, in which one party serves as the instrument of another whose will or wish cannot be immediately ascertained. On this account, third parties are to exercise the incompetent patient's *actual* (rather than presumed or inferred) wish.

What of cases in which no such actual wishes can be acted on? What, in short, of cases that resemble *Quinlan*? In such instances, the court argues, there is room for inferring the patient's wish from the formerly competent patient's lifestyle and values. *Eichner* articulates core ideas behind the idea of *inferred* choice. But even here the court's concerns are qualified in interesting ways. For cases in which a patient's competent, express wishes do not exist, Mollen writes, we look particularly to a close family relative, a spouse, parent, child, broth-er, sister or grandchild . . . as an appropriate person to initiate, as committee of the incompetent, the process of reaching . . . a decision. Such an individ-ual who has known and loved the patient personally, presumably for years, can best determine what that patient would have wanted under the circum-stances. It is a decision we trust that will derive from a deep and abiding re-spect for the patient as an individual. But more important, we believe that it must be based on the assumption that the patient would have wanted it that way. This approach seeks to fulfill what would be deemed to be the dying patient's own wishes, and reaffirms notions of self-determination.[61]

Eichner is quick to add, however, that the proxy's authority is not absolute. Should there be any questions about the representative's decision, that deci-sion, "under particular circumstances, can always be tested as to whether it is in the best interests of the patient."[62]

As with *Quinlan,* and to a lesser extent *Saikewicz, Eichner* attempts to hold together considerations of privacy, autonomy, and self-determination, on the one hand, with considerations of medical interest, on the other. In *Eichner,* striking that balance can mean one of two things. It may mean that there are grounds for state scrutiny if an incompetent patient's representa-tive might be caught in a conflict of interest, unable to voice the patient's presumed wishes in a disinterested fashion. Or it could mean that a deci-sion that runs against the patient's apparent medical interest bears a heavier burden of proof than one that does not. I hasten to add that Mollen does not clarify which of these interpretations the court is recommending; nor does he specify the "particular circumstances" in which a representative's ac-tion may be scrutinized. At the very least, the court does not assign an ab-solute right to a representative who seeks to divine an incompetent patient's wishes.

In *Eichner,* we meet once again a feature of mandate theory insofar as wishes and interests are presumed to be connected. A representative who acts on an incompetent patient's inferred wishes is presumptively acting in behalf of that patient's interest. The court does not prohibit itself from ex-amining proxy decisions in which a wedge between presumed wish and ac-tual interest might exist. In short, there is no unqualified affirmation of patient autonomy.

Quinlan, Saikewicz, and *Eichner* draw from contexts in which the norms of autonomy and beneficence frame an understanding of patients' rights and direct the behavior of spokespersons of adult patients who are unable to provide informed consent regarding whether to begin or continue treat-ment. All three cases have served as legal and moral precedents for ascertaining how proxy consent might be provided for voiceless patients. Each case provides grist for refining proper standards of proxy consent, and we do well to draw together some insights before proceeding to cases involving children.

For cases in which formerly competent patients have provided prior, clear, and explicit instructions about the desired course of treatment—for example, in a living will—the first line of argument in *Eichner* is correct: A proxy should function as "a megaphone or mirror" of his or her ward's wishes. In this respect, spokespersons honor the value of the patient's autonomy and capacity for self-determination. Such a proxy is not a representative, strictly speaking, but "a servant, a *delegate,* a subordinate substitute for those who sent him."[63] Such is the task that Philip Eichner sought to exercise for Brother Fox.

Where incompetent patients have *not* provided clear and explicit instructions about the proper course of treatment, but others are in a position to infer what that patient would want, proxies are to honor the value of patient autonomy by reconstructing the patient's wishes from what that patient has competently expressed in word and deed. Here the third party acts in what is closest to Pitkin's model of a *representative,* rendering present what is absent. Joseph Quinlan represented his daughter in that way, however convoluted *Quinlan*'s description and authorization of such action happens to be.

When incompetent patients have provided neither competently expressed instructions nor competently expressed actions and values from which a decision can be reconstructed, third parties have no substantial autonomy to protect. In such cases, they must decide in light of what can reasonably be understood as the patient's interests. Individuals who are responsible for rendering a decision in these cases, as Pitkin argues, act as *guardians,* not as delegates or representatives. That should have been the way in which the *Saikewicz* court understood the responsibility of Patrick Melnik, Saikewicz's guardian *ad litem.*

REPRESENTING COMPETENT AND INCOMPETENT CHILDREN

The landmark cases of *Quinlan, Saikewicz,* and *Eichner* enable us to sketch broad lines for delineating the responsibilities of proxies who must consent to or refuse treatment for incompetent wards: *Delegates* lend voice to a patient's prior express, competent wishes; *representatives* infer the patient's wishes by reconstructing those wishes from prior competent actions and comments; *guardians,* lacking either competent statements or patterns of behavior from the patient on which to rely, decide in behalf of the patient's basic medical interest.

In pediatric contexts, the question is how these duties can instruct those who are responsible to care for a child's basic medical interests. That question is immediately complicated by the obvious fact that children differ in degrees of competence. As I noted at the outset of this chapter, adults' responsibilities must be calibrated according to the level of a child's maturation. Recalling the three broad groups of children to which I referred (with important caveats) in Chapter 3, the following cases and responsibilities suggest themselves.

First is the class of emancipated minors, mature minors, and adolescents who are at least fifteen years old. As I noted in the previous chapter, persons in these groups are presumptively competent and ought to be treated on the model of adult care. Accordingly, these ought to find themselves in the regime of presumptive antipaternalism, wherein health care professionals shoulder the burden of proof in establishing a patient's incompetence. Patients who are able to express their preferences have a right to have their wishes heeded. They need no delegate, representative, or guardian, and no question of "proxy ethics" pertains to these patients.

Patients who are unable to communicate their preferences are obviously different. In the standard argot, they are "incompetent" owing to factors that have diminished their deliberative and communicative capacities. In such instances, it is vital to recognize that the term *incompetence* can function in confusing ways and that such confusions might easily translate into unwarranted paternalistic conduct by families or medical professionals. That is to say, the temptation might arise to treat such an individual as a child, on the model of *incompetence* as *protocompetence*—that is, as insufficiently mature to make a medical decision. To prevent this confusion, it is necessary to distinguish between two kinds of incompetence in the case of children: *Incompetence* as *immature* (protocompetence) and *incompetence* as *inaccessible*. A sixteen-year-old patient who is incompetent in the second way should not automatically be considered incompetent in the first way as well.

Presumptively competent adolescents who are *incompetent as inaccessible* have a right to be treated on the model of adult patients. Here the *Eichner* court's opinion is directly instructive. Patients who have provided clear, competent expressions of their preferences, when those preferences pose no threat to third parties, have a right to have their wishes heeded. Here the task of the proxy is to serve as the patient's *delegate,* functioning as a megaphone of the patient's wants. That is to say, proxies are to make present the actual (absent) wishes of the patient.

If a patient in this age group has not expressed a clear preference for one kind of treatment or another, or for nontreatment, the proxy's task is to be the *representative.* He or she is responsible for inferring what that patient would want from that patient's competently expressed statements, values, and commitments. Here the task is that of constructing presumed wishes, following the model of Joseph Quinlan. Given what is intimately known of the patient's background, values, lifestyle, and commitment, the proxy is to produce what can reasonably be believed to be that patient's preferences.

With many patients in this age group, it may be that neither competent, express statements nor a critical mass of competent behavior can be relied on to craft a basis for proxy consent. In such cases, the task of the proxy is to function as a *guardian*, deciding on the patient's basic interests. Here the idea is that some patients have not produced enough evidence to guide delegates or representatives. Assuming that what would benefit a patient is what that patient would wish, the guardian is to proceed with an eye to patient welfare.

Second is the class of children roughly between the ages of eleven and fourteen years. Children in this category are presumptively incompetent, lacking sufficient maturity to express wishes that should be heeded in medical decision making. Here we shift regimes from presumptive antipaternalism to presumptive paternalism. Accordingly, these children shoulder the burden of proof to establish their competence and decision-making authority.

Parents or caretakers for children in this second group can be seen in several ways, depending on circumstances. When a child has established competence, the proxy's responsibilities are those that I have defined for young persons in the first group. In the more frequent instances in which the presumption of incompetence is not rebutted, the model of expressing or securing the patient's informed consent is not relevant. Rather, proxies are to safeguard the patient's basic interests. Following the philosophy of Pitkin, we can say that such proxies are to function as *guardians*. Children in need of caretakers are not represented, strictly speaking; nor may they assign the duty of delegate to their proxies. Their basic interests are real and objective.

When such patients are communicative, a guardian's additional duty is to seek the child's assent, to solicit the child's feelings and judgments, where appropriate. But recalling the error of *Saikewicz*, we should not confuse consent with assent. Failure to provide assent should not be seen as requiring proxies to protect a child's privacy rights in medical decision making. Attempts to construct the child's decision on the model of substituted judgment as understood by *Saikewicz* is to extend confusion into another population of patients.

The third class of patients are those under the age of eleven years. As I noted in Chapter 3, the presumption of incompetence cannot be rebutted in treatment decisions for these children. As a result, they rely on others to safeguard their basic interests. Here, parents or caretakers are to function as *guardians,* seeking to protect and promote the child's basic interests and seeking, when appropriate, the child's assent.[64]

Delineating the responsibility of parents and caretakers in this way is designed to accommodate concerns for children's welfare and children's developing powers of self-determination according to patterns of child development. The goal is to provide a more fine-grained understanding of children in order to adjust expectations of their competence and avoid two broad extremes: assuming that children are little adults, to be treated on the model of adult medical decision making; and assuming that children are all incompetent and that pediatric medical care is, or ought to be, thoroughly paternalistic. Two court cases illustrate how tempting each of these extremes can be. I want to conclude this chapter by discussing each.

In the Matter of Martin Seiferth, Jr. (1955)

Martin Seiferth was a young boy with a cleft palate and harelip, a condition that is normally treated at a very young age, whose father held strong convictions against medicine and surgery.[65] Martin's father believed in mental healing and in allowing "the forces of the universe to work on the body," and he refused surgery for his son.[66] In 1953, when Martin was twelve, a petition was filed in Erie County Children's Court by William Mosher, deputy commissioner of the Erie County Health Department, to declare Martin's father negligent, to transfer custody of Martin to the commissioner of social welfare of Erie County, and to authorize surgical and orthodontic repair of the boy's palate and harelip. At the trial, Martin, his father, and their attorney met in the chambers of Judge Wylegala after physicians presented information to all of them about the risks and benefits of remedial surgery. Martin indicated that he was pleased by what the doctors had showed him, but had come to the conclusion that he should try to close the cleft palate and harelip himself through natural forces. Impressed by Martin's level of maturity and the fact that he had clearly formed convictions of his own, Wylegala denied the petition and allowed matters to stand, thereby leaving Martin's father as his proxy.

Subsequent to that decision, an appellate court reversed Wylegala's opinion and granted the petition, assuming authority over Martin's medical interests and requiring him to undergo surgery. In 1955, when Martin was fourteen, a subsequent appeal was taken up by the New York Supreme Court, which reversed the immediate lower court's decision and reinstated the Children's Court dismissal of Mosher's petition. Wylegala's earlier decision was thus reinstated and Martin's father resumed authority to refuse corrective surgery.

Although this case precedes the rise of modern bioethics by ten years, the majority opinion in *Seiferth* contains seeds of moral wisdom about representing young persons that we do well to examine. Noteworthy in this regard is the court's effort to strike a balance between the goods of respect and welfare when representing the overall interests of adolescent patients. The dissenting opinion, by Judge Fuld, illustrates the difficulties of maintaining that balance when matters of patient welfare and a child's future interests appear to be unambiguous. Let us consider both the majority opinion and Fuld's dissent.

After noting that Martin's problem was not an emergency and posed no serious threat to his health and life, the majority opinion calls attention to two practical aspects of Martin's case that connect to considerations of autonomy and beneficence in proxy consent.

First, in order to benefit from surgery, Martin must cooperate with his surgeons and then comply with his speech therapists at his school. The majority court writes, "It will be almost impossible to secure his cooperation if he continues to believe, as he does now, that it will be necessary 'to remedy the surgeon's distortion first and then go back to the primary task of healing the body.' This is an aspect of the problem with which petitioner's plastic surgeon did not especially concern himself, for he did not attempt to view the case from the psychological viewpoint of this misguided youth."[67] Here the court attempts to take into account subjective aspects regarding Martin's situation, aspects that bear on his autonomy.[68]

Second, *Seiferth* considers whether state intervention can serve the interests of a patient's or family's decision-making processes. In the court's judgment, the good of privacy is imperiled when a state imposes its interests in others' domestic affairs. That is not to say that state intervention is wrong, only that it shoulders a considerable burden of proof in light of other goods that surround family privacy. For *Seiferth*, "less would be lost by permitting the lapse of several more years, when the boy may make his own decision to submit to plastic surgery, than might be sacrificed if he were compelled to undergo it now against his sincere and frightened antagonism."[69] Martin acknowledged that he might later accept treatment, and his father agreed not to interfere with any decision that Martin might make "in a few years."[70] The court here expresses the judgment that, on balance, state coercion is less in Martin's interest than allowing his father to decide on his behalf, however "misguided" that decision might seem. In effect, the court made a judgment about the merits of state intervention in light of the requirements of beneficence. It concluded that, proportionately speaking, Martin's interests were better served by liberty than by coercion.

On this second point, the court indirectly allowed for an overall *quality-of-life* judgment. *Seiferth* reasoned that Martin's overall interests were better served by state nonintervention, even if nonintervention might compromise his medical welfare. According to the court majority, Martin's medical interests must be factored into judgments about his overall interests, and those interests are better served, on balance, if the decisions are left to him and his family. The effect of the argument is to weigh and balance factors that are relevant to the application of beneficence as it bears on the protection of individual and family privacy. Martin and his father are better off if left alone by the state.

Taking these two claims together, we can see that *Seiferth* weighed and balanced the norms of autonomy and beneficence without trying to squeeze either norm into the mold provided by the other. Indeed, Martin's case illustrates how autonomy and beneficence can sometimes enjoy a reciprocal synergism without compromising their distinctive features. Regarding autonomy, the court recognized that Martin's willingness to undergo treatment was vital to its effectiveness. Without free cooperation, Martin cannot benefit from treatment. Regarding beneficence, the court reasoned that Martin and his family are better off if their privacy interests are honored. State intervention is likely to do more harm than good.

Judge Fuld's dissent is premised on the idea that each child "has a right, so far as possible, to lead a normal life."[71] Parents who endanger that right, Fuld maintains, may have their authority overridden on their child's behalf; they are illegitimate proxies. Martin's afflictions "not only grievously detract from his appearance but seriously impede his chances for a useful and productive life."[72] A child's rights impose on the court the duty to protect that child's welfare, regardless of whether that child consents to state or medical action. "We should not permit," Fuld writes, "[Martin's] refusal to agree, his failure to cooperate, to ruin his life and any chance for a normal, happy existence; normalcy and happiness, difficult of attainment under the most propitious circumstances, will unquestionably be impossible if the disfigurement is not corrected."[73] Martin's parents are guilty of neglect, and Martin's cooperation in that neglect is irrelevant to the question of his parents' culpability. As a practical matter, that means that the court should order treatment for Martin, "and leave to the good sense and sound judgment of the public authorities the job of preparing the boy for the operation and of getting him as adjusted to it as possible."[74]

It is tempting to read Fuld's dissent as an example of an illiberal decision, imposing a normative account of normalcy on Martin and his family in violation of their freedom. Matters are more complicated, however. Fuld has two lines of argument available, even though he did not use them.

First, Fuld could argue that, on the one hand, Martin established his competence during the initial proceedings when he expressed his sincere convictions in Wylegala's chambers. By using the language I introduced earlier, we might say that Martin overcame the presumption of incompetence that is appropriate when dealing with fourteen-year-olds and showed that he can stand on his own as a medical decision maker. Nonetheless, Fuld could argue, Martin cannot provide valid informed consent because his metaphysical and empirical beliefs are wrong—he lacks knowledge of relevant scientific facts. Moreover, Martin fails to understand and appreciate the reasonably foreseeable implications of his refusal: As he gets older, the benefits of surgery decrease, and therapy becomes more difficult. Those failures of understanding nullify his claim to provide informed consent. Overriding his decision is therefore justified.

Second, Fuld could argue that Martin's right to an open future is being seriously compromised by his family's beliefs, and that Martin's future interests outweigh his present interests in being respected.[75] In Fuld's judgment, the fact that Martin might later decide to accept treatment is not enough to protect his future interests. Fuld's dissent underscores the difficulty of coordinating a child's primary goods of welfare, respect, and future interests in the attempt to balance the more general norms of beneficence and autonomy in medical decision making. Rather than back away from that challenge, Fuld concludes that Martin's present and future welfare interests outweigh his present liberty interests.

However plausible it might be to reconstruct Fuld's dissent in this way, I find this reasoning unpersuasive. The problem is one to which I referred when I turned our attention away from *Quinlan, Saikewicz,* and *Eichner* to *Seiferth*. I noted in passing that in matters of proxy representation of children, it is often tempting to regard all children as incompetent and to assume that pediatric medical care is, or ought to be, paternalistic. We see that temptation in Fuld's dissent, which rests as much on the judgment that Martin is unable to assess his future interests as it rests on a normative vision of a normal, productive life. Testimony to the court indicated that Martin was an excellent student, that he was cheerful and good-natured, and that he was a reliable paperboy. Those data were entirely ignored in Fuld's dissent, which focuses entirely on the objective merits of surgery and therapy.

Recognizing that good arguments exist on both sides of this case, it is my view that the majority opinion was correct to leave matters to Martin and his father, however much I wish that they had provided better reasons for refusing treatment. Procedures regarding Martin oscillated between allowing him to speak for himself (Wylegala), and guarding his basic interests (Fuld). The majority in *Seiferth* sought to render a decision that attempts to balance these sets of concerns.

Here, as with considerations of paternalism, adult authorities are asked to ascertain how to treat patients as children, and when not to do so. The majority court neither treated Martin as a little adult nor ignored his family interests and his interests as a developing individual. Perhaps that is the best that can be done when representing the interests of young adolescents who deliberate about medical matters that do not involve life-and-death decisions. In any event, no algorithm exists to define that balance in advance of examining particulars in the treatment of adolescent patients. By comparison, the representation of young infants should be less complicated because autonomy-based rights to respect are less weighty, if not null. Surprisingly, a subsequent case suggests otherwise.

Custody of a Minor (1979)

In August 1977, a twenty-month-old boy awoke with a temperature of 106°F and was immediately taken by his parents to their physician in Hastings, Nebraska.[76] Suspecting the cause was leukemia, the family's doctor referred them to the Omaha University Medical Center, where that suspicion was confirmed. The child was diagnosed as having acute lymphocytic leukemia. For pediatric cases, the only known treatment was an aggressive three-year chemotherapy program. Left untreated in children, the disease is fatal.

On September 1, the infant began a program of intensive chemotherapy in Omaha. By the end of the month, results of a bone marrow test showed that the leukemia was in a state of remission. Soon thereafter, the family moved to the father's home town of Scituate, Massachusetts, in part because they were averse to cranial radiation, which was a component of child's medical regimen in Nebraska. Soon after arriving in Massachusetts, the family consulted Dr. John T. Truman, the chief of pediatric hematology at Massachusetts General Hospital (MGH) and placed the child in Truman's care. At the consultation, Truman indicated that cranial radiation was unnecessary and acceded to the parents' desire to administer chemotherapy in conjunction with a diet of distilled water, vegetarian foods, and high doses of vitamins. Truman pointed out that the diet could be used in tandem with chemotherapy, but that by itself, the diet would have no beneficial effects in the treatment of leukemia. The child's treatment at the hospital included injections of vincristine and spinal injections of methotrexate; at home, the parents were to administer a 6-mercaptopurine tablet daily. Bone marrow tests in November showed that the leukemia was in complete remission.

The parents then stopped administering 6-mercaptopurine tablets to the boy, although they did not inform the physicians at MGH of that fact. In November, they asked Truman what would happen if they ceased administering medications and learned that terminating treatment would guarantee a relapse. Their monthly visits continued as scheduled, however. In January, Truman noted changes in the child's condition suggesting that the infant might not be receiving sufficient medication. The family stated that there had been no difficulty administering medication at home and requested a refill for the child's prescription.

In February, the parents brought the child to MGH with a cold and fever. Truman noted that the child was pale, that his liver was enlarged, and that he had developed small hemorrhages under his arm. A blood test revealed the presence of 4 percent leukemia cells, indicating that a relapse had occurred. After several conversations with the parents, Truman learned that they had stopped the child's medications more than three months before.

During the next four days, Truman repeatedly telephoned the parents in an attempt to persuade them to resume the child's treatment. He argued that the chance of a cure, although compromised by the cessation of therapy, still existed, and that their actions generated legal responsibilities for him as a medical provider. Nonetheless, the parents did not resume administering the boy's medications. On February 22, the child was brought to MGH pursuant to an order of temporary guardianship issued by Judge Volterra of the Superior Court of Plymouth, Massachusetts, after a lower court dismissed a petition to assign temporary legal custody to the Department of Public Welfare. Chemotherapy was resumed, and the child's leukemia was again brought into remission.

The Supreme Court of Massachusetts reviewed the Superior Court's decision twice, in 1978 and 1979. The first case was reviewed on the court's own initiative; the second case resulted when the parents appealed that decision, seeking to retain full custody of the boy and to supplement his regimen of chemotherapy with metabolic therapy involving the daily administration of enzymes, vitamins, and laetrile[77] to treat the boy's leukemia. In each trial, the Supreme Court upheld Volterra's decision to assign temporary custody to state authorities. Although the 1979 decision rendered the final verdict, it relied on arguments that are developed more fully in the 1978 decision, and to both of those opinions we should direct our attention.

Noting that prior court decisions, like *Seiferth,* had shown great reluctance to overturn parental decisions regarding the refusal of medical treatment that involved comparatively little risk and great benefit to a child, Judge Hennessey of the Massachusetts Supreme Court nonetheless argues that parental rights are conditional, that "the parental right to control a child's nurture is . . . akin to a trust, 'subject to . . . [a] correlative duty to care for and protect the child.' "[78] Testimony indicated that chemotherapy had been used with substantial success in treating leukemia and that no evidence had been presented showing that an alternative treatment was consistent with good medical practice. The parents had substituted diet and prayer, arguing that "it is more important to us that [the boy's] life be full instead of long."[79] Testimony also indicated that the only physical side effects of the boy's medication were stomach cramps and constipation, which were readily controlled with other medications. On balance, the regimen's benefits outweighed its burdens, and no comparative alternative existed. Upholding the lower court decision, Hennessey argues that the child's medical interests were at risk and that Volterra's argument was consistent with "the applicable interests of the State in protecting the welfare of the children living within its borders, in the preservation of life, and in protecting the ethical integrity of the medical profession."[80]

Much of Hennessey's decision rests on its understanding of the second idea—namely, protecting the welfare of children living within the state's borders. The moral core of *Custody* turns on an understanding of the boy's basic interests and how those interests limit parental autonomy. Strangely, however, Hennessy understands the boy's interests in light of the value of patient autonomy. Specifically, his 1978 opinion connects the idea of the infant's interests to the doctrine of substituted judgment. According to Hennessey, the lower court's decision to assign temporary custody to the Department of Public Health was warranted because that court "applied the doctrine of substituted judgment" in the attempt to safeguard the interests of the child.[81]

Not surprisingly, the court leaned heavily on its verdict in Saikewicz; five of the seven judges in *Custody* (including Liacos) had been at bar in the *Saikewicz* decision. Citing *Saikewicz*, Hennessey observes that a judge who applies that doctrine on behalf of an incompetent person "must first attempt to 'don the mental mantle' of that person, so as to act on the same motives and considerations as would have moved [the individual]."[82] Hennessey adds, "By requiring a court to ascertain as nearly as possible the incompetent person's 'actual interests and preferences,' the doctrine of substituted judgment seeks to ensure that the personal decisions concerning the conduct of individual affairs remain, to the greatest extent possible, with the individual. In this way, the free choice and moral dignity of the incompetent person are recognized."[83] Although there are appreciable differences between some incompetent adults and this child of "tender years," *Custody* maintains that "the substituted judgment doctrine is consistent with the 'best interests of the child' test."[84] The court is to focus "on the various factors unique to the situation of the individual for whom it must act."[85] With that in mind, Hennessey concludes that the two standards for proxy action are identical: "As a practical matter, the criteria to be examined and the basic applicable reasoning are the same."[86]

Hennessey thus provided the right verdict for the wrong reasons. Two problems with his argument combine to make the decision in *Custody* a lamentable one. First, *Custody* wrongly assumes that protecting the interests of an infant must include considerations of patient autonomy. Hennessey has a misguided understanding of the primary goods at stake, assuming that both medical welfare and respect must somehow be specified and co-ordinated in the treatment of infants. But it makes no sense to "don the mental mantle" of a two-year-old, so as to act on "the same motives and considerations as would have moved [the individual]." Nor is it plausible to require "a court to ascertain as nearly as possible the patient's 'actual inter-ests and preferences' " when that patient is a baby. Indeed, it is absurd to go so far as to talk of the "free choice" of the infant, drawing on the paradigm of inferring wishes of incompetent adults from their previous competent wishes.

Second, *Custody* confuses two kinds of incompetence in its attempt to apply the standard of substituted judgment: incompetence as *inaccessible,* and incompetence as *immature.* Hennessey's decision is complicated be-cause the patient in question is incompetent in both senses. The mistake here lies in assuming that the procedure for representing incompetent-as-inaccessible patients likewise functions to guide proxy decisions regarding patients who are incompetent-as-immature. In my discussion of *Saikewicz,* I pointed out why it is a mistake to assume that the same procedure should apply for all proxy decisions on behalf of incompetent-as-inaccessible pa-tients. In *Custody,* we see that error extended into another class of patients —namely, immature patients (infants). *Some* incompetent-as-inaccessible patients, like Karen Ann Quinlan, may be represented in light of the "sub-stituted judgment" doctrine that aims to reconstruct the patient's wishes on the basis of prior statements and commitments. In *Quinlan,* that was pos-sible because Karen was a *formerly* competent person. Other incompetent patients, such as Joseph Saikewicz or the baby in *Custody,* are incompetent in different ways: Saikewicz was a *permanently incompetent patient*; the baby was *incompetent-as-immature.* Applying the substituted judgment doctrine by analogizing formerly competent patients such as Karen Ann Quinlan with Saikewicz and the baby in *Custody* fails to consider morally relevant features of each patient's type of incompetence.

We do better to draw some distinctions that aim to calibrate procedures to the needs and abilities of patients, thereby resisting the idea that the de-mands of autonomy are always relevant in the treatment of patients. Some, like the infant in this case and the profoundly retarded like Joseph Sai-kewicz, should not have such ableist prejudices imposed on them. Instead, those who act as their spokespersons should see themselves as guardians who must act to protect the patient's medical interests, not delegates or rep-resentatives who must work to honor the patient's wishes. Legal (and moral) decision making would be clearer and more helpful if it could resist the idea that protecting patient dignity is always a matter of respecting pa-tient autonomy. In pediatric ethics, it is a vice to assume that all patients should be treated as "little adults."

VARIABLES

The ethics of proxy consent in the care of children turns on several variables, depending on the maturity and accessibility of the patient in question. Keeping in view broad norms for representation in political contexts, I have attempted to identify three roles for patient proxies in pediatric contexts and to highlight two extremes that role morality must try to avoid: treating children as incompetent en masse, and treating children as "little adults." The dissent in *Seiferth* and the opinion in *Custody* remind us how tempting each extreme can be when considering the needs and wants of adolescents and infants, respectively. As with matters of paternalism, matters of delegation/representation/guardianship turn on how best to calibrate adult responsibilities to the circumstances of the child.

Throughout this discussion, I have tried to walk gingerly through the complicated terrain marked by the norms of beneficence and autonomy. My chief aim has been to focus on how to weigh and balance considerations of children's freedom, when appropriate, in light of their basic interests. Lurking in the background of our discussion thus far, but left untouched, are quality-of-life questions in the care of children. *Seiferth* called attention to quality-of-life considerations in decisions that are not matters of life and death; *Custody* posed the same issues when it rejected the mother's statement that "it is more important to us that [the boy's] life be full instead of long."[87] In the next chapter, I will bring those background issues to the foreground. My aim will be to call attention to another set of (correctable) confusions, and to sketch, roughly and in outline, normative presumptions about basic interests and the care of children.

FIVE

Basic Interests

Our pluralistic beliefs about child-rearing do not lead to a
uniform interpretation of the best interests standard.
—*Hillary Rodham*[1]

PERPETUAL MOTION

While visiting a children's hospital in the Northeast, I encountered an intriguing sculpture of sorts, half art and half science, housed in a large glass encasement. Named *Perpetual Motion,* the sculpture is a colorful contraption of metal, wood, rubber, and plastic. Mechanical activity begins in one corner, where a machine-driven pulley lifts brightly colored balls, one at a time, to the top of the sculpture and propels them down a long, circuitous metal runner. As each ball proceeds along its route, it drops through baskets, rings a bell and chimes, knocks on wooden blocks, sends a pendulum swinging to strike a gong, and bounces along a xylophone, creating a gentle cacophony throughout the day. Each ball travels down and through the sculpture's maze for about forty seconds before it finds its way to the bottom runner and back to the pulley to begin another journey. No family passes by without stopping to watch and listen; children of all abilities, races, ages, and ethnic backgrounds find *Perpetual Motion* fascinating.

The sculpture is symbolic, but not in the usual sense that art is symbolic. By appealing to children with diverse needs and backgrounds, *Perpetual Motion* is an analogy for a primary good. The architecture and artistry of *Perpetual Motion* draw universal attention, joining people from a wide range of beliefs and customs. As a site of shared admiration, the sculpture represents the idea that some goods cut across cultures and needs, that some goods are basic to a child's interests. Pediatric care is premised on the idea that certain needs and interests are not final goods but rather are instrumental to a child's pursuit of other, more comprehensive goods, whatever those latter goods might be. In pediatric care, basic interests are not generally in dispute, and these interests (like *Perpetual Motion*) provide a center around which to concentrate talent, energy, imagination, and hope.

A child's basic interests are the proper object of an adult's duty to care. In this chapter, I want to pursue that idea and the challenge it poses to medical ethics. To prepare for that discussion, I want to review some of the ideas we have examined thus far.

At the outset of this book, I noted that medical ethics has devoted considerable attention to the norm of patient autonomy, in large part to ground the idea of patients' rights and to protect patients from medical power and paternalism. As a limit on the value (and exercise) of beneficence, respect for autonomy may trump medical providers' recommendations and may require providers to tolerate patients' decisions that are contrary to their medical interests. In adult medicine, what poses as beneficent treatment must be acceptable on the patient's own terms. Antipaternalistism and respect for patient autonomy are laudable ideas, but, as I noted in the Introduction, developing their moral contours can crowd out attention to equally important issues in medical contexts for patients who cannot exercise substantial autonomy. Our discussion of pediatric paternalism and representing patients in the last two chapters should help us see how that is so; there, I aimed to identify classes of patients for whom autonomy-based rights make no sense and whose dignity must be protected on other terms. These incompetent patients have not provided a basis for others to function as their delegates or representatives. Such patients need guardians to make decisions for them on the basis of their basic interests.

Who are such patients? Here our focus is on children and adolescents, and they fall into four groups.

First are *previously competent patients* who are inaccessible as a result of infirmity or accidental trauma, and who cannot provide express or presumed wishes regarding treatment. This group includes patients for whom insufficient information exists to invoke explicit wishes or the mechanism of substituted judgment, despite the fact that they were formerly competent. Some mature minors, emancipated minors, and older teenagers who are rendered unconscious by infirmity or trauma fall into this class.

A second class would be *presumptively competent patients* who are communicative, but whose competence is rebutted on psychological or other testing. In this class would be fifteen- to seventeen-year-old patients who lack sufficient maturity to shoulder the burden of competence.

Third are *presumptively incompetent patients* who are unable to override the rebuttable presumption of their incompetence. In this group we find eleven- to fourteen-year-old patients.

The final category comprises patients who are *unrebuttably incompetent*, namely, children who are ten years old or younger.

In all of these cases, the idea of respecting patient autonomy has no place in the determination of decision-making authority. True, for patients in the second, third, and fourth groups, there is a need for adults to nurture freedom and responsibility. My focus in this chapter is on decision making apart from these developmental concerns—decision making that aims to protect the dignity of patients who lack sufficient autonomy to provide informed consent at the specific moment when a decision must be made. In those instances, decisions must be guided by these patients' basic interests. Stated more abstractly, for these patients the good of beneficence does not compete with the value of autonomy; the latter cannot function as a side-constraint on parental or medical authority.

That is not to say that the value of autonomy is entirely absent from cases involving these patients. As I noted in Chapter 2, strong reasons exist for valuing parental autonomy and family privacy, reasons that involve the family as a source of the child's experience of love and affection; the parents' knowledge of their child; the experience of authenticity and responsibility in decision making; and the role of the family as the principal social unit in which individual identity is forged. Therein lies reasons for our first revision of the pediatric paradigm: Professionals' commitment to care can be modified by respect for a family's customs and beliefs. But once again we must recall that the value of family privacy is constrained by considerations of the child's welfare. As Judge Hennessey remarks in *Custody of a Minor,* "the parental right to control a child's nurture is . . . akin to a trust, 'subject to . . . [a] correlative duty to care for and protect the child.' "[2] In pediatric care, the idea of mediated beneficence means that professionals and parents must ally to secure the welfare of the child. Therein lies the simple but important goal of forging a therapeutic alliance.

In this chapter, I want to deepen our understanding of protecting a child's basic interests as the core feature of that alliance. Throughout the discussion, we will be recalling some of the basic points I developed in Chapter 2, in which I discussed the duty to care and the obligation to provide for the child's primary goods of welfare, respect, and the right to an open future. Here I will begin by addressing the complaint that basic interests, however they are understood in medical ethics, are indeterminate—that we cannot agree on what it means to act on anyone's basic interests because we cannot agree on a vision of the good life. Without a socially shared vision of what it means to flourish as a human being, it is impossible to determine how to protect a patient's interest. What is "good" for a person is up for grabs in a culture that lacks a shared understanding of the ends of human life, for without the idea of such ends we cannot determine how to promote that person's interest. The problem of moral pluralism will thus be our first topic, for unless it can be adequately addressed we cannot properly advance any understanding of a guardian's duty to protect a patient's welfare. Given that there are many patients within the four classes I have mentioned, the stakes are considerable if we cannot speak coherently about envisioning and protecting patient well-being. More generally, if the idea of patient well-being is seriously to be doubted, then the general priority of beneficence to autonomy in the pediatric paradigm makes no sense.

After considering those problems, we will turn to how the idea of protecting a patient's interests connects with quality-of-life considerations, for here, too, we must address the challenge that pluralism poses to decision making in medical contexts. No less than patients and their families, ethicists differ about the terms that should guide medical decisions. After considering the problem of pluralism in general, we will turn to that problem as it bears on criteria for evaluating quality-of-life considerations that hover in the background of medical decisions putatively made in patients' interests.

We will then draw from these concerns about pluralism, patient interests, and quality-of-life criteria to examine four cases that involve judgments about what ought to be done in a young patient's interests. I will conclude by garnering insights from these cases to distinguish the norms of autonomy and beneficence as these pertain to decision making in adult and pediatric medical contexts.

Before beginning our discussion of pluralism and patient welfare, however, we must first recall an important qualifier from my discussion of beneficence and benevolence in Chapter 2. Here, as before, I will speak of a child's *basic interests* rather than best interests, despite the fact that the latter category is typically used in court decisions, public policy, and medical ethics regarding young patients. As I argued earlier, obligating parents or care providers to protect a child's best interests asks too much of them, for such interests compete with other goods that justifiably vie for attention and respect. The duty to care means that children have claims to the beneficent action of their caretakers, and the denial of such claims can violate a basic set of rights. That is not to say, however, that children have a right to the maximal level of caring action that others might be able to provide, for we must accommodate children's claims within a complex array of other duties and virtues. Parents or guardians must weigh responsibilities to one child against obligations to other family members when appropriate, and must weigh responsibilities to children against other domestic, civic, professional, economic, and social commitments. Moreover, parents or guardians have duties to themselves, and they may be unable to discharge their other responsibilities without appropriately attending to their own needs. As a matter of fairness to parents or guardians, other family members, and society at large, children do not have the right to maximal care from their parents. For that reason, it makes more sense to talk of children's basic interests, rather than their best interests, when considering medical welfare in pediatric contexts.[3]

THE CHALLENGE OF PLURALISM

In medical settings, seeking a child's basic interests involves evaluating a number of treatment options, including nontreatment, in order to determine which offers a balance of benefit over burden. In contrast to reconstructing or expressing a patient's wishes, the idea of seeking a person's basic interests requires us to examine the merits of treatment on objective grounds. The main idea is that patients' wishes occasionally fail to accord with their welfare, or that it is impossible to divine their wishes. In either case, it may sometimes be necessary to protect patients' welfare independently of their subjectivity.

Doubts exist in Western, liberal societies about whether it makes sense to speak normatively of patients' basic interests. Those doubts derive from the fact that individuals in liberal cultures have different ideas of what is good for them—about what is in their basic interests. Definitions of health and the value that individuals assign to health differ widely from person to person. Some persons judge moderate corpulence to require medical attention, sometimes surgery; others see moderate corpulence as the sign of a lively, robust life. For some persons, health is less important than travel, gourmet cooking, or intellectual stimulation. Given the diversity of lifestyles and values, what seems essential to the health of one person may be entirely insignificant to another.

In Ezekiel J. Emanuel's mind, this fact of pluralism should be worrisome because it undermines the idea of basic interests and the correlative norm of patient welfare. Ezekiel argues that we lack an objective, socially shared criterion for determining how best to measure relative benefits and burdens. That is because estimations of patients' welfare are inextricably bound up with considerations of their quality of life, and liberal societies lack consensus about what a good life should look like. The moral fact of pluralism subverts any effort to talk about the proper ends of medicine in normative terms. Ezekiel writes,

> Determining what is a benefit and what is a burden is inextricably linked to a particular conception of the good life. We can only tell if some situation or thing is valuable or harmful by relating it to a more encompassing conception of what is meaningful and worthy. The possibility of using the best interests standard becomes a question of whether there is an objective, socially shared conception of the good life. For only with such a conception of the good life could there be an objective, socially shared standard of benefits and burdens.[4]

Consider two patients with laryngeal cancer, for which the removal of the larynx is one option. Emanuel observes, "Two patients being treated by the same physician at the same hospital may opt for very different treatments. One may value his speech more and accept a shorter life, while the other may value longevity over having the ability to speak."[5] The first patient would thus choose nontreatment, whereas the second would choose surgery, chemotherapy, radiation, or some combination of these. Medical providers are not in a position to declare which decision is desirable or accords with an objective account of the patients' best interests because what is desirable is relative to each patient's commitments and values.

Compounding this problem of moral pluralism is liberalism's methodological neutrality, its desire to craft principles of fairness that are not implicated with any particular understanding of the good life. We saw aspects of this neutrality when discussing Rawls and his idea of the original position in Chapter 2. For Rawls, liberal political theory must attempt to articulate an understanding of justice that is not beholden to any "comprehensive" theory of the good—for example, Eastern Orthodoxy, Mormonism, Pure Land Buddhism, utilitarianism, Vaishnavism, liberal Catholicism, or secular humanism. A comprehensive theory makes metaphysical claims about agency and selfhood, and purports to provide an account of the moral life that relies on a theory of ultimate truth or reality.

Related to this aspiration to neutrality is the distinction between liberalism as a *political* theory and liberalism as a *comprehensive* theory. As a political theory, liberalism seeks to develop a doctrine of justice for political and social institutions, and set the boundaries for the proper conduct of the state. It thus eschews liberalism as a more ambitious comprehensive theory, which focuses on metaphysical questions about human agency and the moral life, and typically esteems the value of autonomy. As a political liberal, Rawls seeks to fashion principles with which reasonable persons would agree when deliberating according to the constraints imposed by the veil of ignorance. In that way, liberals like Rawls develop duties and virtues of social justice that can function within societies that allow for widely different beliefs and lifestyles. In Rawls's language, liberalism as a political theory "stays on the surface, philosophically speaking,"[6] thereby avoiding philosophical debates about ultimate truth. The procedure is neutral not in the sense that it cannot be normative, but in the sense that its normativity does not depend on any particular vision of the good.

For Emanuel, liberalism's aspiration to neutrality prevents liberals from articulating the kind of vision necessary to make sense of weighing benefits and burdens when considering patients' interests. That is because estimations of benefits and burdens cannot be considered independently of a more general account of the good life. No neutrality regarding comprehensive ends is possible. Any normative vision of the good life, however, would violate political liberalism's aspiration to avoid implicating its account of justice within particular traditions or comprehensive visions. If,

for example, treatment decisions were made on the basis of maximizing patients' capacity for free choice and minimizing the impediments to exercising choice, then that decision would endorse a vision of personhood that
privileges the good of self-determination, and that affirmation runs contrary to Rawls's desire to stay "on the surface, philosophically speaking."
Or, treatment decisions that seek the patient's interests principally on the
basis of pain alleviation privilege a hedonistic account of human well-
being, and this approach, too, is contentious and particularistic. More worrisome is the fact that liberalism seems unable to adjudicate between the
merits of either approach without becoming one more comprehensive doctrine.

As I have suggested, if Emanuel is correct, then much of what occurs in
medical care is either unintelligible or illiberal, because several classes of patients exist for whom treatment decisions *must* be made on the basis of
basic interests. If such decisions are putatively made without reference to
some understanding of patients' overall good, then they are unintelligible.
If they *are* made with reference to patients' overall welfare, then such decisions impose a normative vision of the good on those patients and thus appear to violate political liberalism's promise of neutrality. Given the fact that
parents and pediatric medical professionals routinely act as guardians and
expect to make decisions on behalf of children's basic interests, we must ask
whether Emanuel's worries hold up.

The answer is that they fail on two counts, both of which derive from
misunderstandings of liberal theory. The first problem centers on Emanuel's faulty understanding of neutrality in liberalism and his inability to recognize the special duty to care along with the principles of paternalism as a
product of the veil of ignorance. The second, related problem is Emanuel's
failure to see how such principles generate the duty to provide primary
goods to persons in need. This latter point allows individuals to guard others' basic interests, when necessary, without having to worry about imposing
a comprehensive vision of the good on their wards. It is entirely conceivable, in short, for political liberals to authorize beneficent action without violating the aspiration of neutrality or turning their theory into another
comprehensive doctrine. Let us take each point in turn.

It is true, as Emanuel observes, that liberalism as a political theory as-
pires to a certain kind of neutrality, which must be understood in a very
precise way. Sometimes it is assumed that neutrality prohibits liberal doctrine from passing any judgment on various comprehensive commitments.
However, that inference would deny liberalism any normative bite, and liberal neutrality is misunderstood if seen in that way. Rather, liberalism is
"neutral" in the sense that it attempts to craft principles of justice on terms
that do not rely on particular religious and philosophical doctrines. In
Rawls's more recent formulations, the idea is to build on an "overlapping

consensus" of comprehensive visions of the good life, what Rawls calls a consensus that "consists of all the reasonable opposing religious, philosophical, and moral doctrines likely to persist over generations and to gain a sizable body of adherents in a more or less just constitutional regime."[7] Principles of justice developed in this way remain neutral to the extent that they do not derive their authority from any particular set of comprehensive doctrines; justice-as-fairness hovers over those doctrines, as it were, compatible with their more "thickly textured" visions of the good life, but beholden to no one vision exclusively. When such principles remain "on the surface, philosophically speaking," they avoid an exclusive association with a particular tradition or vision of human well-being. Such "neutral" principles can then be deployed to evaluate the moral quality of social institutions and public policy.

The critical question for Emanuel is whether this neutrality prevents political liberalism from talking about "the good," and the answer is yes and no. The answer is yes if such talk implicates political liberalism in a comprehensive vision of the good; the answer is no insofar as political liberalism can coherently presume the duty to provide primary goods. Heeding the demands of methodological neutrality, political liberals avoid connecting exclusively with a "thick" theory of the good. But such neutrality does not rule out talk of a "thin" theory of the good, or the duty to provide such goods to others, and herein lies the second error in Emanuel's account.

To see this point, let us retrace some steps. I noted in Chapter 2 that Rawls's theory generates principles of paternalism to protect us "against the weakness and infirmities of [our] reason and will in society." Such principles, crafted from behind the veil of ignorance, authorize some persons to act on others' behalf when they cannot look after their own good. If we are to construct principles of fairness without knowing our social position, age, or gender, we would produce principles that would ensure that we are not abandoned if infirm or dependent once the veil of ignorance is lifted and we learn about our actual position or condition in society. Principles of paternalism aim to guarantee that as a matter of fairness, infirm or dependent persons would be treated according to norms that are rational and caring, aimed to protect their wishes, if possible, or their fundamental welfare. Behind the veil of ignorance we would fashion principles that would encumber some to respond to the needs of others who cannot care for themselves. In other words, from within the constraints of methodological neutrality, it is possible to construct duties to care. Liberalism is not unable to produce obligations of beneficence or the obligation to assist in another's' welfare. Quite the contrary: Given the fact of human finitude and vulnerability, it would be irrational not to encumber ourselves and others with the duty to care. If we failed to do so, we would leave each other victim to the arbitrary forces of the social and genetic lottery.

The key point for Rawls is that such principles become pressing when an individual cannot pursue his or her own good and cannot communicate his or her wishes. In such instances, "we act for him as we would act for ourselves from the standpoint of the original position. We try to get for him the things that he presumably wants whatever else he wants."[8] In that way, principles of paternalism generate the obligation to provide primary goods for an infirm or dependent person, goods that are instrumental to a wide variety of comprehensive visions of the good. As we saw in Chapter 2, primary goods are goods that one needs whatever else one wants. Such goods are instrumental to the ends of human life, assuming that such ends can vary as much as they do in liberal societies. Regardless of what individuals want or will want, we can assume that there are various things that they will prefer more of than less.[9] Children in possession of these goods can generally be assured of greater success in carrying out their intentions and advancing their aims, whatever these aims happen to be or become.

So much for the duty to care as a feature of liberalism, compatible with its aspiration to neutrality. Let us consider that duty within medical settings, where Emanuel believes liberal tenets cannot support substantive judgments about what constitutes a patient's interests. We have observed throughout this book that when the norm of patient welfare and its corresponding virtues and duties are brought to bear on medical interactions between professionals and competent adults, they are (or should be) qualified by the side-constraint of autonomy. That value is institutionalized by the mechanism of informed consent. A physician may thus be required to treat two patients with laryngeal cancer in quite opposite ways, for each patient may privilege different values—longevity or vocal communication—that require treatment or nontreatment, respectively. Each adult patient's decision stands within, and is rendered intelligible by, different overarching visions of the good life. But what of patients, such as children, for whom questions of autonomy are less pressing or irrelevant? What of cases in which such patients' overarching vision of the good has not materialized? Does that mean that considerations of these patients' basic interests are indeterminate?

When it is not possible to ascertain a pediatric patient's comprehensive goods and corresponding values, we are left with the family's or professionals' therapeutic judgment about how to balance benefits and burdens when determining the patient's basic interests. As I noted in Chapter 2, that means coming to terms with the goods of physical, intellectual, and emotional welfare; respect; and the right to an open future. Families and medical professionals may differ as to how such goods are to be weighed and balanced; such differences are generally differences about how to specify the duty to care. It is not necessary here to rehearse how these tensions might be presumptively sorted out.[10] What is important to note is that liberal theory supports a determinate idea of what constitutes pediatric patients' basic interest—that liberalism can produce norms for evaluating decisions that are putatively made in children's interest. Primary goods are both open ended —compatible with different visions of the good life—and determinate, providing normative guidelines for assessing practical decisions by parents and professionals in behalf of children who cannot decide for themselves.

Taken together, these points about liberalism's ability to encumber us with the duty to care and to attend to others' claims to primary goods demonstrate that liberals are able to talk of social policy or professional practice that aims to "do good" for others, so long as we understand "good" in a thin rather than thick sense. Contrary to Emanuel's claims, liberal doctrine can readily affirm the idea that it is a good thing to protect others' basic needs. That idea compromises neither liberalism's methodological neutrality nor its recognition of pluralism. Those who act as others' guardians can do so justifiably. Their task is to determine as best as they can what is beneficial for their wards in light of the goods of physical, intellectual, and emotional welfare; respect; and the rights to an open future.

STANDARDS OF QUALITY OF LIFE

A theory of primary goods allows us to speak coherently about seeking a patient's basic interests in a liberal, pluralistic culture.[11] What I have said thus far about primary goods is somewhat abstract; here I wish to speak more concretely about such interests and take up another feature of the problem of indeterminacy that Emanuel provocatively puts before us. In addition to the fact that patients express different preferences as a result of having different values, we must take account of various *criteria* for evaluating medical decisions. As I have noted, considerations of basic interests are tied to quality-of-life judgments insofar as the latter provide an overarching rationale for making sense of patients' medical interests, and this connection appears problematic because no socially shared vision of the good life exists in liberal cultures. Emanuel deepens his challenge to medical ethics by noting the differences between normative terms for evaluating patients' decisions. That fact sharpens the problem of indeterminacy insofar as it points to a general lack of *theoretical* consensus about how to evaluate patients' decisions, adjudicate disagreements between patients and professionals, and construct medical policy. Most troubling is the fact that liberalism appears unable to evaluate the relative merits of any such standard.

Emanuel identifies six criteria for making quality-of-life decisions. Without purporting to exhaust all possibilities, he accurately names those that have functioned most prominently in the literature of medical ethics: the physical, hedonistic, relational, autonomy-based, economic, and utilitarian conceptions of quality of life.[12] Emanuel lists and describes these standards as damaging evidence for liberal doctrine, because their relatively peaceful coexistence in medical decision making reveals how toothless liberalism is as a blueprint for policy and social institutions. That is to say, the fact that liberalism tolerates such widely divergent standards reveals how difficult it can be to forge social consensus about the ends of medical treatment.

Let us first rehearse these six criteria and then turn to a liberal assessment of them. Throughout this discussion it is important to keep in mind the idea of primary goods as goods that name a patient's basic interests, and that such goods are fully compatible with liberal doctrine. It is also important to remember that liberalism functions to provide a permissible range of activities and choices, setting the outer boundaries beyond which human behavior or social policy is judged as unjust. Given these two features of a liberal medical ethics policy—affirming primary goods, and setting the outer limits of acceptable policy—what can be said about the six criteria for evaluating quality-of-life decisions? Which, if any, can be judged as standing outside acceptable practice and policy by liberalism's lights?

Consider first the physical conception, which claims that life itself is an absolute good, regardless of its "quality." Often known as either "vitalism" or the sanctity-of-life position, this conception holds not only that life is sacred or a supreme value, but also that all human life is equal and that attempts to draw distinctions between one person and another on the basis of different endowments is a form of unjustified discrimination. On this view, a so-called defective child should be kept alive, regardless of his or her prospects, using all available medical therapies and technologies. All persons have an equal right to life; preventable death is an unmitigated evil.

The second conception is hedonistic, which understands a person's quality of life in terms of the avoidance of pain. In medical contexts, this conception produces the rule that withholding treatment is justified only when it promises to reduce the patient's physical or psychological pain. Here the focus is obviously not on the self's physical life per se, but on the self as a locus of sensations.

Third is the relational conception, developed most notably by the Jesuit moral theologian, Richard McCormick. On this view, physical life is seen as an instrumental good, "a value to be preserved only insofar as it contains some potentiality for human relationships."[13] Rather than focus on physical life as an end in itself or the self as a locus of sensations, McCormick insists on a social understanding of the self and measures the prospective merits of treatment accordingly. Drawing on biblical and theological materials, McCormick argues that "our love of neighbor is in some very real sense our love of God. The good our love wants to do Him and to which He enables us, can be done only for the neighbor." Hence, McCormick argues, "the meaning, substance, and consummation of life are found in human *relationships,* and the qualities of justice, respect, concern, compassion, and support that surround them."[14] Patients who seem able to experience love and communication and who can interact with others satisfy this criterion. The key is not to focus on life itself, but on the connection between physical life as an instrumental good and a fully human life, viewed relationally. McCormick writes, "When in human judgment this (relational) potentiality is totally absent or would be, because of the condition of the individual, totally subordinated to the mere effort for survival, that life can be said to have achieved its potential."[15]

The fourth conception focuses on autonomy as the principal index for assessing quality of life. This idea emphasizes not social relationships but individuals' capacity to form, evaluate, and revise their ends. The core value is individual self-determination, especially emotional and intellectual independence. The model self in this regard has capacities of thinking and judging, deliberating about aims and objectives, ascertaining what particular acts will achieve those chosen ends, and acting on those deliberations.

On this point it is important to distinguish between autonomy as a side-constraint and autonomy as an end state or ideal of personhood. James F. Childress, following Robert Nozick, understands this distinction well. As a *side-constraint,* Childress writes, respect for autonomy "limits the pursuit of goals such as health or survival; it even limits the pursuit of the goal of the preservation and restoration of autonomy itself."[16] In this way, autonomy places a negative check on what one person may do for another, even (but not only) when such action involves treatment that may enhance a person's autonomy. In medical settings, autonomy as a side-constraint establishes a firewall that protects patients against professional power and paternalism. Conceived as an *ideal of personhood,* in contrast, autonomy is an end state to be achieved. In this formulation, the ideal of unfettered self-determination is seen as a comprehensive good, a final end that defines human well-being. This ideal may justify limiting patients' decisions when those decisions risk impairing the exercise of self-determination.

Fifth is the economic conception of a person's quality of life, according to which one's "quality" is a function of being able to engage in socially meaningful work and living independently. Productive persons who interact in society and the market enjoy a better life than those who are economically dependent or unable to work.

Finally is the utilitarian conception. Not unlike the fifth conception, this standard looks to the overall social good that a medical decision will be likely to produce. Here we are to focus not on the quality of individuals' lives for them, but on the net balance of pleasure and pain that will result from deciding to treat patients one way rather than another. The relevant good is seen neither individualistically nor relationally in McCormick's sense. Rather, the merits of a decision are determined in light of its contribution to the larger social whole. On this view, if keeping the demented or incurably infirm alive does not contribute to the aggregate good, then medical treatment may be justifiably withheld or withdrawn from such patients.

Obviously these standards would produce different decisions about the same patient. On the first conception, Karen Ann Quinlan's respirator would not be withdrawn; according to the relational or utilitarian conceptions, strong justifications for withdrawing treatment are easily imaginable. At the same time, notable differences beyond the physical standard are clear. A relational standard appears to establish a lower threshold for continuing treatment than the autonomy conception because the latter emphasizes ableist qualities such as independence and self-sufficiency. Each standard can conceivably produce different treatment decisions about moderately retarded and dependent persons. As a result of these kinds of differences, Emanuel concludes that we are left without a rudder when guiding medical practice and policy, that "in a liberal polity there will be no agreed-upon standard and hence no way of publicly defining *the* best interests of a patient."[17]

Yet here it is important to distinguish between actual social arrangements and liberal doctrine, and not to impute features of the former to the latter. The fact that widely different views of quality of life operate in medical contexts is not necessarily damaging to liberalism as a *theory*. There is a difference, in short, between the theory and reality of liberalism, and Emanuel courts confusion by citing aspects of the latter to indict the former.

As I have noted, liberal theory functions in part to carve out a sphere of permissible activity and to draw boundaries for practice and policy. I also argued that the primary goods of physical, cognitive, and psychological welfare; respect; and the right to an open future provide a normative understanding of basic interests along liberal lines. How can these two points relate to the six criteria I have summarized?

The physical conception would clearly fall outside the bounds of acceptable policy or practice, for physical life as an ultimate good goes beyond the value assigned to physical well-being as a primary good. This point might be best understood by noting that, in liberal theory, primary goods relate to other goods in ways that resemble McCormick's understanding of physical life as an instrumental good. For McCormick, physical life is a value insofar as it connects with and contributes to a life that has the potential for human relationships. That same logic constrains the way that primary goods should be conceived: They are goods we need whatever else we want. As conditional and instrumental, they are relative, proximate ends. Although their value can be understood independently of the *substance* of a particular end, they do not have value independently of a *connection* to more encompassing human ends. To elevate a primary good to supreme value is to misconstrue its fundamental nature as relative and subordinate to the realization of final goals. Without any final goals in view, the value of primary goods becomes moot. If physical life is the only value being protected by medical treatment, then treatment may be terminated. Because a primary good is relative, the duty to preserve it is limited.

A similar argument would constrain appeals to the hedonistic conception. One can plausibly argue that minimizing pain is a primary good insofar as it is necessary for the realization of other goods. Although some persons may choose lives that, for whatever reason, burden them with encumbrances or extraordinary challenges, the person who chooses pain as an end in itself is typically pathological. Minimizing pain as a relative good functions to aid persons in the achievement of their values and commitments. One of the key traditional goals of medicine, after all, has been to reduce pain and suffering. Treatment decisions premised on the value of pain minimization as a relative good are thus acceptable on liberal grounds. Treatments that involve enormous suffering toward a reasonably achievable end may thus be ruled out as unacceptable or "extraordinary means" according to a theory of primary goods. That is to say, treatment in which the benefit is disproportionate to the suffering involved in treatment need not be mandated by considerations of the patient's basic interests.

Third is the relational conception. Here we are not considering a good that can be viewed instrumentally or relatively, but an end to which other values are subordinated. Note that this conception differs from the first two: It does not suggest a relative value that might be absolutized. "The potential for human relationships" must be thought about as part of a comprehensive vision, not a relative or instrumental end. Liberals might thus think of the relational conception as one end to which their account of primary goods can link. For political liberals, primary goods are compatible with a relational standard for measuring a patient's quality of life insofar as the goods of patient welfare, respect, and the right to an open future are instrumental to the good of human sociality and intersubjectivity.

We should also note that McCormick's relational criterion is qualified in ways that render it compatible with liberal ideas. His account can allow for only a conditional acceptance of the relational criterion—a point that can easily be overlooked by moralists and social critics who esteem relationships in unqualified terms. McCormick speaks about relationships in which parties have the capacities to give and receive love, but the language of love can mask parental self-justification for untoward decisions. As we shall see in the next chapter, an unqualified appeal to relationships can open the door to decisions that may require excessive sacrifices from one of the parties. Hence, it is important to recall that McCormick emphasizes the good of relationships *along with* "the qualities of justice, respect, concern, compassion, and support that surround them."[18] This qualification captures in broad strokes the kinds of conditions imposed by a thin theory of children's medical interests. So long as the relationships that are valorized by the relational conception heed children's needs, respect their wishes (when appropriate), and allow for an open future, that conception is compatible with the normative constraints implied by the principles of paternalism. The relational criterion stands within the boundaries marked off by liberal theory insofar as the criterion is qualified by the requirement to provide primary goods.

Fourth is the autonomy conception. Here we meet a value that clearly connects with liberalism *as a comprehensive doctrine*; philosophers such as Kant and Mill place supreme value on capacities of reflective self-determination. As I noted in Chapter 2, this conception provides one, but only one, basis for a theory of primary goods. The values of physical, cognitive, and emotional well-being, respect, and the right to an open future make sense to the extent that they are instrumental to the process of self-determination in one's adult years. Accordingly, liberalism as a *political doctrine* may affirm autonomy as a legitimate end for measuring patients' basic interests. But political liberalism cannot elevate autonomy as a necessary criterion for making such assessments without violating its aspiration to neutrality. As my brief treatment of the relational conception suggests, primary goods can contribute to more than one conception of patients' overall interests.

The fifth and sixth conceptions, the economic and utilitarian, are similar enough to be treated together. Both base the value of treatment on the patient's ability to contribute to the overall social good. Each conception is ruled out by the notion of primary goods as denoting a patient's basic interests because these conceptions understand a patient's quality of life in comparative rather than individualistic terms. That is to say, each assumes an idea of "quality of life" as social worth rather than personal worth, as worth to society rather than as worth to the individual in question. Insofar as political liberalism is antiutilitarian, aspiring to protect the rights of persons on terms independent of their contribution to the social aggregate, both conceptions stand outside the fundamental tenets of liberal political philosophy.[19]

Understood as denoting a patient's basic interests, the idea of primary goods can thus lead to a reasonable reduction of criteria for assessing a patient's quality of life without reducing all options to comprehensive liberal ideals. Primary goods provide a qualified protection of physical health and the minimization of pain, a qualified endorsement of the relational standard, an endorsement of the autonomy conception as one candidate for quality-of-life decisions, and no authorization for either the economic or utilitarian conceptions. As such, the idea of patients' basic interests as expressed in primary goods rules out the physical and hedonistic standard, when these are viewed as sufficient bases for determining quality of life, and it rules out economic and utilitarian conceptions altogether. It thus provides a reasonable pluralism that allows for goods other than autonomy. Liberal doctrine provides pluralism but not indeterminism, variety but not normlessness.

CASES AND PRIMARY GOODS

If I am correct in reconstructing the idea of a patient's basic interests according to a theory of primary goods, then we can see how such an account functions in light of concrete examples. The relevance of such goods to quality-of-life judgments can occur in four types of cases: pointless treatment; beneficial but painful treatment; beneficial, relatively painless, but unwanted treatment; and withdrawing treatment when burdens outweigh benefits. Each of these cases can be found in court precedent or in my clinical experience at Baylin.

Henry the Corpse

It would seem obvious that a medical professional does not have a responsibility to treat a dead person. Beauchamp and Childress write, "Treatment is not obligatory when it offers no benefit to the patient because it is pointless or futile. . . . For example, if a patient is dead, although still on a respirator, he or she can no longer be harmed by cessation of treatment."[20] Those authors add that definitions of death can vary across beliefs and traditions: "If heart and lung function can be maintained, some religious traditions hold that the person is not dead, and the treatment is not futile, even if health care professionals deem it futile."[21] As a result of differing beliefs, conflicts can arise about whether medical treatment accords with a putatively dead patient's basic interests.

The case of Henry Gucci in Baylin's intensive care unit (ICU) provides an apt illustration and is complicated in ways that standard approaches to medical ethics often omit. Henry was a seventeen-year-old adolescent who, along with a friend, broke into an apartment with plans of setting a fire. Their scheme was foiled when the home's occupant entered and discovered them. The occupant, a karate expert, chased the young men down the street, caught Henry, and kept him in a choke hold while waiting for the police to arrive. A vigorous struggle ensued; Henry was asphyxiated and experienced cardiac arrest. He was brought to Baylin early on a Saturday morning, unconscious, breathing, and in neurological distress. Over the weekend, his brain proceeded to swell; he remained unconscious. On Tuesday, a computed tomographic (CT) scan revealed increased fluid in the skull; on Wednesday, he stopped breathing and was put on a respirator. At that time, an initial flow study of his brain was inconclusive; two subsequent exams indicated that brain death should be declared. On Thursday night, Baylin's neurology team declared Henry brain dead. His mother refused to accept that diagnosis and insisted that he be kept on a respirator.

According to Baylin's house staff, Ms. Gucci embarked on a "barrage of aggression" in the unit, "screaming and [becoming] hysterical."[22] After one "blood-curdling scream," she fell to a fetal position on the floor and required attention from members of the psychological–social team who were summoned to the scene. Members of that team learned that Henry's mother had a history of anxiety and depression and had been prescribed antidepressants more than once. During Henry's admission, she was a constant source of aggravation. In addition to verbally intimidating nurses on the floor, she brought in as many as twenty teenagers to keep a loud vigil at Henry's bedside. Remarked Marcia Padroni, the outcomes manager at the time, "Mom used them to keep her miracle hope alive and put pressure on the docs and nurses."[23]

Ms. Gucci's responses to Henry's condition were partially fueled by beliefs that do not easily cohere with scientific criteria and terminology. When pregnant with Henry, she was told by physicians that he would be stillborn. When he was seven months old, he contracted meningitis, and she was told that he would be severely retarded. That neither of those predictions came true was a function, in her mind, of miracles that had occurred for her and Henry. Those inaccurate predictions also gave her pause about the merits of medical expertise. In addition, her first pregnancy resulted in a stillbirth, and she believed that Henry was the reincarnation of that child. She shared all of these thoughts with nurses and attending physicians during the week.

On Friday, Michael DeVries, one of the ICU's attending physicians at Baylin, agreed with Ms. Gucci that Henry would be kept on the respirator over the weekend and that house staff would continue to administer standard care. No do not resuscitate (DNR) orders were issued; nurses were required to administer cardiopulmonary resuscitation (CPR) if Henry experienced another cardiac arrest. In his conversation with Henry's mother, DeVries added that medical support would be withdrawn by noon on Monday, regardless of her wishes. The goal of keeping him in the hospital over the weekend was to provide time for his mother to consult with another neurologist and her lawyer. At it happened, Ms. Gucci contacted the state's Department of Social Services, claiming that Baylin was abusing her son, and notified one of the state's two senators about her situation.

It is tempting to view this as a case in which the value of respecting parental autonomy conflicts with the patient's basic interests. House staff were asked to honor Ms. Gucci's request for treatment that was, in DeVries's words, "violative of [Henry's] dignity."[24] In effect, ICU nurses were asked to provide counterfeit care—medical treatment that did Henry no good. However, at a meeting in which house staff were debriefed about the case, the problem turned less on the tension between parental autonomy and patient welfare, however helpful those ideas are for sorting out some of the moral issues in Henry's case. Rather, DeVries imposed on the staff the problem of having to care for a corpse in a situation of emotional and professional adversity. Specifically, the nurses' complaint turned on the fact that they were required to act outside a therapeutic alliance with Ms. Gucci. As Claire Hawthorne noted, it is not unusual for nurses to attend to a corpse in certain cases: "We've done that for organs, for forty-eight hours. It's for another's good, but we all buy into that good. [In this case, we acted] for the mom's good. People felt ambivalent about whether it was for her good."[25]

Henry's case illustrates instances in which pediatric care providers must work as much to treat family members as they to do treat their patients. A commitment to Henry's basic interests would mean that all would have agreed to discontinue the respirator and medications when the neurology team declared him dead, for no further therapy was required to forge an alliance among the professionals and family members. The duty to care generally ceases when no further medical benefits are possible. Sometimes an alliance is difficult to forge with parents whose beliefs are deeply implicated in their child's lives. A therapeutic alliance was nonexistent in Henry's case, and his basic interests were compromised for several days as a result of DeVries's decision to heed his mother's wishes. House staff felt professionally diminished by the request to follow the demands of someone whose good they didn't "buy into." As it turns out, Ms. Gucci agreed to the withdrawal of treatment on Monday; she never pressed charges or pursued her complaint with the senator's office. In granting her wishes, Baylin's house staff avoided what would have been a violent and uncontrollable situation. As I will indicate below, the deeper problem is that Ms. Gucci pushed the value of autonomy well beyond its appropriate limits.

Aaron's Request to Die

A second kind of case turns not on treating dead patients as if they were (or might become) alive, but on the fact that death may be preferable to medical treatment—even treatment that provides some hope for medical success. Here the decision is that patients' interests cannot be served, on balance, by medical treatment, given the burdens that such treatment imposes. In asking them to endure medical treatment, they are being asked too much. That idea lies at the heart of the distinction between ordinary and extraordinary means of care.

The story of Aaron Wolfe provides one illustration of a patient for whom the burdens of treatment outweighed its prospective benefits. Aaron was a ten-year-old with a history of recurrent medulloblastoma (brain tumor) owing to a genetic deficiency that prevented his body from suppressing tumors (Gorlin syndrome). He also had suffered from meningitis, migraine headaches, and skin cancer. Adding to his woes was Aaron's Stevens-Johnson disorder, a rare condition characterized by severe blisters and bleeding in the mucus membranes of the lips, eyes, mouth, nose, genitals, and rectal area. Those symptoms can be treated with corticosteroids, analgesics, fluids, and sedatives. Aaron was admitted to Baylin's ICU after experiencing a bout of seizures accompanied by increased skin rashes, breathing difficulties, mucositis, and a high fever. A veteran of medical care, Aaron had already undergone numerous surgeries. At admission to Baylin, his lips were swollen, his eyes and mouth secreted mucus, and his upper extremities, face, back, and rectal area were covered with lesions and rashes. While in the hospital, he was at high risk of infection and in constant pain. Over the early course of his admission, he began to experience increased respiratory distress. The fact that his skin was sloughing off his cartilage and bones made intubation virtually impossible.

In a family meeting with Aaron's parents, the physicians were beseeched by a sobbing, exhausted, and grief-stricken mother: "Whatever we decide, please don't let him be in any more pain. Please, please, no more pain for him. He's suffered enough in life." That request was repeated at least three times, with increasing distress, during the parents' forty-minute session with their son's medical team. Aaron's parents then agreed to a DNR and DNI (do not intubate) status for him. Baylin's neurologists indicated that Aaron was not dying, but that it was not clear what could be realistically done to improve his condition; at best, he would return to a life of constant seizures, recurrent surgeries, and the fires of an epidermal hell.[26]

Within a day, Aaron's condition clearly deteriorated. He became incontinent and urinated on his rashes, aggravating his already considerable discomfort. His mouth had loose flesh in it, raising further concerns about his ability to breathe. Christopher Martin, the attending physician (as well as the ICU's director and a member of the hospital's ethics committee), authorized Aaron's parents to regulate his comfort level by allowing them to release morphine by way of a patient-controlled analgesia (PCA) device, a bedside mechanism that normally allows patients to administer a restricted amount of pain relief to themselves. In Aaron's case, "the parents could push the PCA device with no lock-out. They wanted it to end quickly. They released 90 mg of morphine in a couple of hours. It went a lot faster than I expected. Starting in the morning, they pushed every five minutes."[27]

According to Jaime Rogers, one of Aaron's nurses, "He asked his dad permission to die. It was an open dialogue with them [the parents] and the kid." With the approval of Martin, Aaron's request was granted. "Theoretically," remarked Jaime, "he could have survived. But it was okay to let him go."[28] The burdens of ongoing medical treatment were extraordinary.[29] Remarked another ICU nurse about these kinds of cases, "A kid at [a cancer clinic] ran away. He wanted to die comfortably. He went to Florida. 'I'm not coming back,' he said, 'because you'll throw me in a hospital.' "[30]

In the Matter of Kevin Sampson

In 1970, the Commissioner of Health in Ulster County, New York, brought a neglect proceeding against Mildred Sampson for failing to provide adequate medical and surgical care for her son, fifteen-year-old Kevin Sampson.[31] Kevin had von Recklingshausen disease, an illness that left him with a large facial deformity that caused his entire right cheek, the corner of his mouth, and right ear to drop down, "a massive, grotesque, repulsive . . . disfigurement of face and neck."[32] As a result of his appearance, Kevin had been excused from school since the age of nine years and was virtually illiterate. The staff psychiatrist of the Ulster County Mental Health Center, after a psychological examination, reported that Kevin showed signs of delayed development, a high level of dependency on others, and "inferiority feeling and low self concept."[33]

The unanimous recommendation by all of those who dealt with Kevin was that steps should be taken to correct his condition through surgery, even though he was not at risk of death or in need of surgery to improve his hearing or eyesight. Surgery could not cure Kevin of his affliction or even produce what doctors described as a "normal face."[34] Moreover, the risks of surgery were considerable; the operation would take six to eight hours and would involve a considerable loss of blood. The overall goal of the surgery would be to alleviate Kevin's condition and improve "his chances of growing up into a normal adulthood."[35] As such, the benefits of surgery would be more psychological than physiological. Judge Elwyn of the Ulster County family court writes, "The massive deformity of the entire right side of his face and neck is patently so gross and so disfiguring that it must inevitably exert a most negative effect upon his personality development, his opportunity for education and later development and upon every phase of his relationship with his peers and others."[36] This disfigurement, Elwyn adds, "constitutes such an overriding limiting factor militating against his future development that unless some constructive steps are taken to alleviate his condition, his chances for a normal, useful life are virtually nil."[37]

At issue was Mildred Sampson's agreement to permit the surgery but not a blood transfusion, as she was a devout Jehovah's Witness. Without that permission, the operation would have been impossible, as it would have involved what one physician described as "much, much, much" loss of blood.[38]

Noteworthy in this case is the presence of quality-of-life considerations for a patient who is neither terminally ill nor comatose and incommunicable. Instead, the court faced the question of how to consider the basic interests of a child in a case involving beneficial but unwanted treatment. Specifically, the *Sampson* court was asked whether a parent's religiously based refusal to provide beneficial medical treatment outside of an emergency situation constituted neglect, and if so, whether the court was authorized to intervene on behalf of the child's interests. The surgery in question included considerable risks and promised only to alleviate, but not cure, Kevin's condition. Recognizing that Mildred Sampson's decision was premised on religious convictions, the court asked itself how to balance "the potential good to be attained against the risks to life necessary [sic] involved in so dangerous a surgical procedure and consideration of the validity of the religious objections which have been raised to the administration of blood transfusions."[39]

Sampson invites immediate comparison with *In the Matter of Martin Seiferth, Jr.,* which we examined in the previous chapter, insofar as both cases concern whether to mandate treatment that is not meant to resolve a life-or-death situation but to improve an adolescent's quality of life. Recall in *Seiferth* that the court refused to override parental objections to potentially beneficial surgery and subsequent therapy for Martin Seiferth, an adolescent with a cleft palate and harelip. *Seiferth* considered the merits of an operation with fewer risks and greater benefits than Kevin would be likely to experience. If *Seiferth* decided in such a low risk/high benefit case to yield to parental authority, then all the more reason to think that the *Sampson* court would follow that precedent to resolve a case involving higher risks and fewer obvious benefits.

But Elwyn sharply distanced this case from *Seiferth,* arguing that *Seiferth* had been decided fifteen years earlier and that subsequent legislation in New York had conferred on judges broad discretionary powers to protect the basic interests of minors. The effect of these facts was to cast doubt on the validity of *Seiferth* as binding precedent. Instead, Elwyn drew directly on the dissent of Judge Fuld in *Seiferth*. Fuld had argued on behalf of state intervention to override the refusal to repair Martin's cleft palate and harelip, stating that each child "has a right, so far as possible, to lead a normal life."[40] Parents who endanger that right, Fuld maintained, may have their authority overridden on their child's behalf; they are illegitimate proxies. Martin's afflictions "not only grievously detract from his appearance but seriously impede his chances for a useful and productive life."[41] According to Fuld and Elwyn, a child's rights impose on the court the duty to protect that child's welfare, regardless of whether that child consents to state or medical action. "We should not permit," Fuld writes, "[Martin's] refusal to agree, his failure to cooperate, to ruin his life and any chance for a normal, happy existence; normalcy and happiness, difficult of attainment under the most propitious circumstances, will unquestionably be impossible if the disfigurement is not corrected."[42]

The prospects for a "normal, happy existence" were likewise at stake in Kevin Sampson's case. For Kevin, Elwyn argued, some risk must be taken to produce such prospects. Elwyn thus decided to override Mildred Sampson's refusal, placing Kevin in her custody but putting her under the supervision of the county's Commissioner of Social Services for a year on the condition that she cooperate with his order to have surgery performed on her son. (The cost of the surgery and hospital care would be shouldered by the county.) Delaying a decision until Kevin was old enough to settle the matter for himself—as was considered in *Seiferth*—"totally ignores the developmental and psychological factors stemming from [Kevin's] deformity which the court deems to be of the utmost importance in any consideration of the boy's future welfare."[43]

I observed in my discussion of *Seiferth* that the court's permission of parental refusal was a quality-of-life judgment that settled that matter in light of an overall estimation of Martin's basic interests. In *Sampson* we likewise meet quality-of-life judgments, but those judgments lead toward the opposite conclusion—in favor of state intervention rather than against it. That fact bids us to compare the cases in order to determine whether different conclusions that derive from quality-of-life considerations point to the indeterminacy of the standard.

There are three notable differences between Martin Seiferth's and Kevin Sampson's cases. First is the fact that Kevin, unlike Martin, showed no opposition to the proposed surgery. The sole obstacle in Kevin's case was his mother's refusal to permit a blood transfusion, but her refusal finds no additional support in anything Kevin said or did. Nothing in the court records indicate that Kevin would fail to cooperate with medical professionals. Martin, in contrast, was unlikely to comply with the proposed surgery and subsequent therapy; he considered the physicians deluded. Second is the fact that Kevin, unlike Martin, showed considerable lack of psychological development as a result of his affliction. Martin Seiferth was active in school, had a paper route, was highly regarded, and presented himself well to others. Kevin, in contrast, suffered from "low self concept" and was illiterate as a result of missing six years of school. Third, and related to this second difference, is the weight that should be accorded each boy's wishes. Kevin's delayed development suggest that his wishes should have far less weight than Martin Seiferth's, who was articulate and affable. Even if Kevin had expressed some resistance to the idea of surgery, his autonomy appears to be diminished when compared with Martin's.

Stepping back from these particulars, we can see that in *Sampson* the primary goods of respect and the right to an open future were handled differently from *Seiferth*. Martin Seiferth expressed his wishes in ways that call for some measure of respect because his cooperation would be vital to the treatment's effectiveness. Kevin Sampson did not express similar wishes and made no bid to an independent set of claims or desires. Any presumptive competence that might be assigned to persons of his age was clearly rebuttable. He needed someone to act as a guardian of his future interests considerably more than Martin, who showed no evidence of delayed development or diminished autonomy. Moreover, Kevin had suffered more psychologically and educationally, and his prospects for future development were considerably more limited than Martin's. The boys' claims to respect and rights to an open future differed in the balance: Martin's claim for respect was stronger than his right to an open future, whereas Kevin's right to an open future found no counterweight in claims to respect.

Each case was decided correctly, but we would be wrong to think that *Sampson* simply developed a line of argument from Fuld's dissent in *Seiferth* to protect the basic interests of a neglected adolescent. Rather, in both cases, the courts were asked to put the prospect of medical treatment in the balance with primary goods—claims to respect and the right to an open future—and in each case, that balance came out differently owing to morally relevant features of each boy's circumstances.

Ahmet Ali

Ahmet Ali was ten-month-old boy admitted to Baylin twice in the spring of 1998 for surgeries to repair his cleft palate and clubfeet. Born to observant Muslims who were first cousins, Ahmet had an atrial septal defect (a hole between the two atria in the heart), was hearing impaired, had one abnormal kidney, and depended on a tracheostomy tube to breathe. Neurological studies indicated that he lacked a connective band of fibers that hold together the hemispheres of the brain. Hospital records note "decreased visual acuity and unusual eye movements." Ahmet "seems alert, does not smile on initial exam. Parents report that he moves his extremities a lot but does not roll or sit." At the age of two months, he was admitted to the hospital for respiratory distress and shock; at five months, he had a cardiac arrest, requiring aggressive cardiopulmonary resuscitation. Within a six-month period, he underwent three surgeries: one to correct his heart defect, a second to repair his hernia, and a third to correct an abnormality of the penis in which his urethra opened on the undersurface. Ahmet suffered from obstructive sleep apnea, leading to pulmonary edema—excess fluid in his lungs—and was fed through a tube that was inserted into his abdomen. While in the hospital, he was also treated for bronchospasm, a narrowing of pulmonary airways. As a result of illness and respiratory distress, Ahmet had been home less than one month during his first ten months of life. In his small bed in the ICU, his body wiggled in a dark and silent confusion as nurses, attending physicians, residents, and fellows circled around him.

Cases like Ahmet's are some of the most difficult in pediatric medical ethics. He was not dying or terminally ill; not indigent (his parents financed his medical care); and not admitted to the hospital (this time) under emergency conditions. His many congenital anomalies pose the following questions: Does his quality of life justify ongoing treatment? Is it in Ahmet's basic interest to undergo a life of surgery, with little hope of connecting with his family or developing interpersonal relationships? What would be the best course of action (or inaction) if Ahmet's condition deteriorated and medical professionals had to make a decision about whether to perform CPR or to intubate him?

House staff in the ICU indicated that Ahmet's parents refused to consider decisions about whether to withhold or withdraw treatment from their child. The parents upheld a sanctity-of-life position, avoiding hard questions about their boy's overall quality of life. But Islam does not adhere strictly to a vitalistic ethic, requiring caretakers to do all that is necessary to save physical life. Treatment of Ahmet is thus gnarled by religious and philosophical difficulties.

Muslim teaching allows a more permissive approach than vitalism. According to Aziz Sachedina, professor of Islam at the University of Virginia, decisions about Ahmet's care should be informed by Muslim teaching in ways that are open to quality of life considerations. Sachedina writes, "There are two rules that a Muslim ethicist would apply to Ahmet's case: 'Removal of probable harm' (*daf' al-darar al-muhtamal*) and 'no harm and harassment' (*la darar wa la dirar*)." Either rule would permit withdrawal or nontreatment. In personal correspondence, Sachedina adds:

> The first rule requires a risk-benefit analysis in undertaking treatment that might or might not alleviate the suffering of the patient. As a matter of principle, Muslim law requires to do everything possible to cure a sick person. This excludes mere prolongation of suffering wherein there is no lasting benefit to the sick. Rejection of harm ('*usr wa al-haraj*') is a duty in Islam. Therefore, removal of probable harm can be evoked to stop further treatment of the patient, who by all medical standards, is simply buying time.
>
> The second rule raises the question of the quality of life. Is life under these medical circumstances worth prolonging? How about the harassment caused to the child and to the people connected with the child? No individual is seen detached from the immediate people related to [him or] her. Hence, in this situation, Ahmet's condition has not shown any improvement. Quite to the contrary, complications are multiplying. The family is

empowered to make a decision, in this and similar cases, when the patient is not competent to remove harm from himself or herself, to end the treatment and allow nature to take its course.

In effect, in Islamic teaching the norm of nonmaleficence opens up considerations of whether treatment is in a patient's overall basic interests. Caretakers are required to consider whether ongoing treatment contributes to any improvement in a patient's condition. If not, it is seen as a harmful act, prohibited by Muslim teaching. About these difficult matters, Sachedina adds, "Only God is best informed of matters that we humans undertake to interpret."[44]

Philosophically, the problem with Ahmet's treatment is that it absolutizes the value of physical life. More precisely, it values the primary good of physical existence as if it were a final good, ignoring the fact that in Ahmet's case it is disconnected from other goods. As I indicated above, the principles of paternalism would not condone such a view on one of two counts.

First, the sanctity-of-life criterion values the primary good of physical life as a final good. Recall that primary goods are goods we need whatever else we might want. As conditional and instrumental, primary goods are relative, proximate ends. Although a primary good's value can be understood independently of the *substance* of a particular end that it serves, it does not have value independently of a *connection* to more encompassing human ends. In Ahmet's case, it is not clear what connections exist between the primary good of physical existence and the final ends that give life meaning and purpose.

A second reason, premised on the relational criterion, proceeds according to the formal logic of the first: Ahmet shows no potential for engaging in human relationships; the good of physical existence is not serving higher, intersubjective ends. He will always depend on others to attend to his most basic needs; he is unable to develop powers of communication and communion. Here McCormick's words are instructive: "When in human judgment this (relational) potentiality is totally absent or would be, because of the condition of the individual, totally subordinated to the mere effort for survival, that life can be said to have achieved its potential."[45] Given Ahmet's level of dependence, cognition, and infirmity, his potential for relationships would be subordinated to the mere effort to survive. According to the relational criterion, it would not violate Ahmet's basic interests to allow him to die.

One difficult question is how this permission can influence interactions between parents and professionals in the health care setting. A general presumption of tolerance, nondirection, and respect for parental autonomy often allows families to decide about treatment in nonemergency situations.

Those presumptions were often adhered to in my observations at Baylin. Although many nurses shook their heads about Ahmet's operations, no one questioned his parents about whether to subject him to future surgeries and intensive care.

Here we encounter the tension between the values of parental autonomy and a patient's basic interests. As I noted in Chapter 2, this tension is often resolved in favor of respecting family privacy given the fact that parents or guardians must shoulder the burden of decision making about treating or not treating their child. Introducing quality-of-life considerations into a family's deliberations, especially in nonemergency settings, seems intrusive and moralistic. Pediatric medical ethics, guided by the idea of mediated beneficence that aims to protect a child's basic interests, would counsel professionals and counselors to initiate conversations that do not doom a child to treatment decisions premised solely on the physical criterion. Unfortunately, that hope may be as remote as the prospect of an improved quality of life for children like Ahmet.

THE ASYMMETRY BETWEEN AUTONOMY AND BENEFICENCE

Cases like Henry's and Ahmet's illustrate how the norms of beneficence and autonomy impose different kinds of demands on families or health care providers who are in a position to make a medical decision about whether to treat a patient. We do well to linger over that difference here, if only to shed light on confusions that can materialize in moral disputes about the limits of medical care.

Respect for patient autonomy functions negatively, imposing restraints on a medical professional's prerogatives. That is to say, in medical care respect for autonomy generates a negative right rather than an ideal of personhood. Recall that respect for autonomy as a *side-constraint* "limits the pursuit of goals such as health or survival; it even limits the pursuit of the goal of the preservation and restoration of autonomy itself."[46] Respect for autonomy as *ideal of personhood,* in contrast, values autonomy as an end state to be achieved. I have already indicated why liberalism as a political theory cannot privilege autonomy conceived in this way: Political liberalism's methodological neutrality prevents it from invoking the authority of a single particular vision of the good life. As a practical matter, it would be paternalistic to impose such a vision of the good life on patients who do not want their autonomy maximized. Respecting autonomy (only) as a side-constraint avoids that problem, for it allows patients to make decisions for reasons that need not include the value of autonomy as a comprehensive ideal.

For our present purposes, the more important contrast is between autonomy as a side-constraint and the norm of beneficence. That latter norm can generate positive or negative obligations on the conduct of a family or health care provider. Normally beneficence grounds the practice of care, establishing positive duties to attend to the suffering and needs of others. But it can also generate negative duties—for example, the duty not to treat. In these latter cases, the idea is that it would be contrary to patients' basic interests to subject them to medical intervention.

Coordinating these negative and positive aspects of beneficence and autonomy produces some important distinctions. In adult medical care, as I have indicated, the standard picture is that the medical provider's positive duty to care may be held in check by the patient's right of refusal, functioning as a side-constraint. The paradigm is that (professional) beneficence as a positive duty is constrained by (patient) autonomy as a negative right. In pediatric medical care, however, the more pronounced place of beneficence in the overall moral equation produces a different picture for professional ethics. That difference is of two types.

First, parents or guardians cannot morally refuse treatment that is in the basic interests of their child. That is to say, respect for parental autonomy is conditional on the family's commitment to their child's basic needs. In pediatric care, the norm of autonomy does not have the same strength as a side-constraint that it does in adult contexts. Stated differently, in pediatrics the professional's positive duty of beneficence can trump the negative right of parental autonomy.

Second, medical providers might disagree with families about the meaning and implications of beneficence. What might appear as a tension between parental autonomy and a professional's duty to care can mask a deeper tension between two incompatible visions of the patient's basic interests. I suspect that this is where most conflicts between families and professionals occur: Each has a different understanding of how properly to care for a child in need. In some cases, one party might see beneficence as enjoining medical intervention, whereas the other party sees beneficence as enjoining nonintervention or the withdrawal of treatment. Forging a therapeutic alliance means arriving at a shared perception about how to care for a child's basic interests. Before that alliance is achieved, beneficence may be functioning positively (for one side) and negatively (for the other).

In this way, the norm of beneficence differs from respect for autonomy in medical ethics. We should note that asymmetry here. Beneficence can either require or prohibit medical treatment in ways that autonomy cannot. Parents or guardians (like Ms. Gucci) who believe that professionals are subservient to their wishes misunderstand the liberties that autonomy provides. Professionals who heed demands for medically unwarranted treatment, thinking that patient or parental autonomy limits their prerogatives, can make one of two mistakes: Either they see autonomy as a positive rather than as only a negative right, or (in pediatric settings) they see it as unqualified rather than as qualified by the value of patient care and the duty to protect the patient's basic interests.

Having examined the duty to care, paternalism, representation, and patients' basic interests, we have moved "roughly and in outline," as Aristotle would say, regarding normative matters in bioethics and pediatrics. But cases like Henry Gucci's, Kevin Sampson's, and Ahmet Ali's involve the place of religion in a young patient's family life, and I have said little about religion directly. Religion can complicate interactions between care providers and families, raising difficult issues of faith, identity, and cultural pluralism in the medical treatment of children. Generally, liberal philosophy seeks to bracket religious beliefs, along with other comprehensive doctrines, in fashioning basic principles of public justice. That fact has led to a woeful inarticulacy among liberal theorists about the place of religion in public life. Often in response to that inarticulacy, religious theorists not only assign a privileged place to the claims of piety, they consider them sufficient as a basis for social criticism. I will avoid both of these tendencies, seeking neither to privilege nor to ignore religious tenets in medical ethics. Rarely do medical professionals have the liberty to champion their religious beliefs, and even less rarely are they entirely free to ignore the religious beliefs of their patients.

At the same time, the culture of biomedicine has its own worldview and ethos, and these can comprise a set of comprehensive beliefs that clash with the cultural backgrounds of patients and families. Thus, in the next several chapters, I will turn to cases that aim to track the place of religion and culture (including the culture of biomedicine) in medical care, hoping to deepen our understanding of the responsibility of parents and professionals in the treatment of patients who are young and sick.

Part II

PRACTICAL CASES

SIX

A Fighter, Doing God's Will:
Technologically Tethered, Retaining Fluids,
on Steroids, Sedated, and Four Years Old

BILLY RICHARDSON

It is commonly thought that health care providers experience their patients' deaths as a failure, a defeat in the battle to provide health and life. Seeking to inform the healer's art, William F. May writes of the metaphoric parallels between medicine and war:

> The metaphor of war dominates the modern, popular understanding of disease and determines in countless ways the medical response. We see germs, viruses, bacteria, and cancers as invaders that break the territorial integrity of the body; they seize the bridgeheads and, like an occupying army, threaten to spread, dominate, and destroy the whole. . . .
> Further, the language of war describes the mounting counterattack. We refer to the *armamentarium* of drugs, the bombardment of tumors with radioactive substances, to say nothing of wielding the hand-held weaponry of burning iron and knife.[1]

The images of battle and war are particularly apt in an intensive care unit (ICU), in which health care providers often commit themselves to an all-out attack against disease and death. Yet when four-year-old Billy Richardson died in the spring of 1998, house staff in Baylin's ICU breathed a collective sigh of relief. For them, and for this intrepid patient, the war was over. Billy had come to Baylin to undergo a bone marrow transplantation (BMT) procedure to treat his Hurler syndrome, a rare, inherited metabolic disorder caused by an enzyme defect that produces an abnormal accumulation of mucopolysaccharides in the body's tissues. Affected children develop cardiac abnormalities; umbilical hernias; skeletal deformities; and enlarged tongues, livers, and spleens. Physical and mental growth are impaired, and children acquire features that give the condition its former name of gargoylism. Many children with Hurler syndrome do not live more than two years, and they often die from pneumonia or cardiac arrest.

Billy had several of these conditions and more, requiring multiple hospitalizations before his arrival at Baylin the previous autumn. At six weeks of age, he stopped breathing, and his father administered cardiopulmonary resuscitation (CPR) by taking directions over the phone from an emergency medical service. In 1994, he developed hydrocephalus—an excess of cerebrospinal fluid in the skull—requiring a shunt for drainage. In 1995, he had an umbilical hernia, and a year later, he acquired pneumonia. Billy's heart was weak, and his renal insufficiency required regular dialysis. He was developmentally delayed, able to sit up by himself but not walk. Billy communicated with some single words, signs, and babbles. His diet consisted of pureed and baby foods, and rice milk.

Billy's allogeneic BMT at Baylin was his second. The first, unsuccessful attempt was carried out in another region of the country when he was thirteen months old, and his parents came to Baylin after several other hospitals declined their request for a second try. Aware that the procedure was risky and that the chances of success were remote, Baylin's oncologists nonetheless agreed to the Richardsons' request. The hope was that new marrow would provide a continuing source of the enzyme that Billy lacked. That treatment would not cure Billy, but it would improve his quality of life by addressing some of the metabolic issues caused by his enzyme deficiency.

BMT patients do not necessarily require intensive care, but Billy required mechanical ventilation soon after he was irradiated and injected with new marrow. It was in Baylin's ICU that I met and interviewed Michelle Richardson, Billy's mother; joined family discussions about Billy's condition; and observed meetings among care providers and counselors about how to approach the Richardsons regarding Billy's ongoing and increasingly futile treatment. Only slowly did I sort through the complexities surrounding Billy's case. What materialized is an example of a child's basic interests being held hostage directly by parental indecision and indirectly by medical professionals' respect for family privacy in a situation complicated by medical ambiguity and the need for scientific research. Billy's case was further complicated by the fact that his parents acted on religious principles, requiring professionals to grapple with the family's piety as it informed their decision making. That requirement is no small challenge in modern medical (or other) settings in which it is assumed that religion plays a special role in persons' identity and can lend special gravity to their deliberations.

Billy's body was socially constructed according to different perspectives, in which religious, medical, and political idioms all circled around him and defined his situation in quite different ways. Those idioms, as we shall see, found common ground in the value of respecting liberty, which has developed in modern medicine as a defense against professional power and expertise. The value of patients' and families' autonomy is both a product of and a contributor to the nondirective ethos of modern medicine. Respect for freedom provided the backdrop for Billy's body to become a battleground for multiple and contested interests, none of which guarded him from aggressive treatment or embraced the substantive value of his medical welfare. As we will see, the irony in Billy's case is that parents' liberty to decide for their children, far from resisting care providers' and researchers' interests, might have played into them.

AGGRESSIVE TREATMENT

When I first saw Billy lying on his bed, he appeared much larger than most four-year-old children. Billy was enormously overloaded with fluids; his swollen body was bright pink with patches of rash; and he was connected to a series of technologies to feed and sedate him, monitor his heart rate and blood pressure, and assist his breathing. Billy regularly received X-rays to observe his lung fields; he had undergone a tracheotomy to ease mechanical ventilation; and he required occasional blood transfusions. Because of the danger of infection, he was kept in one of the unit's glass-enclosed rooms, and he was cared for by members of the elite rank of the ICU's nurses—those with the greatest seniority and experience with challenging situations. Billy remained in that room for two more months, generating enormous heartache and consuming substantial sums of money, energy, and attention from the ICU house staff, before his internal organs finally gave out.

Billy's situation became morally and medically challenging not because his second transplant failed, but because it showed signs of engraftment. In that respect, the Richardsons' decision to pursue the remote chance of successful treatment seemed vindicated. Their prayers, and those of their church and family members, had been answered. But what was troubling about Billy was that the rest of him did not, as they say in the unit, get on board: He quickly experienced multisystem organ failure. Billy's lungs required increasing mechanical support to push oxygen into his system; his heart needed increased doses of vasopressers to maintain circulation; his kidneys ceased to respond to dialysis; and attempts to diurese him aggressively jeopardized his weak renal system. Billy's fluids leaked from his capillaries into whatever pockets of his body would absorb liquid. He developed sepsis (blood poisoning) on at least three occasions, and it was constantly at risk of recurring. Billy was fed through a nasogastric tube that he usually, but not always, tolerated. He also developed signs of graft-versus-host disease, in which lymphocytes in the donor marrow recognize their new environment as foreign and reject their host. He thus developed a skin rash and diarrhea, and he required regular doses of corticosteroids to prevent rejection. Those corticosteroids, however, also increased the chance of infection because they suppressed Billy's immune system. Mechanical ventilation, while pushing oxygen into his bloodstream, also fibroticized his lungs, turning them into petrified tissue, lifeless and hard. Billy thus required increased settings on the ventilator for greater pressure and volume; by the end of January, house staff remarked that he had "no chance to get off the vent." Two months later, the ventilator pressures were so high that they blew a hole in one of Billy's lungs.

Complicating matters further were Billy's sedation and the ongoing danger of increased tolerance to pain medications, requiring larger and larger doses and making it difficult to calibrate pain relief. Over the course of one weekend, house staff reduced his pain medications, and Billy underwent discernible withdrawal, his arms and legs shaking. "Even though he's asleep, he *senses* where he is in the ICU," remarked his mother. "With Billy we must always go slow in changes."[2] His ongoing treatment required house staff to confer regularly with Billy's parents about how to proceed; his medical file includes twelve different consent forms. And none of his multisystem organ problems could be corrected by the introduction of new, healthy marrow. Keeping Billy alive to allow his marrow time to develop and produce healthy blood cells and enzymes imposed great hardship on the rest of his young body.

Like so many in a hospital, Billy's case was one in which the cure seemed considerably worse than the disease. An entry in Billy's chart in the middle of February summarized the complexities: "A CV [cardiovascular] echo shows new right ventricular dysfunction. It is probably secondary to pulmonary hypertension secondary to a progression in his pulmonary disease from most likely an infectious etiology as well as pulmonary fibrosis on top of ARDS [acute respiratory distress syndrome], as well as his underlying Hurler's syndrome causing his chronic lung disease at baseline."

BILLY AND GOD'S SOVEREIGNTY

Throughout this period, Michelle and Kyle Richardson were unwilling to stop Billy's aggressive treatment, and house staff did little to revise or challenge their views. The Richardsons' reasoning was not entirely obvious. It was not the case, as I initially thought, that they were committed to a sanctity-of-life doctrine—convinced that they must keep their son alive at all costs. At no time did they suggest that allowing Billy to die would be a religiously presumptuous decision on their part, or that allowing a child to die is tantamount to murdering him. Michelle believed that life is sacred, but not that it is an absolute good. She believed that only God had the right to take a life, but she did not think that allowing Billy to die would be taking his life. Rather, if she and Kyle were to decide to withdraw treatment, it had to be on "God's timetable," not the hospital's or the doctors'.

The Richardsons were, in part at least, theological determinists who interpreted their experience as a segment of a larger divine narrative. In some respects, the story of Billy is the story of theocentric piety and fidelity gone awry. For the Richardsons, Billy was a secondary cause through which God was working. That is not to say that they felt incapable of making a decision, or that confidence in God's will made their situation easy. As Michelle remarked, "God's in control, though sometimes I wonder. We've been placed here for a reason. We don't know why. We've seen things and how others have grown. [Still,] there's got to be an easier way."[3]

What was Billy's role in God's plan? According to Michelle, Billy was an invitation for others to grow in neighbor-love. Confronted by Billy's condition, people were faced with the question, Can they love and accept a young child with his condition? Can people respond to Billy's strange appearance, his developmental delay, and the challenge of caring for his many needs? In Michelle's mind, modern society has few resources for overcoming its prejudices and accepting a child like Billy: "Society's value judgments are way off base. . . . Society says, 'The person [like Billy] is not perfect.' But none of us is perfect."[4] Billy thus posed a fundamental question about *our* capacities, the strength of our virtues, our disposition to care, our commitment to equality. For that reason, keeping Billy alive was a response to divine sovereignty—God's direction of history—and an occasion for increasing neighbor-love in the world.

Michelle cited several examples. First, "there was a guy [from their home area] who followed Billy since he was an intern, and he made a career choice because of Billy. He saw the need for expertise in this weird disorder." Billy thus worked to focus and direct the choice of a young doctor's specialization. Others were more immediately affected and moved: "Children in church send cards, prayers, and put Billy's picture on the[ir] refrigerators." Moreover, "COTA [Children's Organ Transplant Association] is raising funds" for her and her husband. These acts are the result of Billy's place in the world, teaching others how to "look beyond themselves."[5] According to Michelle, "[Billy] touched so many people. He changed us. Oh, my God. I've done things I'd never thought I'd do. There's nothing I can't do. He enriched life; day-to-day stuff." Perhaps most important was Billy himself. "Billy is a fighter," Michelle often remarked, as if to recall the combative images to which May alludes. That characteristic of their son helped the Richardsons decide to seek the second BMT. "We wanted to give him the chance to fight it through. If he hadn't been so feisty, we might not have done this." With Billy, "there's always this unknown in there. He doesn't follow the book, for good and bad. Others [with Hurler syndrome] usually die from pneumonia or cardiac [arrest]. Many don't last until two."[6] But with her boy, there is what Michelle called "the Billy factor"—what she would later say is "really the God factor."[7]

When I asked Michelle about her sense of the divine, she told me that she was confident that God was near and active in Billy's case. "God is present. Definitely. That Billy is still here says something for God's presence. He's guiding according to his will, which may not be what we want. . . . God is here, orchestrating, allowing us to go through it all of this. It's his will; we may not like it. That is ultimately what is good for Billy." Charlene Dodson, a chaplain at Baylin, described Michelle's belief that "God is micromanager" in everyday affairs.[8] Yet such piety did not provide many assurances. "I haven't processed all of [it] yet. That is God's will. But there's the parent, the human part." For Michelle, there was faith, but also doubt. In our interviews, she remarked, "I don't know what the ultimate outcome is going to be. I don't think anyone knows for sure. There's a lot of uncertainty. . . . You really struggle."[9]

These beliefs, however qualified they might appear, nonetheless empowered Michelle and Kyle to provide tireless care for Billy. They saw their love as mirroring divine *hesed*, God's steadfast, covenantal love, within a cosmic order that would reward the just. "He *promised*. Look at Romans 8:28: ['We know that all things work together for good for those who love God, who are called according to his purpose.' NRSV] He promised, I'm sorry," she stated with nervous laughter.[10] After Billy died, Michelle remarked that the idea of divine promise meant that "no matter what happened, we would be there, and we were. It was comfort to us that we were both there. We kept our promise that we'd stick with him and physically be there. And we both were."[11] Without the perspective of belief,

> you can't keep losing face for three months and stay together. If I was that way, I couldn't advocate for Billy. I couldn't do that for him. . . . That's hard for docs to understand in the ICU. The doctors are on a different time frame. We've been here before and we've pulled out. But you can't definitely say [for sure]. The folklore of the ICU says, "Kids *do* pull out." Is it the majority? No. Could it be your kid? Yes. No one knows who those kids are.[12]

For Michelle, "God determines whether you make it through this process. I've seen too many second BMTs make it. I know that an experimental drug pulled two kids out. God is sovereign. That's exactly right. Docs can do nothing and kids can pull through. Someone is in control." Even particular medications are part of the larger story: "High-dose steroids haven't done much yet. Does that mean that God cannot flip things around? No."[13]

Michelle and Kyle came from different religious denominations but eventually joined the same Presbyterian church, where Kyle became an active member of the men's group. Although Michelle did not explicitly cite the writings of John Calvin, their views were not far from one strand of Calvin's piety and theology. Of relevance is Calvin's confidence in the providential direction of history and the sense that God has a direct, causal hand in human affairs. In *Institutes of the Christian Religion,* Calvin writes that providence "is the determinative principle of all things in such a way that sometimes it works through an intermediary, sometimes without an intermediary, and sometimes contrary to every intermediary."[14]

Calvin's view of divine sovereignty and freedom are strong, arguably as strong as one finds in the Christian tradition. It is important to pause over this point, if only to underscore the core principle: For Calvinists like Michelle, God either works with, without, or *against* natural causes. Affirming the unfettered freedom of God, Calvin holds that nothing can restrain the divine will, that the order of creation need not restrain the order of redemption, *that miracles are always possible.*

Such piety was central to Michelle's decision making. In her mind, "God can do *anything,* from letting [Billy] go home, to healing him in one day, to the other end of the spectrum. You have to trust that something is happening that isn't yet. That helps you handle the *long* time. It's a marathon. Bone marrow transplantation is a marathon." Michelle added that one of her favorite biblical passages was Hebrews 12:1, in which readers are instructed, "Let us lay aside every weight and the sin that clings so closely, and let us run with perseverance the race that is set before us, looking to Jesus the pioneer and perfecter of our faith, who for the sake of the joy that was set before him endured the cross, disregarding its shame, and has taken his seat at the right hand of the throne of God" (NRSV). She then added, "No one said it was this long. Both in and out of the hospital. It's definitely [a matter of] patience. [But] God has his own timetable. I don't like it right now; it's way too long. But he's got his timetable."[15]

Why wait so long for Billy to improve instead of withdrawing aggressive treatment? According to Michelle, "There's one more day for God to flip it around. Time for a new idea. A new change." What does such piety forbid? "Not giving [God] the opportunity to do what he wants to do. . . . At this point we could turn off the vent and [Billy] could breathe on his own. Would we turn it off now? Absolutely not. Withhold aggressive treatment? CPR? Ditto."[16] All events, even the boy's death, were under God's direction. When Billy died, Michelle remarked, "It was God's decision to let him go when he went. We felt that we didn't want to prevent God from the possibility of a miracle. We knew in our hearts that it was time. But we don't want to count out God."[17]

PARENTAL AND PROFESSIONAL DUTIES

Billy's case ought to focus our attention on two sets of duties in pediatric medicine: his parents' and those of the professionals who were involved in his care. I have yet to say anything about the latter; they are more complicated, and might have involved mixed motives. Consider the Richardsons first.

A week before Billy died, his attending physician noted in his file that the medical teams from oncology and intensive care met and concurred

> that the current condition is ominous and he has significant probabilities of dying. Both teams agree that it would be in Billy's best interest to withdraw support and/or give him DNR [do not resuscitate] status if his respiratory condition does not improve after the high steroid course. This situation was mentioned to the family. They are not ready to make decisions. They thank us for the information but do not wish DNR status or withdrawal of support even if his respiratory condition worsens or remains unchanged.

A week later, a few hours before Billy died, the charge nurse remarked, "Dad was in bed with Billy over the weekend telling Billy that he can go. They're hoping that Billy makes the decision for them." Indeed, the view that Billy was, in some sense, in control, seemed to be at the core of the Richardsons' decisions (or refusal to decide). At ethics rounds in June, Rachel Stevens, another nurse in Baylin's ICU, noted that the Richardsons "desperately hoped that the decision would be taken out of their hands. They were grateful that they didn't have to make the decision to withdraw."[18]

Herein lies both an irony and, I believe, a moral error in Billy's care. For all of the language about God's proximity and activity in this case, the real agent was Billy, for it was Billy who was expected to "decide" about the proper plan of action. Discussing whether to withdraw treatment, Michelle remarked, "The plane is not at the end of the runway. There's [what we talked about earlier]: the Billy factor. He's unpredictable. It's really the God factor. It builds our faith. The docs say that he should have turned around by now, and then forty-eight hours later, he does. God lets him win the battles. [Billy] is a fighter. [People] are waiting for Billy to tell them what he needs." Rather than empowering or encumbering the Richardsons with parental duties, the idioms of faith allowed them to defer their role as guardians for their son's basic interest. The burden of decision was put on his young shoulders, relieving them of that responsibility.

To be fair, the Richardsons were wrestling with an overwhelming reality: the death of their child after four years of treatment, anguish, relocation, fatigue, and physical ups and downs. As I noted in Chapter 1, a child's infirmity poses horrific challenges to parents. "It's been almost a five-year battle," Michelle commented after Billy died.[19] No parent can be expected to deliberate in cool reason when confronting his or her child's death. But Billy's steady decline and his increasingly aggressive treatment were sufficient signals that his course was irreversible. The Richardsons imposed on Billy the duty of "telling people what he needs," and that was too much for them to ask.

The language of Billy's agency is curious in another way. Not only did the Richardsons' piety allow them to avoid questions about his basic interests, they imputed to Billy a level of autonomy that is unusual by anyone's lights. For all of the talk about divine power and steadfast care, the Richardsons found the language of freedom, autonomy, and self-determination more compelling. Religion meant less about caring for Billy's basic interests than about constructing for him a zone of privacy and noninterference, as if Billy were competent to communicate—indeed, fight for—his needs.

In provocative and odd ways, then, the Richardsons were liberals of a sort, for it was Billy's liberty interests that they sought to protect. They did not advocate the kind of liberal ideas that I defended in Chapters 2 and 5 when I spoke about political liberalism and the duty to care; they rather spoke from a more general and diffuse liberal doctrine, which privileges freedom and self-determination as human ends. In this regard, they illustrate a problem in pediatric medical ethics that I have discussed earlier in these pages: They imputed a level of competence and responsibility that is normally reserved for much older children and adults. Their conduct reflects our culture's desire to protect patients' rights against the medical establishment, to resist the imposition of others' values and the power of expertise in its several varieties. As Michelle stated, the doctors' timetable was not to be determinative. Billy's case illustrates a more general tension between respecting the value of autonomy and heeding medical authority. In contexts regarding competent adults, the value of autonomy is presumptively weightier than the value of medical expertise. But applying a model of adult care and decision making to the care of very young children is a temptation that should be resisted. The fundamental question is not only a *procedural* issue of who should decide (Billy? God? his parents? the doctors?). There is also the *substantive* question: What course of treatment (or nontreatment) is in Billy's basic interests? *His physical welfare, not his liberty interest, was at stake.*

There is also the fact that Michelle Richardson sometimes spoke of Billy in quite nonliberal terms, as someone who existed for others' benefit. Billy was a channel through which God was present and active, challenging others to grow in neighbor-love. Yet instrumentalizing Billy stands in obvious tension with the line of argument I have just rehearsed, for it views Billy not as a subject with liberty interests but as an object who serves the moral needs and interests of others. This perspective, too, is problematic, for it made Billy serve others, as if he were not already enduring enough hardship. Billy was asked to do work for himself and others. Both kinds of work imposed on him expectations that were too much to ask.

What about the medical professionals involved in Billy's care? What responsibilities should they have been expected to assume? On the one hand, house staff expressed the understandable desire to respect parental autonomy. As we saw in Chapter 2, that value has presumptive merit given the fact that families are the primary social unit responsible for protecting a child's welfare. Without a zone of privacy, parents or guardians cannot enact their responsibilities. As Jolene Johnson, one of Billy's nurses, remarked at ethics rounds, "I didn't agree with the family. But it was their child. And they have to live with how this went. It is critical that we create a situation that families can live with." Here the idea is that the family must bear the consequences of its decision. Those expectations imply a respect for freedom that is the condition of responsibility. Hence the note in Billy's record the day before he died:

> Billy's face and head remain very edematous, with the eyes swollen shut and the chest wall edema so thick that heart tones are barely audible. Breath sounds are minimal and very distant, and chest X-ray shows almost complete opacification of all lung fields. We continue to support Billy per his parents' wishes.

To be sure, respect for the Richardsons' prerogatives was not without moral tensions, and several in the ICU disagreed with the Richardsons about their conduct. As Jolene remarked, "We don't meet the needs of the family at the expense of a child's comfort. . . . We couldn't put brakes on ourselves. . . . We have duties to put limits on what we do. [Even at the end] we bagged him on the same settings he was on with the ventilator."[20] Those limits are usually defined by what the patient needs, not what the family wants. Thus, Billy's care providers were forced to consider not whether the parents *generally* ought to be respected, but *to what extent* they ought to be respected. As I noted in the case of Henry Gucci, there are limits to what families can demand of medical professionals in cases of futility.

This understandable concern for limiting a family's prerogatives was nonetheless complicated by three other considerations: first, that Billy was not in pain; second, that Billy's case was providing valuable medical information; and, third, that overriding the Richardsons' decisions might not be the best way to express disagreement with them.

These concerns came together in one set of responses during ethics rounds. When reviewing Billy's case, John McDowell, Billy's oncologist, put the matter this way:

To override their decision would have been a sad outcome. It was a risky procedure. Other parents would not have brought him to a second transplant. Having enabled them to do that, and *then* to reverse that would have been functionally abandoning them. Rather than working with them, we say, "Have a nice life."

We didn't harm Billy. We gave a high-risk therapy that no one forced them to accept. That's how we learn about things so that the next group of patients will benefit. There was a tacit agreement: "We will see this through with you even though we see the risks." It's different from a drowning.

It was a gray area clinically. No one could look into his eyes and say he was 100 percent dead. We're trying to push the envelope; we've never had a patient like Billy. We can't say we've had 80 patients like Billy and they've died. We couldn't say he's going to die and it's in his best interest . . . Uncertainty is the proper premise here.[21]

McDowell's point is that Billy's case was not simply a conflict between parental autonomy and a pediatric patient's basic interests. It was rather a matter of trading off a *commitment to the parents* against Billy's interests in a situation of medical ambiguity. Because Billy was not in pain, he was not being used for the sake of the family.

On McDowell's description, then, house staff was not yielding to parental autonomy but acting covenantally—to honor a "tacit agreement." Had Billy been in pain, the matter would have been different—there would have been a conflict of interests to adjudicate. To be sure, on this description, Billy's interests were secondary to the family's. But given the hospital's promises and the expectations that they generated, the alternative of overriding the parents' decisions and withdrawing treatment would have been to *abandon* Michelle and Kyle during their difficult time. Hence McDowell's reasoning: Billy's interests did not override the value of supporting his parents' interests, given that he was not physically suffering and not "100 percent dead." Honoring the duty of nonmaleficence allowed house staff to honor other duties as well.

Moreover, McDowell considered Billy an experimental subject, providing information that might be helpful for future cases. Here the question is whether Billy's treatment was entirely therapeutic, and whether nontherapeutic treatment imposed undue hardship on him. Often in an ICU, therapeutic and nontherapeutic treatment are not sharply or easily distinguished. Once again, the fact that Billy was not in pain seems crucial to the McDowell's argument. But it raises a new and different question: Was Billy being instrumentalized for the hospital's own aims?

Putting together all the elements from the Richardsons and McDowell, we arrive at a potentially volatile elixir, in which medical professionals may have yielded to parental autonomy out of mixed motives. Hence my question: Did the medical service tolerate the Richardsons' failure to withdraw aggressive treatment in order to acquire information from Billy for future cases? Was parental autonomy truly *respected,* or was it subsumed by the hospital's need to acquire potentially valuable medical information?

I can only raise this question about the physicians' motives. I have few data to support the suspicion that it implies, and *I raise it less as a worry about Billy's case in particular than as a worry about therapeutically ambiguous treatment in research hospitals more generally.* In Billy's case, one feature suggests that such a suspicion is not entirely speculative: The oncologists and intensivists never strove to steer the Richardsons toward a decision to withdraw. Jack Buckley, one of Billy's attending physicians, wrote the following in Billy's medical chart two weeks before the boy died: "Overall I think Billy remains critically ill with essentially no chance of meaningful survival." Yet this statement was not conveyed in any of the meetings I attended, nor did Michelle indicate that it had been conveyed in any private meetings she had with house staff. The physicians' interactions with Michelle and Kyle might have taken advantage of the Richardsons' desires to leave the matter in Billy's hands. If that is true, then Billy was doing work not only for God and his parents, but for medical science as well.

Billy was a fighter playing several roles: an instrument of the divine will, an agent with liberty interests, and (perhaps) an experimental subject. His third role might well have been unintended but foreseen, a by-product of medical care carried out in a research hospital. If that is true, then moral considerations would turn in part on the principle of double effect. According to that principle, untoward consequences of an acceptable act or intention must be proportionate to the good that is sought by that act or intention. That principle would allow professionals to acquire information from Billy's case if those benefits were not out of balance with his hardships. But it is by no means obvious that the research benefits derived from Billy's treatment were proportionate to the treatment to which he was subjected, or that this balance was openly considered.

In any event, in none of Billy's three roles—as divine vessel, agent with liberty interests, or research subject—were his medical interests given first rank among the values honored by others involved with his care. I want to conclude by commenting on Billy's roles and the issues involved.

First, as instrument in God's providential activity: In contrast to the Richardsons' piety, we cannot let religion trump a child's basic medical interests. At times religion must bow to common morality, and in pediatric medical contexts, that means honoring a patient's basic interests. In theological terms, the order of redemption does not nullify the order of creation. Christians have a duty to be charitable, to exercise steadfast love and care for others. But that duty does not entail aggressive medical treatment for patients such as Billy.

Theologians such as Calvin, despite his remarks about miracles and divine sovereignty, might be invoked to argue for withdrawing treatment rather than continuing aggressive treatment. Calvin's view of sovereignty is meant to call attention to the limits of the human will—to the conditions of finitude in which human action must situate itself.[22] On that reading, talk of God's will is meant to call attention to human limits and our inability to control the course of human events. According to Calvinists, we are to accept gracefully and respond charitably to contingencies over which we have no control. On that account, the Richardsons exhibited a kind of medical works-righteousness, in which they refused to heed the limits of human willfulness and sought to provide a space in which Billy was expected to save himself. The Richardsons' language of divine sovereignty and their hope for a miracle, rather than expressing respect for God's will, provided an idiom according to which they allowed their indecision to function as the (controlling) decision to continue their son's treatment. Instead, they might have considered the fact that they had met the limits of finitude and the boundedness of Billy's embodied existence.

Other resources within the Western theological tradition develop these concerns more directly. Once again we are invited to consider the goods of creation in relation to the goods of redemption—what some call the relation between nature and grace, or justice and love. On these terms, the lesson of Billy reminds us that there is what Thomas Aquinas calls an *order* of charity, in which natural patterns, processes, and regularities have their own integrity and value.[23] Aquinas poses various questions about how we are to be fair when we sort through the loves required by charity: fathers more than mothers, relatives more than strangers, parents more than spouses (as objects of reverence), spouses more than parents (as sources of intimacy and affection), fathers more than children (as objects of reverence), children more than fathers (as sources of union and affection). Indeed, Aquinas adds that loving one's body less than one's neighbor—a demand imposed on Billy—is not required by charity, "except in a cases where [one] is under obligation to do so; and if one willingly offers oneself for that purpose, this belongs to the perfection of charity."[24] In all of theses cases, Aquinas relies on data from his view of nature to inform how we are to resolve conflicts of duties in our various loves.

To be sure, Aquinas's view of what nature teaches reflects medieval (and patriarchal) values that are unacceptable to egalitarian social critics. Whatever we might make of Aquinas's specific claims about the order of charity, his main point is worth preserving: The pursuit of goodness cannot violate natural patterns and processes that provide structure and coherence to everyday life. Nor can love override the demands of justice that natural regularities impose on those who seek to do good. To ignore those patterns in the name of the divine will is to allow too much room for religiously informed parental authority. It allows for a kind of religious fanaticism.[25] If Billy teaches us anything, it is that children have basic interests, including respect for their bodies and the limits of those bodies, that supernatural piety might not adequately protect.

Aquinas's position might seem far afield from our present concerns, but his position is similar to the one I developed in Chapter 2, in which I specify primary goods within the duty to care. Those goods—physical, emotional, and intellectual welfare; psychological respect; and the right to an open future—are basic values that no commitment to beneficence and benevolence can justifiably ignore. Whatever particular ways that a family might say that it loves and cares for a child, those ways must be disciplined by basic claims of justice. Primary goods as I have outlined them function in ways that parallel Aquinas's understanding of the order of charity. Love that fails to heed primary goods borders on fanaticism and serves interests that are not the child's.

I am not saying that the Richardsons' conduct was wrong because it was religious. It is not the fact of piety, but the supernaturalism, to which I am objecting. I am saying that their particular convictions misguided them. Their piety would be appropriately challenged by other religious convictions, like Calvin's or Aquinas's, to settle Billy's case differently. Indeed, thinking that we can resolve this case by removing religion from the equation is to overlook the details of Billy's story, and that strategy would leave medical professionals untutored about the specific idioms of faith that inform parents' and families' decision making.

In practical terms, these thoughts about Calvin and Aquinas bear on the work of the chaplains in Billy's case. Not infrequently the Richardsons consulted Charlene Dodson, Baylin's head chaplain and a theologically astute member of the ICU's psychosocial team. Like her team members, Dodson worked to support families who were coping with trauma, stress, fatigue, and grief; she was part of a therapeutic counseling mission. Engaging religious beliefs directly, although not impossible (as we will see in the next chapter), runs against the grain of tolerance and pluralism in modern hospital settings. Providing chaplains the freedom and confidence to raise questions about a patient's or family's piety requires reforming the moral culture of medical care.

Then there is the second issue I mentioned: focusing on Billy's liberty interests, his role as decision maker. However valuable we might think it is to nurture children's freedom and to impart a sense of self-care in medicine, it is clear that Billy had no competence in matters bearing on his treatment. The language of decision drew on the value of freedom in ways that are inappropriate. As I noted in Chapter 3, evidence from developmental psychology draws the line at fifteen as the earliest age to presume competence in medical decision making. Billy's youth, medical status, and developmental delay indicate that he could not competently express his wishes. Others responsible for Billy's well-being should have been expected to decide in his behalf, to guard him against medically unnecessary treatment.

The fact that his parents failed in this task brings us to our third concern: the duties of medical professionals involved in oncology and intensive care. It is true, as McDowell notes, that overriding the Richardsons' decision would have been unfortunate given the promises that the hospital conveyed when taking on Billy for a second BMT. But in the debriefing about Billy, it was hardly clear how far those promises can go, or what limits can be placed on the professionals' conduct. The fact that Billy was not in pain seems to leave that matter entirely to the provision of analgesia and appears to draw from the hedonic criterion for quality-of-life that I discussed in the previous chapter. The question that Billy raises is not simply whether he was harmed, but whether he was wronged by imposing aggressive treatment that became increasingly detached from any hope for success. Moreover, if it was indeed true that Billy was being instrumentalized for research purposes as a foreseen but unintended by-product of his treatment, then that fact should have been disclosed to the Richardsons.

FREEDOM, SUPERNATURALISM, NONDIRECTION

Billy was a fighter on several fronts: for God, for freedom, and perhaps for medicine as well. Note that none of these causes were his own. Whatever alliance the Richardsons were able to forge with the house staff at Baylin drew from the value of liberty: Billy's freedom to decide, and the Richardsons' freedom to protect his liberty interests. As if to illustrate more general theories of religious projection, those liberties seemed to mirror God's absolute sovereignty—God's own unfettered freedom. For the Richardsons, divine freedom provided the overarching framework within which their protection of Billy's liberty was understood; freedom, so important to their protection of Billy's liberty interests, characterized their account of ultimate reality as well.

Attention to the value of patient and family freedom is not always adequate to guide decisions in pediatric settings. It may well be that freedom is a value worth preserving in the extreme in cases of adult medical care. But in pediatrics I hope that at appropriate times we can see beyond one value and into another, caring for young children so as to preserve their basic interests according to a commitment to charity that is disciplined by a comparable commitment to (natural) justice.

SEVEN

Respecting Jackson Bales's Religious Refusal: On What Grounds?

Ask a medical school class whether physicians should respect
the wishes of a competent adult who is a Jehovah's Witness
to be allowed to die rather than accept a blood transfusion,
and the immediate and unanimous response is yes.[1]

Pediatricians are not used to being powerless.

—*Dr. Sarah Radford, a resident at Baylin*[2]

CALIBRATION AND SPECIFICATION

I noted in Chapter 4 that one challenge in pediatrics is to calibrate expectations of patients' decision-making authority to their age and maturity. I argued for drawing the line earlier than the age of eighteen when presuming competence of adolescents and said that care should be adjusted to honor the primary good of respect when appropriate. We do well to recall that mediated beneficence means acknowledging the laws of nature and recognizing that they have physiological as well as psychological dimensions. Ignoring children's wishes, seeking to produce a good for them, can injure their developing self-esteem and might produce more harm than good. More generally, children's developing powers of self-determination focus our attention on two norms in medical ethics, beneficence and autonomy, which apply in different ways depending on the age, maturity, and capabilities of the patient in question. Let us call this the challenge of *calibration*.

When adults are called on to serve as a young patient's proxy, a related kind of challenge can materialize—namely, how to interpret the meaning and implications of patient welfare. Such a challenge can produce conflicts when professionals and families have different understandings of how the duty to care should be specified when treating young patients. As I noted in

Chapter 5, disagreements can surround what it means to care for a young patient: One party might see beneficence as requiring medical intervention, whereas the other might see beneficence as requiring nonintervention or the withdrawal of treatment. Each party connects its judgments to a broader account of the patient's good. One challenge in forging a therapeutic alliance is arriving at a shared perception about how properly to care for children's or adolescents' basic interests. The tension between parental autonomy and a professional's view of beneficence might mask a more fundamental disagreement about a young patient's good and how that good is to be specified when deciding about treatment. Let us call this the challenge of *specification.*

The case of Jackson Bales illustrates how difficult these tasks of calibration and specification can be in even the best of medical settings, and how these challenges can be complicated by a patient's religious beliefs. Jackson was admitted to Baylin for acute respiratory distress and severe chest and back pain as a result of blood clogging in his lungs and compromising his oxygenation, a symptom of his sickle-cell disease. Standard therapy is to assist oxygenation with a blood transfusion, seeking temporarily to replace hemoglobin S, an abnormal type of hemoglobin that lies at the root of sickle-cell disease, with healthy hemoglobin. But Jackson had recently become a Jehovah's Witness, and his religious beliefs now prohibited such treatment. A recent immigrant from Haiti, Jackson's mother had died two years earlier, and around that time, he accepted the beliefs of his father, Harold. Jackson's refusal of blood products put his life in immediate danger, generating a tense ethical debate among house staff about whether, and on what basis, to respect his decision.

Jehovah's Witnesses are a Christian millennialist group founded in Philadelphia in the late nineteenth century and now number about three million members worldwide. Witnesses adhere literally to the Bible and are best known for evangelizing door to door and for their polemical tract, *The Watchtower*. They are also known for embracing two tenets. First, they refuse to acknowledge any earthly power and thus refuse to pledge allegiance to the flag or take an oath of loyalty. Witnesses will not serve in the military, and in the United States, they have secured the right to be exempt from wartime conscription. Second, they refuse to accept blood products, drawing on biblical passages that they believe prohibit blood transfusions for therapeutic reasons. The main text that supports this belief is Acts 15:19–21, in which the leaders of the Christian church in first-century Jerusalem ordered Gentile converts to obey Jewish law only insofar as it commands abstinence "from things polluted by idols, from fornication and from what is strangled and from blood." Jehovah's Witnesses decline blood products because, on their view, this scriptural passage forbids taking blood into the body by any route whatsoever. Unlike religious believers who are "faith healers," Jehovah's Witnesses seek out medical treatment, but their views limit the treatments that adherents may accept.

Complicating matters for Jackson was the fact that he had recently turned eighteen and was thus no longer a minor. More than a few admissions to Baylin's intensive care unit (ICU) were legal adults. Of those, most had a history of childhood illness and treatment at Baylin, and they returned as adults to maintain continuity of care. Treating a legal adult, or someone close to the age of majority, was hardly anomalous at Baylin, reminding us again that pediatric care providers routinely treat patients across a broad developmental range. We should examine the case of Jackson Bales, then, because the professional world of pediatricians sometimes includes patients who are adults, or who are near the age of majority. *The distinction between pediatric and adult care providers does not parallel the distinction between children and adult patients.* Indeed, given my arguments in Chapter 3, it matters little whether Jackson was eighteen or sixteen: In either case, he would be presumptively owed the same kind of respect that an adult deserves.

Jackson's case involved two attending physicians at Baylin who disagreed about whether and how to respect his wishes. Their differences reveal competing grounds for respecting religious beliefs, and those grounds imply different limits for respecting another's piety. Moreover, those grounds had direct implications for the challenges I mention above, namely, calibrating expectations of decision-making authority and specifying the meaning of care. I hope to show how gnarled these challenges can become when they intersect with patients' and families' religious identities. The case of Jackson Bales teaches us, among other things, that respect for religious beliefs is not a sufficient basis for heeding a patient's decisions and that different grounds for respecting religion can lead to very different courses of action.

To see this point, we must first turn to some basic ideas in political philosophy about grounds for respecting religion in public life. With those ideas in place we will return to Jackson's story to see how different bases for respecting religion led to different role responsibilities for and decisions by medical professionals. Once those roles are sketched, I will track their implications for calibrating and specifying care in the treatment of young patients, focusing on the difficulties of balancing respect for patient freedom and benefit when these values conflict.

RELIGIOUS LIBERTY: CHOICE OR CONSCIENCE?

When discussing grounds for respecting religion, Michael Sandel draws the instructive distinction between religious liberty as a matter of *choice* and a matter of *conscience*. Often in liberal society, Sandel argues, we view religion on a voluntarist model, according to which the self is prior to its ends, free to adopt or reject goods that provide meaning and texture to identity. The choices of such "unencumbered selves" are respected not because they are morally praiseworthy, but because the autonomous self that underlies such choices has a dignity that inheres in its capacity to choose. Respect for choice is neutral about the merits (or lack thereof) of another's piety; it rather esteems the freedom that provides the conditions of any choice. Respect for religion is secondary and subordinate to the good of autonomy and the related values of liberty and equality. On this model, Sandel writes, "religious beliefs are 'worthy of respect' not in virtue of what they are beliefs *in*, but rather in virtue of being 'the product of free and voluntary choice,' in virtue of being beliefs of a self unencumbered by convictions antecedent to choice."[3]

Sandel's alternative model focuses on "encumbered selves"—those who experience religion not as a matter of free choice but as a matter of conscientious obligation. Drawing on the ideas of Jefferson and Madison, Sandel notes that American public philosophy once viewed religious liberty as freedom to exercise religious (or nonreligious) convictions—"to worship or not, to support a church or not, to profess belief or disbelief—without suffering civil penalties or incapacities."[4] On that account, religious freedom refers to the "right to exercise religious duties according to the dictates of conscience, not the right to choose religious beliefs."[5] In contrast to the voluntarist conception, Jefferson held that "the opinions and beliefs of men depend not on their own will, but follow involuntarily the evidence proposed to their own minds."[6] Respecting the religious freedom of encumbered selves means respecting "duties they cannot renounce, even in the face of civil obligations that may conflict."[7]

What, then, are the *grounds* for respecting religious beliefs on this second model? Those grounds cannot be the fact that beliefs derive from free and autonomous choice. Rather, respect must derive from a judgment about the actual merits of the beliefs and duties in question. Unfortunately, however, Sandel is vague about how criteria for such judgments are formed and justified. He writes, "What makes a religious belief worthy of respect is not its mode of acquisition—whether by choice, revelation, persuasion, or habituation—but its place in a good life or, from a political point of view, its tendency to promote the habits and dispositions that make good citizens."[8] To earn respect, religious belief must first be subjected to the substantive evaluations of others. In the political realm, the case for religious liberty is thus premised on the idea that respect for religion assumes that "religious beliefs and practices are of sufficient moral or civic importance to warrant special constitutional protection."[9]

On this second account, respect for religion must enter into potentially controversial judgments about the extent to which a particular set of beliefs occupies a place in a good life or makes for good citizens. Refusing to assimilate religious freedom to freedom more generally, this approach scrutinizes the merits of piety according to standards that derive from a (vague) account of the good life and political citizenship. That means that there are *limits* to what may be respected. In the judicial realm, where piety and politics sometimes conflict, "judges must discriminate, at least to the extent of assessing the moral weight of the governmental interest at stake and the nature of the burden that interest may impose on certain religious practices."[10]

Those who view religious liberty as a matter of choice and those who see it as a matter of conscience detect liabilities with the other's criteria for respecting religion. To those who see religious belief as an expression of autonomy, respecting religion on the condition that it is part of a "good life" opens the door to ethnocentric evaluations of others' religious beliefs and customs. Such judgments are liable to be parochial, bigoted, or self-serving. Those who see religious belief as worthy of respect if it is part of a good life obviously view matters differently. For them, respecting religion because it flows from an autonomous, free agent is patronizing because it avoids substantively engaging another's actual convictions. It assigns "respect on demand," as if another's freedom or authenticity were a virtue in its own right.[11]

Sandel's argument works less to sort out these more general cultural tensions than to explain why the Constitution singles out religion for special protection.[12] If religious freedom is only a species of privacy rights, then it would make little sense to carve out special constitutional protections for religious belief such as those found in the First Amendment. Viewing religious liberty on nonvoluntarist premises, in contrast, explains why Jefferson and Madison sought to craft protections on the assumption that religion played a special role in American public life: Religious belief informs individuals' sense of duty and, in general, infuses virtues that contribute to the moral strength of the commonweal. Seen in that way, restrictions on religious liberty in order to protect state interests are not a matter of weighing the general value of freedom against the importance of social goods or necessities. Rather, such restrictions are to be weighed in light of how religion's general contribution to the moral fabric of the commonweal compares to other state interests that might hang in the balance.

The importance assigned to religion by the Constitution has symbolic importance that carries over into nonlegal contexts, and Baylin is no exception. A patient's or family's religious convictions were often seen as important and sensitive matters, as central to conscience and not merely a species of privacy rights. In Jackson's case, however, the grounds for this respect were never clearly articulated, and that lack of clarity produced confusion surrounding his care. Professional decisions about how to respond to Jackson's wishes oscillated between viewing religion as a choice and as a matter of conscientious duty. As a result, Jackson's caregivers experienced some confusion about whether, and to what extent, his wishes should be respected.

RELIGION, COMPETENCE, AND AUTONOMY

At admission to Baylin's ICU, Jackson's first attending physician was Michael DeVries. DeVries spoke at length with Jackson and Harold to make sense of Jackson's decision and the religious beliefs that informed it. DeVries came to accept Jackson's refusal of blood products, drawing largely, but not exclusively, on the idea that Jackson had the right to decline treatment as a competent adult.

When Jackson's case was discussed at an ethics rounds among residents, DeVries chose not to attend, believing that it was an easy one. At those rounds, Sharon Johnston, Baylin's Director of the hospital's Ethics Advisory Committee, summarized the case as a basic dilemma: "On the one hand, you have to honor the patient's wishes. And he was competent. On the other hand, there's the duty to help the patient as one of his care providers. It's a clash between the principle of autonomy and the principle of beneficence."[13] The question, however, is how and to what extent each of these principles can inform practical decision making and action because each makes strong claims on the professional's conscience. For DeVries, it was important first to endorse Jackson's competence, as he noted in the medical chart:

> He is a competent 18 yr. old adult and has the right to refuse blood component therapy. . . . I had multiple conversations again w/ him overnight and into this morning, and again [he] insists that he cannot receive any blood product and will not consent to any blood product infusions. . . . I told him directly that I was concerned that he could die. Throughout these conversations, Jackson was awake, alert, and coherent. He consistently and persistently maintained that the did not wish any blood component therapy, but did desire other maximal support.

DeVries indicates that Jackson's refusal was not premised on the voluntarist conception of the self when he states that Bales "*cannot* receive any blood product." Note that he does not say that Jackson "chooses not to receive any blood product": Jackson acted on a duty of conscience, and DeVries's summary captures that sense of obligation. Out of respect for a religiously based imperative, and noting that Bales is a competent adult, DeVries saw little difficulty in heeding his patient's refusal. DeVries's judgment mixes a respect for religion as a duty with an understanding that a competent patient's autonomy justifies his right to refuse medical therapy, even conventional therapy. Perhaps because he was operating in a pediatric setting, DeVries declined to respect Bales's decision solely on the basis of the young man's autonomy. DeVries calibrated his understanding of Jackson's decision-making authority to his status as a legal adult, but his respect for Jackson's decision drew in part on a judgment that Jackson's refusal was a matter of conscientious duty. He thereby avoided the patronizing approach of respecting Jackson's religion as a matter of "respect on demand."

We might understand DeVries's position as specifying beneficence rather than as respecting autonomy, especially if we see patient benefit as including patients' understanding of their overall good. On that description, DeVries broadened his understanding of Jackson's welfare to subsume Jackson's own views of his basic interests. As Albert R. Jonsen writes, in cases regarding Jehovah's Witnesses' refusal of blood products, "the belief that impedes competent care is part of the patient's firm conviction about the good life. The physician who acts against that belief does not benefit the patient." The core idea is to collapse the norm of patient autonomy into the norm of beneficence, following Mill's general refusal to separate objective and subjective interests.[14] Jonsen continues, "to act toward a person in a way that does not contribute to his conception of the good life is not benefitting him. Since the physician's sole moral obligation is to benefit the patient, the physician has no obligation to override the clearly expressed refusal of blood by a competent adult Jehovah's Witness."[15] Matters of medical responsibility thus turn on "the wider meaning of benefit" and whether medical treatment contributes to the good life "as the patient conceives it."[16]

One problem with this view, however, is that it requires health care providers to determine whether a patient's views are truly "part of the patient's *firm conviction* about the good life." For that reason, they must probe the strength of a patient's convictions, reopening concerns about that patient's autonomy. Not all decisions enjoy the same degree of resolve—in medicine no less than elsewhere. And it is precisely the issues of conviction and freedom that vexed Alyce Sheridan, DeVries's replacement as attending physician after his two-week rotation. On the first day of her watch, she wrote,

> All of [Jackson's] care givers are quite concerned that this is still somewhat unclear if he is making this decision b/c he is strongly believing in this faith or b/c he is afraid of his father being upset at him if he goes against his father's belief. Jackson has not been baptized into the church; he was Protestant until two years ago and he does not go door-to-door or do pioneering work in the Jehovah's Witness faith. We are trying to find out if he has other friends who would know what his belief had been prior to his admission.

Sheridan generally declined to acknowledge Bales's status as a legal adult and regularly asked him whether he had changed his mind about refusing treatment. According to Sarah Radford, a member of Jackson's care team, Sheridan once "woke him up, while intubated, to ask him again. The team had a lot of trouble with that" (because it was physically painful for Bales).[17] Perhaps Sheridan thought that criteria for ascertaining Jackson's competence should be more stringent because of the gravity of his decision. Recall from Chapter 3 Brock and Buchanan's idea that competence is task-relative, and that the bar for determining competence should be raised for patients who are making high-risk decisions. Jackson's case illustrates one danger with this idea: It opens the door to paternalism, tempting physicians to ignore legal thresholds and treat adults as if they were incompetent. Sheridan's conduct yielded to the pediatrician's temptation of infantalizing patients and failing to adjust treatment according to patients' age and level of maturity. Radford acknowledged the general problem. She noted that no judge would force a seventeen-year-old to accept a transfusion. "Still," she added, "we felt like we just lost him [to majority status]."[18]

Radford's comment would be challenged by my account of paternalism in Chapter 3 because it appears to use the age of majority to mark the boundary between what I have called presumptive paternalism and presumptive antipaternalism. Radford suggests that if Jackson had been below the age of majority, house staff might have been justified in treating him with fewer limits on their authority, rather than as an adult. Once again, we meet the challenge of calibration.

For now, I want to concentrate on a different point: Sheridan's actions were premised in part on the judgment that Bales's refusal was not necessarily worthy of respect—that however dutiful his refusal might be, it did not really serve his own good. She might have decided that Jackson's beliefs could not connect with a vision of the good life because they bordered on something like preventable suicide.[19]

In Sheridan's mind, there was no warrant for folding Jackson's subjective interests into an understanding of his overall welfare; she kept the two distinct. It was not obvious, in other words, that "to act toward a person in a way that does not contribute to his conception of the good life is not benefitting him."[20] For her, to fold the good "as the patient conceives it" into "the wider meaning of benefit" was medically dubious. Her description of Bales's situation is noteworthy for assigning responsibility for his problem to his religion and not his sickle-cell disease. On the fifth day of his stay in the ICU, she wrote, "Jackson has stabilized. However, he is not actively improving from his acute chest crisis secondary to the fact that he is a JW, refusing transfusions." In her mind, Jackson's sense of duty was the cause of his illness, and whether that merited respect and cooperation was not obvious. Thus she repeatedly asked Jackson if he had changed his mind about refusing a transfusion. Sheridan also actively sought confirmation from Jackson's visitors. In the medical chart, she wrote, "Multiple meetings w/ parent and elders of his JW church. They were quite adamant that they did not want him transfused, and that they would rather that he die than be transfused b/c they strongly believed that his only hope for redemption and a better life is in the next life." Over the course of the next few days, Jackson was put on nitric oxide, and his condition briefly improved before quickly deteriorating. On the third day after his admission, it seemed very likely that Bales would die from a preventable illness under Sheridan's watch. That fact violated her sense of professional obligation: to promote a patient's welfare.

When I spoke to Sheridan about Jackson's case, she expressed uncertainty that his convictions were sincere and firm. She recounted a conversation, " 'Would you sign this refusal form?' the hematology team asked. He declined to do so. They took that as ambivalent. 'Are you a Jehovah's Witness?' he was asked. 'My dad is,' he said." She recalled that before his mother's death, he was a member of a mainline Protestant denomination, that he was not formally baptized as a Jehovah's Witness, and that he had done no proselytizing—"no door-to-door activity." She added, "That to me is fishy." Hence her judgment: "I'm not saying for sure that's what he really wanted. I'm not saying we're wonderful because we supported his beliefs."[21]

The caregivers were also concerned about whether Jackson could express his views with Harold and the church elders at his bedside. "His dad wouldn't leave . . . I have family members who are Jehovah's Witnesses. I consider it a pseudoreligious cult type of thing. There's lots of coercion involved. The kid might have been trapped. He has nowhere else to go. If he's transfused then his dad will shun him. He had no other support outside of his family." In her mind, Jackson had little room to express his views freely. "It's like a pregnant girl with a mother who's a Roman Catholic, who wants an abortion. You don't ask her in front of her mom." For Sheridan, Jackson's case raised important moral issues of confidentiality. Transfusion "should not have been discussed with him in front of his father. His father didn't need to know. To me this is coercion."[22]

By raising this question of confidentiality, Sheridan shifted matters from whether Jackson's substantive views were worthy of respect to whether the procedures for securing informed consent were adequate. She was worried that one of the conditions of informed consent—voluntariness—was lacking. Focusing on informed consent enabled her to avoid awkward questions about whether her judgments about Bales's religion were intolerant and thus presumptively paternalistic. Attending to proper procedure allowed her to sidestep charges that she had treated him paternalistically, allowing her to equivocate about whether she saw him as a "kid" (her word) or as an adult. Before she accepted an adult's decision, she could say, she needed to determine whether the decision was free from coercion. For Sheridan, one problem with Jackson's care was that "we didn't give him an out. We didn't ask him in a way that assumes confidentiality." When I asked her if she thought that Jehovah's Witnesses were wrong, she replied, "I don't agree with the degree of coercion. It's very exclusive: others can't be a 'bad influence.'" House staff, she added, "need to know a little theology. They need to know what makes a cult: isolationism and coercion."[23]

Whether Jehovah's Witnesses indeed constitute a cult is less important than the fact that Sheridan saw Harold's conduct as "cultish." Those worries led her to think that proxy decisions about Jackson's care would not reflect his own deeper commitments. Hence the effort to "find out if he has other friends who would know what his belief had been prior to his admission." Stated in terms that recall our discussion of patient representation, Sheridan was concerned that Harold had served less as Jackson's *delegate* than as his *guardian*. Whatever views Harold might express must heed Jackson's truest wishes and beliefs. Whether she was acting to protect Jackson's autonomy or his conscience was irrelevant to the paramount duty to protect him from proxy decisions that had not consulted his own wishes.

REFLEXIVE PATERNALISM

Proxy decisions might be handled differently. Consider the case of seventeen-year-old John, also a Jehovah's Witness, as described by Kathleen Lawry, Jacquelyn Slomka, and Johanna Goldfarb.[24] When he was fifteen years old, John was paralyzed by gunshot wounds to his lumbar spine. Surgery was now recommended to treat his chronic osteomyelitis, which had arisen from pressure sores that were the result of his relative lack of movement. Osteomyelitis is an infection of the bone and bone marrow, and in chronic cases, it causes constant pain in the affected area. Surgery is required to remove the infected bone, sometimes followed by a bone graft.

How John's case was handled poses an instructive comparison to Jackson's. Like Jackson, John refused potentially life-saving blood products. Preoperative screening revealed that John was anemic and that he needed a blood transfusion before surgery to increase his red blood cell count. Citing his religious beliefs, John refused a transfusion. His surgery was canceled, and he was sent home with a prescription of iron that he was to take orally. Soon thereafter, John was admitted to an emergency room; he had lost considerable weight and had contracted a fever, a probable symptom of an underlying infection. He was informed that his anemia was serious and that both surgery and a transfusion were medically indicated. Again, he refused a transfusion, but he added that he "didn't want to die."

In John's case, health care providers reached a solution that was briefly considered and rejected in Jackson's treatment. Recognizing that John faced a dilemma between wanting to live and being required by conscience to refuse blood products, a physician befriended him to discuss his situation. Which wish reflected John's true desire: to avoid dying, or to avoid being shunned by his community for violating one of their beliefs? For the doctor, the key was to arrive at a solution that would allow John to express himself without jeopardizing his standing in his religious community. Knowing that John would be ostracized by his fellow believers, John's physician realized that he was being forced to choose between biological death and social death. The doctor thus proposed to convey his own convictions and to offer his services as John's confidential proxy. Lawry et al. write:

> After much consideration the physician told John that he had thought very carefully about their discussions and that even though he respected John's religious beliefs, his own moral position was that he would have to transfuse him if it was a question of life or death. He asked John to decide, if knowing this, he wanted him to continue to be his primary physician. . . . John told the physician that he wanted him to continue as his primary physician. John could not make a decision to accept or refuse a transfusion, but he could decide whether he wanted this person to be his primary physician, knowing he would transfuse him if he felt it was medically indicated. Posing the question in this manner enabled John to exercise his autonomy and to make a decision.[25]

In the minds of Lawry et al., this solution avoided viewing matters as Johnston had when she presented Jackson's case at Baylin—as a conflict between autonomy and beneficence. It was rather premised on recognizing that choosing between biological and social death is only an illusory choice, beyond anyone's capacities. "Instead," Lawry et al. write, "the physician presented a choice that the patient was actually able to make—a choice to maintain or to abolish their relationship." John and his doctor negotiated a course of treatment, and such negotiations "can occur only within a mutually respectful physician–patient relationship and within a health care system that places this relationship as primary."[26]

This solution appears to respect a patient's religion as an encumbrance of conscience rather than as an expression of voluntary choice. As such, it appears to exemplify Sandel's second model for respecting religion and avoids "respect on demand." But does this solution resolve ethical issues about who ought to make decisions in medical settings? The basic question is whether John's physician acted paternalistically. Lawry et al. argue that reframing John's case in terms of choosing whether to maintain or end a relationship and negotiating the proper course of action dissolves any concern about paternalism. What John sought to preserve was his friendship with, not his subservience to, his doctor. Because the course of action was negotiated, it did not reflect values that were the physician's alone. Respect for John's freedom was the overriding concern; the goal was to provide a feasible set of alternatives among which he could choose. In this way, John's physician seems to have found a solution that combines respect for persons with the norm of beneficence.

But this solution is misleading, and we do well to understand why it was justifiably rejected at Baylin. Let us begin by recalling the distinction between *unreflexive* and *reflexive* paternalism to see how John's case illustrates the latter. Recall from Chapter 3 that an unreflexive paternalist acts on behalf of another without regard for the other's presumed or stated wishes. The act is unreflexive not because the paternalist is unconscious or unreflective, but because the paternalist is assuming authority to make specific decisions without the beneficiary's express consent. A reflexive paternalist acts on the basis of the potential beneficiary's prior voluntary decision to waive his or her rights of autonomy in order to authorize a second party to protect the beneficiary's interests without additional, specific consent. Reflexive paternalists decide on authority that has been transferred to them by autonomous beneficiaries. The decision is paternalistic insofar as putatively beneficial acts occur or decisions are made that lack the beneficiary's express consent. In (medical) reflexive paternalism, patients assign broad powers to medical professionals to act on their behalf, without securing consent for specific procedures that may become necessary in the course of treatment. Such an arrangement is paternalistic because patients assign responsibilities to health care providers to make specific decisions for the patients' good, but those decisions lack the patients' express consent.

John's case has less to do with the importance of maintaining a relationship with a doctor than with reflexive paternalism, for John transferred decision-making powers to his physician in the event that he needed a transfusion. In this respect, both parties took advantage of a perceived ambiguity in Witness doctrine and practice: Is the prohibition of receiving blood products one of *strict liability* or *consent*? The question is meant to distinguish between material and voluntary acts. If the prohibition is one of strict liability, then receiving blood products in any circumstances, even against one's will, implicates the recipient in an evil deed. The very fact of receiving blood products taints the individual with wrongdoing. On the other hand, if the prohibition pertains to voluntary acts, then individuals are implicated in an evil only if they consent to receiving blood products. On this latter account, one may not expressly consent to transfusions but may consent to allow others to authorize a transfusion.

A recent statement by the Jehovah's Witness Public Affairs Office seeks to resolve this ambiguity. According to a June 2000 statement, members who are transfused against their will, or who accept transfusions in moments of stress and fear but regret their actions later, are not to be removed from fellowship. A member who "willfully and without regret accepts blood transfusions . . . revokes his own membership by his own actions."[27] On that account, John may have escaped his dilemma, for he did not consent directly to a transfusion. By transferring decision-making authority to his physician, John did not sin and thus avoided having to choose between biological and social death.

Still, the solution was paternalistic, for it allowed a proxy to act on John's behalf without John's express consent. The solution of Lawry et al. is less about preserving relationships than about specifying autonomy: John may freely transfer responsibility for making decisions about his care. This route was wisely rejected at Baylin in Jackson's case because house staff saw the idea of "preserving relationships" as disingenuous, for it allowed a patient to circumvent moral responsibilities implied by his religious tradition. Religious duties are not respected in this approach; they are avoided. Witnesses who allow a doctor to decide to transfuse them are less involved in negotiating substantive values than in determining how to generate a *process* that allows others to settle matters of medical welfare. John consented to a transfusion by consenting to someone else who promised that he would authorize that plan of action.

FREEDOM AND DUTY

Jackson Bales survived his course of treatment in Baylin's ICU, and when he left the hospital, he was grateful for the quality of care he received. The fact that he survived shows that treatment that physicians describe as "medically indicated" may not be the only available or effective treatment. Apart from Jackson's good fortune, his experience leaves a mixed precedent for treating similar cases. DeVries and Sheridan each confronted the task of treating an older patient in a pediatric setting. It bears repeating that in the moral world of pediatric care, not all patients are children; the distinction between pediatricians and adult care providers does not parallel the distinction between children and adult patients. Confronted by the challenge of dealing with a patient who was presumptively competent, both DeVries and Sheridan isolated important issues and liabilities.

DeVries's response to Bales was, on balance, better than Sheridan's, but not without problems. Recall that DeVries saw Jackson as a competent adult who consistently and persistently refused medical care. He characterized this refusal as a duty of conscience that Jackson could not ignore. On that description, DeVries mixed respect for Bale's status as a competent adult with respect for Bales's duty of conscience. He refused to assign Jackson "respect on demand."

The question here—debated during the ethics rounds at Baylin—is whether professionals should assign a privileged place to religion when they evaluate competent patients who make high-risk decisions. Suppose, for example, that Bales had a twin brother, Sean, who also has sickle-cell disease but who is not a member of a religious group. Suppose, moreover, that Sean is admitted to Baylin for acute chest syndrome that requires intubation and that he competently refuses mechanical ventilation because he has an aesthetic aversion to machines. He tells house staff that he would rather die than be placed on a breathing apparatus because he opposes the idea of being tethered to technology, and that he has thoroughly considered his decision. Despite all of the professionals' attempts to inform him that intubation would be both effective and temporary, and despite his clear understanding of its risks and benefits, he stubbornly declines their recommendation. Should his views be assigned any less respect simply because they do not spring from any identifiable religious reasons?

If DeVries's actions were premised in part on respect owed to the duties of religions conscience, then he might have to treat Sean differently from Jackson. And that fact unfairly discriminates in favor of liberty that is backed by religiously based reasons. In my view, DeVries extended a *courtesy* to Jackson by acknowledging the role of conscience in the patient's decision. He did not merely tolerate Jackson's views but saw a certain dignity in adhering to religious tenets that did not endanger anyone else. But the grounds for extending that courtesy does not justify discriminating between one set of competently expressed beliefs and another. Respect for autonomy as a side-constraint includes limits on what professionals can demand from patients in decision-making contexts. Whether professionals admire or merely tolerate a competent patient's decision should not affect the strength of the barrier that protects patients from professional power and authority. Both Jackson's and Sean's wishes should be heeded.

An additional question is whether and when religion is "respected." Suppose that Jackson had made it clear to house staff that he was a Jehovah's Witness, but that after thinking over his circumstances, he had decided to consent to a transfusion. As several residents indicated at the hospital's core conference rounds, it seems unlikely that house staff would have asked him whether he wanted to violate his religious views.[28] The fact that Jackson's adherence to religious beliefs would trigger a set of questions from his care providers, but that his failure to heed religious beliefs would not, suggests that religious believers receive attention only when their decisions conflict with standard therapy. That seems not to "respect" the religion in question because it attends to the merits of religion only in situations of patient disagreement or medical noncompliance.

Sheridan's line of response was more problematic at first glance, but not without some important insights into religiously based decisions. Her actions stemmed in large part from a pediatrician's commitment to beneficence. Whatever attention to autonomy existed in Jackson's case was dependent on and subordinate to broader concerns about how to specify the meaning of care. The challenge of that specification asks us to look at the patient's good and invites judgments about what is in that patient's interest. When religion is seen not as a species of freedom or individual privacy, but as source of conscientious duty, outsiders are invited to consider whether those duties are justified, especially when a patient's decision violates a basic feature of medical responsibility.

That fact might have tempted Sheridan to treat Jackson as (in her words) a "kid." But beyond this paternalistic error lie other important matters. What might have looked like a dispute about calibrating respect for autonomy was in fact a dispute about how to define the patient's good, and whether to see religion as playing a role in that good. Sheridan thus wanted to know whether Bales was *really* encumbered by conscience. She sought to probe his autonomy not as a value in itself, but as a condition for viewing religion as authentic or inauthentic. In her view, DeVries had not sufficiently determined whether Jackson's piety was "deep enough" to warrant respect. In contrast to Sandel, Sheridan argued that sometimes we must ascertain the mode by which another acquires religious beliefs in order properly to respect those beliefs. Such an inquiry proceeds not out of a respect for autonomy in the abstract or as a matter of philosophical principle, but in order to ensure that another's religiously grounded views are authentic. Sheridan thus commented, "You have to know the person; what is happening on the surface may not be the real thing."[29] Some religions that impose clear imperatives are voluntarily acquired, through personal conversion. As Bales's case suggests, the distinction between religion as chosen and religion as a matter of conscience is sometimes impossible to draw. For religious converts, the opposition of freedom and duty, so important to Sandel's analysis, is often uninstructive or, more importantly, nonexistent.

Concerns about Bales's depth of conviction likewise informed Sheridan's attention to matters of confidentiality. That concern (and the danger of coercion it is meant to prevent) isolates a feature of religion that does not receive attention in Sandel's discussion of religious conscience: the possibility of conscientious *dissent*. In Sheridan's mind, a key question was whether Jackson's (possible) desire to depart from his father's views was adequately protected. She believed that Jackson may have felt a duty to refuse religious commands but that his freedom to discharge that duty was inadequately protected by the arrangements in the ICU. However intrusive and intolerant Sheridan might have appeared to her colleagues, her concern for confidentiality turns Sandel's position in another direction: If religious liberty means protecting the right to act on a religiously informed duty, it should also protect dissent from such duties when one's conscience so instructs.

RELIGION IN THE HOSPITAL

Beyond these thoughts about DeVries's and Sheridan's actions, we would do well to conclude by comparing some general features of Jackson's story with those of Billy Richardson's from the previous chapter. Each case involved religiously based decisions within a complex set of medical and social circumstances. Billy's care operated with a situation of relative uncertainty about the outcomes of aggressive treatment, whereas Jackson's care revolved around options with relatively certain life-saving benefits. In Billy's case, religion served to authorize ongoing, aggressive treatment of dubious benefit; in Jackson's, religion served to authorize a patient's refusal of medically indicated treatment of relatively certain benefit. Religion in Billy's case was shaped by an overall commitment to liberty, whereas in Jackson's case religion functioned more as a duty. I hasten to add that both cases show the difficulty of separating the value of freedom from the value of duty when assessing religious piety in others' decisions.

Further differences appear once we consider how physicians calibrated care according to each patient's age and competence. The language of liberty and self-determination in Billy's case meant that he was perceived on terms that, paradoxically, draw from adult medical care. In contrast, Jackson (a legal adult) was treated paternalistically by one physician, as if he were a child.

As we saw in Chapter 3, paternalism is a complicated matter, and several of its dimensions are relevant to interactions between the house staff, the Richardsons, and the Baleses. In Billy's case, had care providers overridden his parents' demands, they would have practiced second party paternalism—in which a third party overrides the competent wishes of a second party in order to protect a ward who is presumably dependent on the care of that party. Overriding the Richardsons' decision would have sent the message that they (and Billy) were better off leaving decisions about Billy to someone else—that "the doctor knows best."

In Jackson's case, and in the parallel case of John, we see examples of unreflexive and reflexive paternalism. Sheridan's treatment of Jackson illustrates unreflexive paternalism, whereas the doctor's "solution" in John's case illustrates reflexive paternalism. Sheridan infantalized Jackson in order to seek a good for him against his competently stated wishes; John's doctor asked him to transfer decision-making authority so that he could avoid making a difficult decision about his medical interests. With Jackson, competently expressed wishes were ignored to protect him from self-harming decisions. With John, arrangements with his care provider secured his good while enabling him to avoid exercising his competence to decide for himself about whether to accept a transfusion.

Paternalistic actions are also distinguished by how paternalists connect their actions to what they think their beneficiaries want. With Jackson and John, physicians sought to practice moderate paternalism, in which one party decides to make decisions that presumably cohere with the beneficiary's wishes, or at least some of those wishes, despite that beneficiary's competently stated desires. Moderate paternalists recognize that the beneficiary has various values, some of which might conflict, and appeals to one set to override or ignore that individual's tendency to decide according to another set. Sheridan sought to practice moderate paternalism by regularly asking Jackson about the strength of his religious conviction to refuse treatment. If his resolve had been ambivalent, then transfusing him might be an act of moderate paternalism, drawing on one set of desires while ignoring others. John's physician did much the same. He explored John's ambivalence in order to open up the possibility of acting on one set of express wishes—namely, that John "didn't want to die."

The stories of Billy Richardson and Jackson Bales illustrate temptations to which pediatric care can be drawn: either presuming that children are "little adults" with well-wrought powers of self-determination, or that young adults are presumptively incompetent, with insufficient powers of judgment or expression. Each of these tendencies constitutes an extreme to be avoided in the pursuit of virtue in pediatric medicine. Billy's story represents the first temptation, Jackson's the second. In the next chapter, I will focus less on how parents and professionals conceive of children's and adolescents' capacities to decide, and more on how professionals acted, and should have acted, in response to a religious demand for unconventional medical care. Pediatric care not only involves calibration and specification when thinking about a patient's decision-making abilities; it may also involve cultural clashes about how to view medicine as a whole. For various reasons, medical care can raise controversies that are physical as well as metaphysical, posing fundamental challenges to a care provider's basic framework and commitment to care. To issues surrounding the culture of biomedicine and nonmainstream alternatives we shall now turn.

EIGHT

Ericka's Sepsis, Lia's Convulsions, and Cultural Differences

The thesis is that our identity is partly shaped by recognition or
its absence, often by the *mis*recognition of others, and so a
person or group of people can suffer real damage,
real distortion, if the people or society around them mirror back
to them a confining or demeaning or contemptible picture of
themselves. Nonrecognition or misrecognition can inflict harm,
can be a form of oppression, imprisoning someone in a
false, distorted, and reduced mode of being.[1]

—Charles Taylor

What we distribute to one another is esteem, not self-esteem;
respect, not self-respect; defeat, not the sense of defeat; and the
relation of the first to the second term in each of these pairs is
indirect and uncertain.[2]

—Michael Walzer

THERAPY AND IDENTITY

Several of Billy Richardson's and Jackson Bales's care providers at Baylin asked themselves whether to cease aggressive medical treatment (Billy) or to introduce standard therapy (Jackson) against the wishes of each patient's family. Those conflicts might conceal a more fundamental level of agreement between the intensive care unit (ICU) house staff and each patient's family regarding the value of conventional medical care. Although these patient's outcomes were uncertain, neither the care providers nor the family members disputed the soundness of the medical data that guided their treatment regimens. Michelle Richardson did not propose nonmainstream alternatives to what the hospital could offer, and Harold Bales did not believe that his religious faith could change Jackson's situation or that it required house staff to use unconventional healing methods.

The Richardsons were especially adroit when interpreting and assessing data regarding Billy's condition, and they did so daily. Like many parents in Baylin's ICU, they were able to understand complicated medical information and were remarkably articulate when speaking in the house staff's technical language about their son's case. Yet to many families, Michelle and Kyle Richardson appear to have been coopted by the medical establishment because they never asked whether high-tech, tertiary medical care was the best way to address their son's condition. These concerns about cooptation point to another kind of conflict that is increasingly appearing in pediatric health care settings, some aspects of which I mentioned when discussing *In the Matter of Martin Seiferth, Jr.*, and *Custody of a Minor* in Chapter 4. Such clashes are culturally based, challenging the merits of conventional medical treatment and the account of the body on which it relies. That is to say, some patients and families are requesting alternative healing methods and natural remedies for chronic and acute ailments. Such methods and remedies typically claim superior effectiveness when compared to standard medical approaches, relying on laboratory or anecdotal evidence. Not infrequently, their use is also linked to a worldview or set of religious beliefs and practices, and failure to appreciate their merits can indict the religious frameworks of which they are a part. No less than illness, therapy can touch on an patient's or family's culture and identity.

In this chapter, I will explore two cases involving alternative therapies and cultural differences in the care of children. The first is a case from a hospital on the West Coast that was presented to me for critical commentary while I was doing fieldwork in Baylin's ICU. Focusing on the story of an infant girl, Ericka, that case concerns whether, and on what terms, care providers should accommodate unconventional therapies and New Age religious beliefs and practices. Second is the story of Lia Lee, a child of Hmong immigrants to the United States, whose epileptic seizures and subsequent brain damage confronted her American doctors with grave medical and cultural challenges. As recounted in Anne Fadiman's stirring ethnography, *The Spirit Catches You and You Fall Down: A Hmong Child, Her American Doctors, and the Collision of Two Cultures*,[3] Lia's story concerns cultural differences in the course of treatment and whether quality-of-life considerations are potentially ethnocentric.

When pediatricians treat patients such as Ericka and Lia, they must consider whether or how to negotiate between the culture of modern biomedicine and cultures outside the mainstream, whether indigenous or transplanted from elsewhere. In such cases it might seem wise to coordinate conventional methods with nonmainstream beliefs and practices, even at the expense of providing optimal care for patients in need. I want to discuss the merits and limits of that idea after examining each account. Let us consider each case in turn, beginning with Ericka.

TREATING ERICKA WHEN THE MOON TURNS FULL

Ericka's story began when she was brought to an ICU on the West Coast with pneumonia and septic shock, a highly dangerous condition in which tissue damage and a precipitous drop in blood pressure occur as a result of bacteria and toxins in the blood. Born a healthy seven-pound, twelve-ounce baby, Ericka developed a runny nose and cough at the age of ten days. Her mother, Melody, continued to breast-feed Ericka, and she gave her some special herbal tea that she had used during pregnancy. Two days later, she brought Ericka to the emergency department because the infant was lethargic, fed poorly, and breathed heavily. A chest X-ray revealed bilateral patchy infiltrates, and bilateral crackles were heard over the lung fields. Soon after her admission to the hospital, Ericka developed moderate respiratory distress and was put on a ventilator with high airway pressures and concentrations of oxygen. Like Billy, Ericka suffered a pneumothorax, caused by high ventilation pressures, for which a chest tube was inserted. Her circulation and blood pressure likewise deteriorated, requiring dopamine and epinephrine after several fluid boluses of normal saline and 5 percent albumin failed to improve her condition.

Within a week of her admission, Ericka showed clear signs of improvement. Yet Melody remained skeptical of the house staff's promising diagnosis, fearing that the baby's immune system remained weak. With that in mind, Melody asked the staff to permit her healer and spiritual adviser, Jonathan, to assist in Ericka's care. Melody and Jonathan had met as part of a group identified in the case presentation as "New Age Religion," and he had treated Melody for her headaches by prescribing a regimen of daily meditation and an herbal tea after she found that her neurologists' prescriptions left her in a confused daze. After a period of deep meditation, Jonathan agreed with house staff that Ericka was improving, yet he sensed that she needed additional treatment to strengthen her immunities. He thus prescribed an herbal preparation to feed Ericka and to be applied to her chest twice a day as soon as the moon became full.

At first the house staff responded to this request sympathetically, understanding the importance of family participation in pediatric care. Yet the nurse to whom Melody gave Jonathan's packet of ingredients could not hide her shock and disgust, and tossed the packet into a drawer after saying that she would inform the ICU's attending physician of Melody's request. At that point, Melody became visibly agitated, screamed at the nurse, and threatened to contact her lawyer and the local newspapers before storming out of the building.

The next day, Melody returned to the hospital calmer and more responsive. She agreed to allow Ericka's doctors to consult with Jonathan. After some discussion, all agreed to a compromise that allowed Jonathan to apply the herbal substance to Ericka's chest while the nurses continued standard ICU care. Jonathan agreed to defer prescribing tea for Ericka to drink until she was older and healthier. The next day, Ericka's doctor ordered that the mother or nurses would apply the herbal preparation four times a day as directed. Otherwise her treatment in the ICU was unremarkable. Ericka steadily improved in the ICU, and she was extubated after fifteen days. Four days later, she was discharged to return home with her mother.

In a written commentary about using unconventional medicine in Ericka's treatment, Dr. Chester Randle poses two ethical questions and answers both affirmatively.[4] The first is whether accommodating unconventional medical practices is morally acceptable when those practices seem potentially harmless to the patient. The second is whether Ericka's physicians adequately responded to Melody's beliefs within the limits of providing adequate care for her daughter. These questions are complicated by the fact that Melody's demands for unconventional treatment implicated religious and cultural values. Ericka's case reminds us that in pediatrics it is often necessary for health care providers to attend to family members' needs in the course of caring for a child. Once again we are reminded that pediatric medicine occurs within the context of forging a therapeutic alliance between health care providers and a child's family.

I want to argue that Dr. Randle's answer to the first question is inadequate, for Randle fails to provide enough information to be confident that applying an herbal substance to Ericka's chest would be harmless. I want to argue that Randle's answer to the second question is wrong, for the doctors failed to ascertain how Ericka acquired sepsis, and they made no attempt to educate Melody about how to avoid such crises in the future. Their compromise formula worked less to benefit Ericka than to appease her mother. As a result, Ericka's physicians failed to respond adequately to the medical implications of their differences with Melody.

Randle's manner of treating the first question blinds him to the deeper challenges of the second question. He tackles the first question by applying principles of biomedical ethics—beneficence, nonmaleficence, autonomy, and justice—to Ericka's case. In many respects, his approach is instructive because it illustrates the grip that a mechanical application of biomedical principles has on health care providers' practical reasoning. Randle applies moral principles in a "top-down" fashion to Ericka's case. That approach handicaps his understanding of the deeper meaning and implications of these principles.

I will argue for greater caution about how Randle answers the first question and attempt to offer a different answer to the second question. My view is that, when circumstances permit, the role responsibilities of pediatric care providers include challenging parental demands and educating parents about possible connections between their habits and their children's health. In this case, Ericka's physicians failed to exercise their responsibility to educate, despite the fact that circumstances were favorable to discharging that duty. To see this point, we need to move beyond a mechanical application of the principles of biomedical ethics to ascertain their meaning and their (sometimes demanding) implications for professional responsibility. We must thus consider each question in turn: the ethics of using unconventional treatment on Ericka, and the challenge of reckoning with Melody's religious and cultural values.

UNCONVENTIONAL TREATMENT

Randle frames his analysis by citing four ethical principles: "beneficence—use treatments based on the benefits they provide; nonmaleficence—consider the potential harm to patients; autonomy—accept the likelihood that different persons may judge benefits differently; and justice—treat similar cases similarly." Reflecting the influence of a "principalist" approach to bioethics and practical reasoning, Randle picks out core ideas of Ericka's case to see if they comply with these general principles. His conclusion is that alternative therapies are not morally required: "Because unconventional therapies usually fail to meet the first two principles, I believe that a physician is not obligated to provide unconventional therapy."

Randle is correct to argue that Ericka's physicians were not obligated to have Ericka ingest tea that was prepared by Jonathan, because Jonathan's remedy was of unknown effectiveness. This judgment is justified on terms that all treatments—conventional or unconventional—must be evaluated. After noting that nonmainstream therapies have a mixed record and that they are widely used by the American population, Randle observes that Jonathan's prescription was an unknown therapy, subjecting her to a "dangerous experiment of one." In his view, "this unconventional therapy failed to meet the standard of nonmaleficence." Ericka's physicians exercised no cultural prejudice by barring Jonathan from having Ericka ingest a tea made from unknown ingredients. Treatment that is not beneficial or is potentially harmful is neither medically nor morally indicated.

Ericka's physicians decided instead to allow Jonathan to apply his herbal tea to Ericka's chest. Yet the basis for this compromise is unclear. Ericka's case report states that her ICU physicians and Jonathan agreed that applying the herbal brew to Ericka's body was not likely to cause harm and could "still allow the infant to receive a form of therapy that [the] mom requested." Immediately we should ask, What was the factual basis for this agreement? Were the contents of Jonathan's tea subjected to laboratory analysis? Was the tea potentially damaging to Ericka's skin, such that it might have caused dermatitis or other forms of aggravation and discomfort? More generally, how do we know that she was not put at risk by this treatment?

I raise these questions because herbal remedies and other forms of unconventional therapy are not subject to the same strict standards that are used to evaluate the pharmaceutical industry in the United States. The Dietary Supplement Health and Education Act of 1994 weakened the authority of the U.S. Food and Drug Administration (FDA) to regulate vitamins, herbal remedies, and dietary supplements by shifting the burden of proving their safety. Promoted heavily by Senator Orrin G. Hatch of Utah, the home of many supplement makers, the law created a new class of products, the "dietary supplement," that would not be subjected to the same restrictions as drugs.[5] Before 1994, the FDA could order a medically suspicious substance off the market until the manufacturer had proved it safe. As a result of the new act, the FDA must now prove a product unsafe before ordering it off the market. Currently, dangerous products may be sold until someone is harmed by them and reports his or her case to medical professionals or government authorities. Under the new law, moreover, consumers have no guarantee that an herbal product contains what its label says it does or that it is free from dangerous contaminants.[6] Little research has been done to examine how herbal products interact with conventional medications. Owing to the current climate of deregulation, risks to public health are not insignificant. In a test of herbal products from Asia, the California Department of Health Services found poisonous heavy metals such as lead, arsenic, or mercury in 83 of 260 samples.[7] In response to reported illnesses, the FDA's actions have not been efficient. The agency took more than four years, more than a hundred reports of life-threatening illnesses, and thirty-eight deaths before it acted against ephedra (sold as the Chinese herb *ma luang*), a stimulant that has untoward effects on people with heart problems.[8]

In fairness to Ericka's physicians, we should note that Jonathan's herbal remedy might have been subjected to laboratory analysis before the compromise was struck. Without wanting to exaggerate this issue, I must note that the case lacks data to assure us on this point. Randle merely states that "the physician and Jonathan were able to develop a therapeutic plan to provide herbal therapy that was unlikely to cause harm and was compatible with conventional medical care." Yet the mere fact that the treatment is unlikely to cause harm does not prove that it is *therapeutic*. Moreover, no data are cited to support the idea that Jonathan's prescription would not harm Ericka. Lacking that information, we cannot be certain that the caregivers have satisfied the duty of nonmaleficence. In accommodating Melody's demands, the physicians might have subjected Ericka to further risk or discomfort.

It appears that the compromise was struck less for Ericka's benefit than for the benefit of Melody and the house staff. Before we conclude this chapter, I will return to this issue of seeking compromises in cases involving alternative therapies. For now, I wish to note that securing Jonathan's and Melody's agreement lessened the emotional tension between Melody and the nurses on the floor and reduced the threat of legal action. Seeking agreement might also have arisen from fears about appearing intolerant or prejudiced about nonmainstream beliefs. But if those are the reasons for the compromise, then the tea was applied to Ericka's skin in order to resolve problems other than her sepsis and respiratory distress. Without further information about why the tea is deemed to benefit Ericka, there is a danger that she is being used for others' benefit. To describe the compromise as one that allows the infant to receive a form of *therapy* that her mother requested is to ignore medical and moral concerns: On what basis can we confidently say that herbal treatment is indeed *Ericka's* therapy?

In raising this question, I do not mean to suggest that nonbeneficial treatment of a child to benefit others is absolutely unacceptable. As I will argue in Chapter 11, some nonbeneficial treatment of children in research settings might be justified according to an ethics of turn-taking and fair play. But in Ericka's case, the use of unconventional procedures is not deemed nontherapeutic, aimed toward others' benefit. It is rather presented as therapy for her, and I have already indicated why we should doubt such a description.

CULTURAL DIFFERENCES

Randle endorses what he calls a "culturally sensitive healthcare system," adding that such a system must be constrained by considerations of patient benefit. He rightly urges flexibility, accessibility, and respect for different cultural practices within the limits imposed by biomedical ethics. Alternative treatments are often presented as part of a holistic approach to health and healing, involving the entire person rather than perceiving the body as a collection of analyzable symptoms. Treating both body and soul is of no small benefit; it focuses on the patient as person. In his view, Ericka's physicians operated within the broad contours of this vision, providing Ericka with medical care while forging a therapeutic relationship with Melody.

In addition, Randle argues, a responsive system "does not imply that patients have unrestricted autonomy." That is to say, respecting the value of autonomy does not mean that patients or parents can *demand* certain forms of medical treatment. In these respects, Randle's claims are correct. As I indicated in Chapter 5, autonomy is not a positive right in health care settings, only a negative one. He writes, "Patients do not have a right to antibiotics just because they want them, or chemotherapy because they are afraid that they might have cancer."

Yet there are additional issues to consider, and herein lies my deeper disagreement with Randle. The most striking omissions concern the cause of Ericka's admission and the requirements of her future care. Both issues might involve Melody's cultural beliefs and practices, which could be harmful to her daughter. Consider Ericka's admission: Apparently, no one asked why Ericka developed septic shock. Was this problem prompted by ingesting the herbal tea that her mother fed her? Might the tea be toxic to Ericka? (Hence another reason to subject the tea to laboratory tests.) Consider Ericka's return home: All have agreed that in due time Melody may feed Jonathan's prescribed herbal brew to Ericka. If so, will this practice expose Ericka to risk? Will Melody's cultural and religious beliefs endanger Ericka in other ways? If so, shouldn't she be dissuaded from acting on beliefs that might affect her daughter adversely?

All of these questions bear on and potentially challenge Melody's cultural and religious beliefs. Critically engaging Melody about her commitments and her treatment of Ericka are clear implications of the duty to care and to avoid harm (beneficence and nonmaleficence). Those duties bear not only on the immediate question of proper therapy in intensive care, but on the cause of Ericka's illness and the prevention of future illness. In neglecting such issues, Ericka's health care providers failed to exercise proper medical responsibilities; the therapeutic alliance they forged with her mother was medically and morally deficient.

In William F. May's mind, the type of relationship between Melody and Ericka's physicians is more "transactional" than "transformational."[9] Recall these terms from Chapter 2 and their relation to the duty to care. A transactional approach involves an exchange of information and the guarantee that goods and services will be adequately provided. But such interactions do not require doctors to instruct patients or parents about how to decrease the likelihood of future illness or how to improve their health-related habits. May argues that a transactional approach privatizes professional responsibility by reducing it to a commodity to be bought and sold on the marketplace. A transformational approach, in contrast, requires physicians to get to the root of their patients' problems, and envisions professional life as part of the larger commonweal. The aim is not to satisfy patients' preferences or to strike compromises in order to reduce emotional tension and the danger of litigation, but to address patients' long-term problems with an eye to preventing illness and protecting public health.

RECOGNITION AND RESPECT

I have stated that the problem with Randle's analysis lies with his method of evaluating Ericka's story, and May's distinction between transactional and transformational dynamics enables us to see how that is so. Randle applies principles of biomedical ethics in a top-down manner to Ericka's case and Melody's cultural and religious beliefs. The goal is to determine whether particular actions can be subsumed within a general principle or to pick out features of a situation to see whether they abide by a more general value. Reflecting a transactional set of assumptions, Randle's analysis is limited to decisions within a narrow time frame—namely, the events in the ICU. Although a top-down approach to practical reasoning and a transactional approach to medical care are not the same, they can enjoy an affinity in institutional settings that prize efficiency. Such an affinity crowds out considerations of causes or consequences—events prior or subsequent to Ericka's admission to the hospital.

A transformational approach requires a more longitudinal perspective, a larger frame of analysis. It thus generates greater expectations of the physicians responsible for Ericka, enlarging the demands of beneficent and nonmaleficent treatment beyond the immediate context of the ICU. These norms require physicians not only to provide care in the ICU, but also to weigh the demands of future health and the prevention of illness. To be sure, such expectations are difficult to meet in intensive care; typically, patients are in and out of such units in a few days. In many, if not most, cases, expecting a transformational approach to patient and family care in ICUs is unrealistic and unfair.[10] But Ericka was in the unit for more than two weeks, enabling physicians to familiarize themselves with her situation and her mother's convictions. Circumstances that would normally excuse physicians from adopting a transformational approach to patient care do not apply to this case.

Randle might respond that my analysis pays insufficient attention to other principles of biomedical ethics, especially autonomy and justice. I appear to overlook autonomy insofar as I fail adequately to respect values that are central to Melody's identity. Randle could point to the irony that a more robust understanding of beneficence in my argument seems to exclude a respect for parental autonomy and the distinct features of Ericka's background. That seems inconsistent, he might continue, for a more longitudinal perspective would seem to imply a more demanding account of all of the relevant principles in medical care. (We will turn to such a perspective when considering Lia Lee.) That is to say, a transformational approach would require us to see Ericka's needs *and* her mother's commitments within a larger narrative. Scrutinizing Melody's beliefs in light of their possible medical implications seems not to grant her the kind of appreciation that is important to her *ongoing* self-respect.

Considerations of identity, respect, and recognition are morally significant in multicultural societies, in which recognition of cultural differences is often seen as a matter of social justice. The citation from Charles Taylor with which I began this chapter makes this point well: Today concerns about recognition and respect are premised on the thesis "that our identity is partly shaped by recognition or its absence, often by the *mis*recognition of others, and so a person or group of people can suffer real damage, real distortion, if the people or society around them mirror back to them a confining or demeaning or contemptible picture of themselves." A person's identity depends in part on internalizing the views that others hold of him or her, and the lack of recognition "can inflict harm, can be a form of oppression," imprisoning that person "in a false, distorted, and reduced mode of being."[11] Cultures that impose such burdens on identity can hardly claim to be just, for they generate the idea that some persons are "naturally" second-class citizens. Given those concerns, my argument fails to recognize Melody's self-defining choices, and that failure raises concerns about justice and equality.

Yet it is important to remember that Melody is not the primary patient in this case. Moral considerations that bear on her needs are derivative on and subordinate to Ericka's needs. If, as this case suggests, Ericka's health is potentially compromised by respecting Melody's self-defining cultural and religious beliefs, the latter must give way to other priorities.

Herein lies a key difference between pediatric and adult medicine: With adults, the duty of care is constrained by considerations of patient autonomy. Physicians must treat a patient with the patient's consent or, if that patient is incompetent, with the consent of a patient proxy who first tries to convey facts about the patient's background and choices. In adult medicine, patients have the liberty to make some medically irrational decisions, and their proxies may represent medically irrational wishes. In pediatric care, however, patient autonomy is a lesser factor and is sometimes irrelevant because many children are incompetent. Those who "represent" children must sometimes guard their best medical interests, not their liberty interests.

Thus we have two responses to the charge of insufficient attention to autonomy and justice as these bear on Ericka's family background: (1) Those norms are relevant to Melody, who is not the primary patient; and (2) Melody must guard her daughter's basic medical interests.

NORM AND CONTEXT

The use of unconventional treatment that is recommended by a parent's cultural and religious beliefs helps us understand some important points about the duty to care for young patients. In pediatric medicine, as we have seen, the duty to care is not constrained by patient autonomy in the same way that it is in adult medicine. Moreover, and equally important, considerations of beneficence cannot be limited to short-term interactions between families and care providers; a more capacious analysis is needed. Stated in terms I developed in Chapter 2, the norm of beneficence should be informed by the virtue of benevolence, disposing care providers to protect a patient's basic interests. If nothing else, Ericka's right to an open future limits what her mother can do to her, however important Melody's religious and cultural practices may be to her own identity and sense of value.

My disagreements with Randle's discussion are thus methodological and substantive, and these disagreements are linked. Methodologically, I have argued for situating ethical judgments within a larger context than Randle's analysis invites.[12] Enlarging the scope of that analysis, in turn, opens the door to substantive concerns about the requirements of responsible medical treatment in the care of children.

The fact that a transformationist approach to medical responsibility generates more robust moral expectations than we find in Randle's analysis points to an important idea in practical reasoning: How we interpret and apply moral concepts relies in part on unarticulated background assumptions.[13] In my view, the duty to care becomes more demanding given what we can infer about transformational dynamics and the corresponding virtue of benevolence. In this respect, the requirements of biomedical ethics are amplified; their range of application is broadened owing to background assumptions regarding the proper responsibilities of health care providers.

ON RESCUING A VAGRANT SOUL

A more taxing set of expectations is called for in Fadiman's ethnography of the cultural clash between Lia Lee's American care providers and Nao Kao and Foua Lee, Hmong immigrants to the United States and Lia's parents. The Lees' fourteenth child, Lia first was admitted to Merced Community Medical Center (MCMC) in 1982 when she was three months old, afflicted by an epileptic seizure. Her recurrent seizures would be the frequent cause of concern for Neil and Peggy Philp, her principal pediatricians at MCMC. Between the ages of eight months and four and a half years, Lia was admitted to MCMC seventeen times and made more than a hundred outpatient visits to the hospital's emergency room and the family practice center. Lia's physicians prescribed a variety of anticonvulsants to allay her symptoms, but as a result of language barriers, Nao Kao and Foua found it difficult to understand Lia's medical condition and to learn how to administer her medications.

Cultural barriers further complicated Lia's case. Lia's American doctors ascribed her condition to the misfiring of her cerebral neurons; her family saw her illness as the result of her soul's meandering. Before Lia's admission to MCMC, her older sister, Yer, slammed the front door of the family's apartment, and Lia's seizures began soon afterward. In her parents' minds, the noise of the door had been so frightening that Lia's soul fled and became lost, snatched up by a *dab*—a Hmong demigod who specializes in kidnaping human souls. The Lees saw Lia's epilepsy as *quag dab peg*—"the spirit catches you and you fall down"—and sought assistance from a Hmong shaman, or *txiv neeb*, to assist in Lia's spiritual healing. Typically, the Lees' shamans sacrificed a cow, pig, or chicken in the Lees' home or in the hospital, believing that the animal's soul could be bartered for Lia's vagrant soul. A sacrificial healing ritual, or *neeb*, was meant to complement the use of conventional medicines in Lia's care.[14] Commenting on Lia's medical and spiritual treatment, Nao Kao remarked to Fadiman, "With Lia it was good to do a little medicine and a little *neeb*, but not too much medicine because the medicine cuts the *neeb*'s effect. If we did a little of each she didn't get sick as much, but the doctors wouldn't let us give just a little medicine because they didn't understand about the soul."[15]

The Lees had great difficulty understanding Lia's treatment regimen. Their daughter's prescriptions were not uncomplicated, and her medications were changed more than once. Making matters more challenging, Lia's medications had notable side effects. Phenobarbital increased her hyperactivity; dilantin caused hair to grow abnormally over her body, and too much of these drugs with Tegretol brought on unsteadiness and unconsciousness. For these reasons, Lia's parents administered her medications inconsistently, often confused about what was really good for her. Lia's nurses and doctors became increasingly worried about what they perceived as the Lees' noncompliance and Lia's recurrent seizures. In 1985, officials at the Merced Child Protection Services (MCPS) determined that Nao Kao and Foua were negligent in Lia's care and had her removed to a foster home.

With the assistance of Jeanine Hilt, a social worker in Merced who took up Lia's cause, Nao Kao and Foua became more familiar with and confident about administering Lia's medications. Progress on that front enabled Hilt to convince MCPS officials that Lia could safely return to her family. According to Fadiman, Jeanine "was determined to try to continue to educate the Lees about Lia's medications so that they could regain custody before twelve months elapsed and they legally lost her for good. Jeanine spent dozens of hours working with Foua."[16] Making Lia's return more manageable, her physicians determined that Depakene was Lia's drug of choice. More easily administered, it was an effective anticonvulsant and had no untoward side effects. Given these changes, hope for Lia (now three years old), seemed real. At the same time, Nao Kao and Foua could see that Lia was developmentally delayed, and they had every reason to believe that her problems could be traced to her American doctors.

The Lees thus stepped up their alternative methods of treatment. When Lia came home from foster care, they brought in a *txiv neeb* to sacrifice a cow, and they had her wear expensive amulets with healing herbs from Thailand. Though unconventional by Western lights, the Lees were by no means uninterested in Lia's health. According to Fadiman,

> Foua inserted a silver coin that said "1936 Indochine Francaise" into the yolk of a boiled egg, wrapped the egg in a cloth, and rubbed Lia's body with it; when the egg turned black, that meant the sickness had been absorbed. She massaged Lia with the bowl of a spoon. She sucked the "pressure" out of Lia's body by pressing a small cup heated with ashes against her skin, creating a temporary vacuum as the oxygen-depleted air inside the cup cooled. She pinched Lia to draw out noxious winds. She dosed Lia with tisanes infused from the gleanings of her parking-lot herb garden. Finally, she and Nao Kao tried changing Lia's name to Kou, a last-ditch Hmong remedy based on the premise that if a patient is called by a new name, the *dab* who stole her soul will be tricked into thinking that she is someone else, and the soul can return. According to Foua, the plan was foiled because Lia's doctors persisted in calling her Lia, thus ruining the subterfuge.[17]

Despite these efforts, Lia's seizures continued, each one longer and more serious. In November 1986, Lia experienced a tonicoclonic seizure that lasted over two hours. (A twenty-five-minute seizure is considered life-threatening.) Neil Philp was on call that fateful evening. After unsuccessfully trying to stabilize Lia, he sent her via emergency transport to Fresno Valley Children's Hospital, a larger and better-equipped facility. Lia was admitted at Valley Children's with status epilepticus and septicemia, a life-threatening condition caused by bacteria in the blood. Her devastating seizure deprived her brain of much-needed oxygen, tragically leaving her with irreparable brain damage. Her infection, we later discover, was probably acquired during a previous visit to MCMC when her immunities were weak. Describing her neurological condition, Lia's medical file in Fresno states that "an EEG [electroencephalogram] was obtained which revealed essentially no brain activity with very flat brain waves."[18] Lia was subsequently discharged from the hospital in Fresno in a persistent vegetative state, to be maintained on artificial life support at MCMC. Soon thereafter, Nao Kao secured her release and brought her home, where everyone expected her to die.

As if to incarnate the Hmongs' firm resistance to Western culture, Lia defied her doctors' prediction that she would die soon. Dearly loved and cared for by her family, she was freed from her epilepsy—it was "cured" by her brain damage. But that liberation came at a high price, for Lia returned home profoundly inaccessible, quadriplegic, spastic, incontinent, and incapable of purposeful movement.[19] Her story concludes with an account of a *neeb* in the Lees' apartment, in which a chicken is sacrificed in hopes of recapturing Lia's lost soul.

Fadiman is not a relativistic champion of Hmong beliefs and practices; she recognizes that Western medicine provides a more reliable way of curing diseases than attempting to capture fugitive souls through animal sacrifice. She confesses having to remind herself that "it was all that cold linear, Cartesian, non-Hmong-like thinking which saved my father from colon cancer, saved my husband and me from infertility, and, if she had swallowed her anticonvulsants from the start, might have saved Lia from brain damage."[20] The key question is how to coordinate the worldview of Western medicine with Hmong worldviews and practices. When, if ever, is it desirable to "fuse horizons" between the culture of modern biomedicine and alternative worldviews and beliefs?[21]

Seeing Lia's story as the tragic result of cross-cultural misunderstanding and miscommunication, Fadiman contacted medical anthropologist Arthur Kleinman for counsel about how to bridge cultural divides in health care settings. Recounting Lia's story in brief to Kleinman, Fadiman solicited three suggestions for Lia's pediatricians. He replied,

> First, get rid of the term "compliance". . . . It implies moral hegemony. You don't want a command from a general, you want a colloquy. Second, instead of looking at a model of coercion, look at a model of mediation. Go find a member of the Hmong community, or go find a medical anthropologist, who can help you negotiate. Remember that a stance of mediation, like a divorce proceeding, requires compromise on both sides. Decide what's critical and be willing to compromise on everything else. Third, you need to understand that as powerful an influence as the culture of the Hmong patient and her family is on this case, the culture of biomedicine is equally powerful. If you can't see that your own culture has its own set of interests, emotions, and biases, how can you expect to deal successfully with someone else's culture?[22]

Fadiman's central claim is that a better understanding of Hmong history and culture might have enabled Lia's doctors to overcome the Lees' resistance to Western medicine and lead them toward a more cooperative set of arrangements. "A little medicine and a little *neeb*," she claims, might have been the correct prescription for Lia. Though that combination would have meant less than optimal care from a biomedical point of view, it might have meant that the Lees would have administered Lia's medications more regularly. Lia's doctors seemed intent on protecting her best medical interests rather than her basic ones.

INSTRUMENTAL ACCOMMODATION

Lia's story account takes a dramatic turn toward its conclusion, when we are told that her doctors in Merced likely made a mistake in diagnosing and treating her. According to Fadiman, Peggy and Neil Philp, Lia's principal pediatricians, failed to diagnose Lia for septicemia because they focused on correcting her seizure disorder. That failure is revealed when Fadiman interviews Dr. Terry Hutchinson in Fresno, Lia's physician during her emergency admission at Valley Children's Hospital. According to Hutchinson, Lia's septicemia, not her epilepsy, accounted for her seizures. Her epilepsy might have predisposed her favorably for a serious seizure, but her septicemia was the main culprit. "The septic shock caused the seizures," Hutchinson remarks, "not the other way around." On his diagnosis, taking Depakene might have lowered Lia's immune system, making her more susceptible to bacterial infection. Hutchinson tells Fadiman, "If the family was giving her the Depakene as instructed, it is conceivable that by following our instructions they set her up for septic shock." He continues, "Go back to Merced and tell those people at MCMC that the family didn't do this to the kid. We did."[23] After reviewing Lia's chart, the Philps agreed with Hutchinson's account.[24] According to Hutchinson and Fadiman, Neil and Peggy focused on neurology and the administration of anticonvulsants to stop Lia's epileptic seizures. They thus overlooked Lia's underlying bacterial infection, for which no cause was ever produced.

Lia's misdiagnosis changes her story into a case of medical error and the likelihood of iatrogenic illness. These are no small worries for parents and children who are admitted to health care settings. My focus here, however, poses a different set of concerns. The fact that Neil Philp overlooked non-neurological causes for Lia's convulsions when she was admitted in November 1986 suggests that overcoming the cultural divide might not have produced better diagnostic outcomes for her. That is to say, it is not obvious that more open or effective lines of communication between the Philps and the Lees would have led to a different set of results for Lia. Fadiman concedes that if the Lees had administered the full regimen of anticonvulsants, then perhaps Lia would not have ended up in a persistent vegetative state. But Fadiman's more important claim is that the Lees' "noncompliance" does not account for Lia's dramatic neurological downturn. That fact might exonerate the Lees somewhat, but it does not bear directly on the claim that resolving their cultural clash would have led to diagnostic accuracy in Lia's case. Put differently, it is not clear that the outcomes for a white, English-speaking child with frequent tonicoclonic seizures and septicemia could have been different from Lia's outcomes, given that the seizures would mask the infection. After all, Lia's seizures began when she was a few months old, requiring frequent trips to MCMC's emergency room. As Bill Selvidge, a physician at MCMC, described the situation: "*No one* at MCMC would have noticed anything but her seizures. Lia *was* her seizures."[25]

This revelation about Lia's misdiagnosis shifts the problem considerably, and Fadiman seems not to notice that fact. Her chief concern is to take up Kleinman's counsel about the importance of dialogue and negotiation when dealing with persons who have quite different beliefs about biomedicine and bodily healing. But that counsel is irrelevant to Lia's final diagnosis. Even if Peggy and Neil Philp had engaged Lia's parents according to Kleinman's prescription, it is not obvious that such a dialogue would have enabled Neil to treat her more accurately, or to diagnose her infection.

The most that Fadiman can claim is that if Lia's health care providers had succeeded in securing the Lees' trust they might have been able to see Lia more frequently, under less urgent conditions. That fact might have increased the chance of diagnosing her septicemia sooner rather than later or have reduced the number of Lia's trips to the hospital, where she was likely to have acquired her bacterial infection. On this general point about communication and trust, Fadiman's critique of MCMC, and modern medical care, is powerful. Wondering whether, or to what extent, matters could have been different, she writes,

> Instead of practicing "veterinary medicine," what if the residents in the emergency room had managed to elicit the Lees' trust at the outset—or at least managed not to crush it—by finding out what *they* believed, feared, and hoped? . . .
>
> Of course, the Lees' perspective might have been as unfathomable to the doctors as the doctors' perspective was to the Lees. Hmong culture . . . is not Cartesian. Nothing could be more Cartesian than Western medicine. Trying to understand Lia and her family by reading her medical chart (something I spent hundreds of hours doing) was like deconstructing a love sonnet by reducing it to a series of syllogisms. Yet to the residents and pediatricians who had cared for her since she was three months old, there was no guide to Lia's world *except* her chart. As each of them struggled to make sense of a set of problems that were not expressible in the language they knew, the chart simply grew longer and longer, until it contained more than 400,000 words. Every one of those words reflected its author's intelligence, training, and good intentions, but not a single one dealt with the Lees' perception of their daughter's illness.[26]

Fadiman's request for greater effort by MCMC's house staff suggests the need for a more expansive approach to beneficence, echoing May's critique of transactional approaches to patient and family care. May, like Fadiman, calls for greater intersubjectivity and communication between professionals and lay persons. Her recommendations, reflecting her ethnographic method, call for a more longitudinal approach to health care.

About the need for greater trust and goodwill between professionals and families, Fadiman is surely correct. For that reason, Jeanine Hilt, Lia's social worker, is one of the story's unsung heroes, for Hilt worked assiduously to educate the Lees about how to administer Lia's prescriptions. Hilt's care was guided by transformational rather than transactional dynamics. Yet it is not clear how far that recipe can take us when seeking to overcome cultural differences, and herein lies one of my disagreements with Fadiman. In Lia's case, securing greater trust with the Lees does not guarantee that their conflicts with the MCMC staff would have ended. Diagnosing septicemia involved drawing blood and performing a lumbar puncture—procedures that (as Fadiman notes) the Hmong generally refuse.[27] Nao Kao thought that a lumbar puncture was "too much medicine" for Lia, and he feared that undergoing that procedure was why she became sicker in Fresno. Fadiman fails to press this problem and its implications for her story. Overcoming one set of cultural differences with the Lees would only have produced another.

Second, and perhaps more important, is the issue of Lia's quality of life. It is remarkable that she does not die, given all that she experienced—although she is described as "essentially brain dead."[28] Fadiman makes it clear that after Lia's dramatic downturn she receives much better care from her Hmong community than an American child in the same condition would receive from American parents, given that Americans would likely shun and warehouse such a child in an institution for the severely handicapped or retarded. Lia is clean, affectionately cared for, and esteemed as potentially having special powers. That said, it remains unclear what kind of quality of life Lia has, or whether doctors would be obligated to continue treating her if she were to face a life-threatening crisis. Fadiman never presses the important question, What should care providers have done had the Lees brought Lia to MCMC in an emergency? Should they save her life, such as it was, if asked?

Richard McCormick has perhaps the clearest response to these questions, but his answer would run against the grain of Fadiman's account. Recall from Chapter 5 that for McCormick, physical life is an instrumental good, "a value to be preserved only insofar as it contains some potentiality for human relationships."[29] He thus writes that "the meaning, substance, and consummation of life are found in human *relationships,* and the qualities of justice, respect, concern, compassion, and support that surround them."[30] Patients who seem able to experience love and communication and who can interact with others satisfy this criterion. But that idea can support nontreatment as well. McCormick writes, "When in human judgment this (relational) potentiality is totally absent or would be, because of the condition of the individual, totally subordinated to the mere effort for survival, that life can be said to have achieved its potential."[31]

For McCormick, then, treatment decisions in cases like Lia's depend on whether patients can connect with their loved ones. On this criterion, Lia does not fare well. Fadiman describes her condition at the age of six in these graphic terms:

> Although Lia was not dead, she was quadriplegic, spastic, incontinent, and incapable of purposive movement. Her condition was termed a "persistent vegetative state." Most of the time her arms were drawn up tightly against her chest and her fists were clenched, a sign of cerebral motor damage. Sometimes her legs trembled. Sometimes her head nodded, not in jerks but slowly, as if she were assenting to a question underwater. Sometimes she moaned or whimpered. She continued to breathe, swallow, sleep, wake, sneeze, snore, grunt, and cry, because those functions were governed by her unimpaired brain stem, but she had no self-aware mental activity, a function governed by the forebrain. Her most conspicuously aberrant feature was her eyes, which, although clear, sometimes stared blankly and sometimes darted to one side as if she were frightened. Looking at her, I could not help but feeling that something was missing beyond the neurotransmissive capabilities of her cerebral cortex, and that her parents' name for it—her *plig*, or soul—was as good a term as any.[32]

At times Lia registered signs of receiving affection, and various people said that she knew how to be loved. McCormick would doubtless wonder whether Lia's condition had exhausted her potential to enter and enjoy human relationships, and whether the goods of relationships and sociality were being subordinated to the quest to protect her physical existence. The Lees seem to adopt a sanctity-of-life position, not a quality-of-life position. In McCormick's mind, there are grounds for saying that Lia should be allowed to die if she presents again with a life-threatening illness: Her quality of life—her lack of relational potential—warrants the withholding of aggressive, life-saving treatment.

In a crisis, would the hospital be required to do everything to keep Lia alive? One of the shortcomings of Fadiman's discussion is that she fails to consider the issue of Lia's nontreatment after Lia is in a persistent vegetative state. In one sense, that fact seems to qualify the cultural clash between the physicians and the Lees. Underlying their many differences was a more fundamental agreement: The need for treatment of some kind was never doubted. True, after Lia returns from Fresno, her doctors at MCMC agree to disconnect her from her life-saving technology and send her home, expecting her to die. But they never forswear a commitment to treat her should she return.

After Lia becomes profoundly inaccessible, a new set of moral questions arises for her parents and care providers. Before that point, the basic problem for the professionals was how to treat Lia in the face of what they experienced as parental noncompliance. The *new* problem, posed by Lia's persistent vegetative state, is not *how* to treat, but *whether* to treat in the event of a life-threatening event. Seen in that light, the question that Fadiman puts before us is this: Are quality-of-life considerations potentially ethnocentric? Supposing that McCormick *is* correct and supposing that the Lees *do* want Lia to be kept alive, would house staff at MCMC be guilty of cultural prejudice if they refused to treat her? Would they be interpreted as saying, "What the Hmong consider to be a life worthy of respect and treatment is not a life that we think deserves to be helped"? Fadiman's recommendation of conjoint treatment—"a little medicine and a little *neeb*"— fails to address this problem.

The issue of conjoint treatment brings us to a third and final point when thinking about multiculturalism in health care settings. Recall that with Lia, as with Ericka, physicians were urged to strike a compromise that incorporated nonmainstream medical practices and remedies. In Ericka's case the compromise involved using an herbal remedy on her chest; in Lia's case, it could involve using shamans in the hospital, along with amulets, coin and egg rubbings, pinching, and the like. The key question is whether such compromises are directly or indirectly beneficial to either Ericka or Lia. *Direct benefits* would be those that directly cause health and healing. (My complaint about Ericka's treatment is that such benefits were not properly considered. My complaint about Lia's case is that these issues were not properly broached once she suffered irreparable brain damage.) *Indirect benefits* would be those that flow from empowering families effectively to attend to their child's basic needs.

Accommodating unconventional methods and remedies in the care of children typically has more to do with a family's background than anything else, and if benefits flow to the child, they do so indirectly. I would like to think that children can benefit when their families' commitment to care is recognized and reinforced by medical authorities. In that way, benefits flow from a family's sense of responsibility, its commitment to care. Compromises in health care settings that recognize a family's cultural or religious heritage may be called for when they help to increase trust between parents and professionals. That trust, in turn, may redound to the child's benefit, for it may enable parents and care providers to communicate more openly and to coordinate treatment regimens more effectively.

COMPROMISES AND PATIENT BENEFIT

Religious belief in pediatric contexts is no small issue for medical professionals, especially when families invoke their piety to refuse treatment for their children. Although legal precedents and moral arguments grant an adult the right of refusal, they do not grant parents or guardians the right to deny medical care to children. In *Prince v. Massachusetts,* the Supreme Court ruled as follows: "The right to practice religion freely does not include the liberty to expose the community or child to communicable disease, or the latter to ill health or death. . . . Parents may be free to become martyrs themselves. But it does not follow that they are free, in identical circumstances, to make martyrs of their children."[33]

Despite this ruling, in 1974 the U.S. Department of Health, Education, and Welfare required states that received child abuse prevention and treatment grants from the federal government to have religious exemptions to child abuse and neglect charges.[34] States quickly enacted exemptions for parents who relied on prayer rather than medical care, or who authorized treatment refusals on religious grounds. A decade later, virtually every state had such exemptions in the juvenile code, criminal code, or both.[35]

In a study of cases of 172 children who died between 1975 and 1995 because their parents relied on prayer or faith healing alone, Seth M. Asser and Rita Swan discovered that 140 died from conditions for which survival rates with medical care would have exceeded 90 percent. Eighteen more had expected survival rates of above 50 percent. All but three of the remaining cases would likely have benefited from medical treatment.[36] The authors conclude, "When faith healing is used to the exclusion of medical treatment, the number of preventable child fatalities and the associated suffering are substantial and warrant public concern. Existing laws may be inadequate to protect children from this form of medical neglect."[37]

The place of religious ritual as a substitute for conventional medical care harks back to the case of Bradley Hamm, to whom I referred in the Introduction. Arguments that I made in Chapters 2 and 3 justify interventions in such instances. The cases of Ericka and Lia are different because their families sought to coordinate religious rituals with mainstream medical practice, not to shun medical care altogether. For care providers who confront those kinds of cases, the challenges are more subtle because the family has entered the health care establishment, albeit on qualified terms. The fact that families' qualified acceptance of medical care is supplemented by religious beliefs and nonmainstream medical practices ensures that their interactions with care providers will be gnarled.

Ericka's and Lia's cases involve two temptations to which care providers (and others) might be prone when considering whether to accommodate nonmainstream beliefs and practices: patronizing tolerance on the one hand, and ethnocentric bias on the other.[38] The first temptation, providing "respect on demand," too readily accedes to nonmainstream beliefs and practices in order not to appear prejudicial; the latter temptation, disavowing the problem of cultural clashes, too readily rejects nonmainstream practices without engaging the persons who hold them. Neither approach is adequate for striking compromises or forming therapeutic alliances in health care settings. A better approach is guided by a basic goal—namely, a commitment to the patient's primary goods that seeks to engage and sometimes transform parents' practices that are not helpful to children.

On my account, multicultural compromises in health care settings are wise only when they are *instrumental* to a child or adolescent's overall good. They are not wise as ends in themselves, as attempts to display liberal tolerance or to recognize nonmainstream worldviews as a requirement of multicultural justice. Accommodating nonmainstream medical practices and remedies must be constrained by the duty to care. Otherwise, as Randle correctly notes, autonomy becomes a positive right, enabling parents and families to make demands that swing wide from a regard for a young patient's basic interests.

Yet neither should instrumental compromises in multicultural contexts be seen as mere expedients, premised on an ethnocentric or dismissive attitude toward parents with nonmainstream beliefs and practices. Compromises are acceptable when they can benefit children indirectly, and finding how to benefit patients indirectly means engaging their families' beliefs and backgrounds. The duty to care thus obligates health care professionals to find ways to enhance a child or adolescent's welfare. That will require medical professionals to reckon with their patients' heritages and customs; medical professionals who fail to do so neglect an opportunity to discharge their professional responsibilities.

The duty to care thus cuts in two directions in multicultural situations. On the one hand, it constrains what a parent may ask of care providers. On the other hand, it obligates care providers to find ways to engage families in ways that might enhance their capacity to attend to their child or adolescent's needs.

Taking these ideas together, three main points are clear. First, when striking compromises or seeking conjoint treatment with families, it is acceptable to use treatments that are not harmful to the child or adolescent, assuming that those treatments are examined in advance. Such compromises are justified by the idea of patient benefit and respect for family privacy and intimacy. Securing the trust and cooperation of parents can redound to the patient's welfare. Second, the basic norm that ought to regulate interactions between care providers and families is patient benefit, understood in light of a child or adolescent's primary goods of well-being, respect, and the right to an open future. Maintaining life support at all costs may not be indicated by a child or adolescent's quality of life. When a patient's physical life is not instrumental to the enjoyment of such rights, then it may be permissible to deny further treatment. Parents who might think otherwise are owed the courtesy of respectful and perhaps time-consuming conversations, but their autonomy rights are not unqualified. And third, when multicultural differences or nonmainstream medical therapies might harm a child or adolescent, professionals have the responsibility to address and educate parents when possible. Seeking patient benefit has longitudinal features, requiring care providers to consider preventive health care measures. This idea is implied by a transformationist approach to patient benefit and the virtue of benevolence, no small features of a therapeutic alliance between care providers and families.

My approach to accommodating unconventional medical practices is largely instrumental, focusing on whether any compromise will contribute to a patient's overall prospects for health and healing. I thus agree with Kleinman when he counsels physicians to "decide what's critical and be willing to compromise on everything else."[39] Yet neither my instrumental approach nor Kleinman's counsel should leave us sanguine about eliminating difficult conflicts. On this matter, Lia's case provides an enduring lesson: Deciding what is critical might only highlight areas of intractable difference between professionals and families when a patient's quality of life is in dispute. Knowing what is critical presupposes an account of a patient's basic interests and the primary goods that surround them, thereby sharpening, but not necessarily eliminating, terms for moral and medical disagreement.

NINE

(Properly) Marginalized Altruism: Screening Organ Donations from Strangers

---

Charity does not necessarily require a man to imperil his own body for his neighbor's welfare, except in a case where he is under obligation to do so; and if a man of his own accord offer himself for that purpose, this belongs to the perfection of charity.[1]

—*Thomas Aquinas*

The benefit came in the giving. That's exactly right. To know that I made a difference, a *real* difference. . . . I spit in the eye of that dragon death. That's enough for me. That was the reward.[2]

—*Joyce Roush, first nondirected organ donor on record*

WE CAN BE HEROES, PERHAPS

In the previous three chapters, I focused on cases that pit patients and their families against medical professionals in situations of moral and political disagreement. Viewing medical cases in that way can be deceptive, however, for it might obscure the extent to which moral controversies are mediated by impersonal institutional arrangements. Given the tradition of individualism in the United States, Americans are prone to focus on individuals and the conflicts that divide them, ignoring ways in which interpersonal differences are situated within wider customs, traditions, and organizational contexts.[3] Personalizing differences between individuals or groups can overlook how "invisible" institutional frameworks exert an influence throughout much of our everyday lives.

In this chapter, I want to shift attention away from what appears to be unmediated interactions between parents, children, and hospital professionals to the self-conscious attempt by Baylin's personnel to consider how the hospital played a mediating role in interactions (and potential disputes) between families and its heath care providers. That kind of reflection was prompted by the need, recognized by members of the hospital's ethics committee, to think about two kinds of cases.

The first comes by way of an *ethics consult,* in which professional personnel contact members of the hospital's ethics committee to help resolve a practical problem for which no clear guidance exists. An ethics consult is requested on an ad hoc basis and typically aims to settle a dispute between members of one of the hospital's services and one patient or family. Sometimes, but not always, that kind of case "grows" into a second kind, in which a problem is so controversial that it requires examination by the hospital's Ethics Advisory Committee at one of its monthly meetings. This latter kind of case might lead to *policy formation* that requires final approval by the hospital's administration. In this chapter, we will examine the first kind of case, in which a practical question, posed to one service in the hospital, had the potential to grow into a policy matter. In the next chapter, we will evaluate a second case that posed explicit political challenges as the hospital's Ethics Advisory Committee sought to form policy in a large medical bureaucracy. Again, in both chapters, we are shifting focus away from specific families and personnel to how interactions between patients, families, and house staff are mediated by the hospital's more general responsibilities (including responsibilities to itself as an institution).

During my initial months at Baylin, the following question materialized: May strangers—individuals unrelated by birth, marriage, or social ties—donate an organ to a specified or unspecified young person in need of transplantation? To my surprise, that question has taken on several permutations. Consider the following examples.

- In 1997, the family of an adolescent with renal failure placed the child on a cadaver transplant list and awaited an organ while the child remained on dialysis. The family's neighbor arranged for a television program to publicize the needy child's situation and provided a phone number for interested persons to call. In response, more than forty individuals offered to donate a kidney to the child. Of these, ten contacted the renal transplant service at Baylin, each expressing willingness to be evaluated for compatibility as an organ donor. (Adult kidneys may match the needs of an adolescent in acute renal distress.) An ethics consult was called at Baylin, bringing together hospital ethicists, social service workers, and renal transplant surgeons, to discuss whether to accept a kidney from an unrelated donor.
- In 1998, Joyce Roush of Fort Wayne, Indiana, approached Dr. Lloyd Ratner of Johns Hopkins Hospital and offered her kidney to any patient who needed it. The offer was eventually accepted, and a year later Dr. Ratner removed Ms. Roush's left kidney and transplanted it into Christopher Bieniek, a thirteen-year-old boy from Aberdeen, Mary-

land. The mother of five children, Ms. Roush claimed that "God tapped me on the shoulder and called me to do this"[4] after she heard Dr. Ratner describe a laparoscopic technique, less time-consuming and painful than standard organ procurement, for removing kidneys. "I knew immediately; there was no second thought for me," she added about her decision to donate.[5] Within days of her surgery, Johns Hopkins received fifteen to twenty calls from people willing to donate a kidney or a part of their livers to unspecified recipients.[6]

- In 1999, the aunt of sixteen-year-old Fondie Foster contacted an Indianapolis television station and asked its broadcasters to publicize information that her niece needed two volunteers, each to donate a lung lobe to Fondie. Born with a damaged liver and diagnosed with cystic fibrosis at the age of five, Fondie had undergone a liver transplant as an infant and a double lung transplant from a cadaver donor at the age of fourteen. A year after the lung transplant, she began showing signs of rejection. After intense publicity in the wake of a hospital's last-minute decision to decline the offer of two live donors for a second transplant, more than ninety prospective donors came forward to volunteer.[7]

- In April 2000, Howard E. Sebree, Jr., published this announcement in the *Indianapolis Star* after seeing a television news program about a girl selling Kool-Aid on the streets to help raise money to pay for the medical bills associated with her father's kidney disorder: "I am willing to donate my kidney to this man or to anyone else in need of one. For many years, my life has been nothing. I just want another chance at life." An inmate at the Wabash Correctional Facility, Sebree had four years remaining on his sentence. He added, "My life begins with praising God first. My gift to someone could be my chance to begin a normal life."[8]

- Starting in August 1999, physicians at the University of Minnesota Medical School began accepting nondirected kidney donations. By March 2000, ninety-eight persons had volunteered, and four were accepted for organ procurement.[9]

What, if anything, is wrong with stepping forward to volunteer? In *The Patient as Person,* Paul Ramsey settles a similar case of organ donation by focusing on the comparative costs and benefits to donor and recipient. For Ramsey, the question turns on the ethics of self-mutilation and, specifically, whether physicians may harm a person without compensatory medical benefit to that person. Ramsey was thinking in practical terms about the limits to care and the proper constraints that ought to be placed on beneficence and benevolence. In his mind, the charity of the donor must be constrained by the value of bodily integrity, preventing altruistic persons from giving organs simply because they want to. It is counterintuitive, Ramsey submits, to presume that someone else "owns" my body parts at least as much as I do. According to Ramsey, making one person ill in order to make another well can be justified only if the prospective benefit to the recipient significantly outweighs the risks to the donor. In effect, Ramsey claims that allowing medical providers to override the duty not to harm is justified only if benefits to others are appreciably greater.[10]

Ramsey rightly sees the case of organ donation as one that approaches the limits of beneficence, requiring us to mark the outer boundaries of charity. Yet it is not obvious that Ramsey's restriction captures the moral complexities of organ donations by strangers, for it overlooks issues of motivation and the effects of risk taking on dependent third parties, among other matters. The effect of his position is to allow altruists to take on risks when the stakes are high for the recipient or low for the donor. Although his view makes general sense as a guide to policy, it begs the question of whether professionals should be party to acts that can compromise persons' welfare, or their dependents' welfare, for reasons that might not be entirely clear, as can happen in cases of very generous offers. Ramsey's rule fails to capture these and other relevant variables, and it is to those issues that I want to focus here.

I initially considered questions of organ donations from strangers during my stint as a participant observer at Baylin, consulting on the first case I mentioned above. (Although such donations are not restricted to pediatric contexts, they first materialized with children as the specified or unspecified recipients.) My initial thought was that donations from strangers presumably spring from altruistic motives—unsolicited, benevolent motives, involving great cost to the benefactor, and seeking no reciprocity or return —and altruism should not be discouraged. Hospitals that accept organs from strangers generate occasions for virtue, a form of "civic agapism,"[11] no small contribution to any society. So long as potential donors are physically and mentally healthy, and so long as they understand the risks of surgery, they are free to offer body parts. Moral heroism seems possible.

Moreover, current transplantation practice imposes no barrier to donations from some *biologically* unrelated donors. In renal transplantation, numerous studies indicate that the rates of patient and graft survival are similar for transplants from living related and unrelated donors, and these rates are appreciably higher than success rates with organs removed from cadavers.[12] More important, a kidney donated by a spouse will have no better chance of survival than a kidney donated by a stranger; in each case, donors are biologically unrelated, and social relation is irrelevant to the chance of success. That fact would seem to provide a clear justification for accepting kidneys from strangers. If current practice allows donations from persons who are not biological relatives, why shouldn't hospitals accept organs from those who are unrelated by marriage or social ties as well, all else being equal? To refuse such offers seems discriminatory because it renders some potential donors ineligible for reasons that appear to be morally arbitrary. So long as organs from unrelated individuals are acceptable, either friends or strangers should be permitted to donate.

Virtues, casuistry, and considerations of fairness apparently converge: Altruistic dispositions, the precedent of accepting organs from biologically unrelated donors, and the norm of equality suggest that hospitals should not impose barriers to donations from individuals who are unrelated by biology, marriage, or community affiliation. A strong presumption in favor of accepting donations from strangers seems justified. What seems needed, then, is not a rationale for procuring organs from strangers, but a set of procedures to ensure the safety of donor and recipient.

INCONGRUOUS, COUNTERFEIT, AND IMPRUDENT VIRTUE

This presumption becomes complicated, however, when we recognize that *who* may wish to donate organs and *why* they may wish to donate are morally relevant variables. Given the risks involved in surgery, it seems reasonable to wonder whether such a supererogatory act is humanly conceivable. Consider other possibilities as well. How would we evaluate the (imaginary) case of a recently employed immigrant who "volunteers" to donate the lobe of a lung to his boss's needy son? What if the prospective volunteer is a parent of six children? Shouldn't health care providers protect donors from themselves, from another's extortion, or from imposing risks on others?

These questions suggest three obstacles to accepting organs from strangers, to which I will return below. For the moment my queries are meant to suggest that considerations of virtue, case precedent, and fairness collide with two other obligations in the professional role of health care providers: nonmaleficence and patient welfare (or beneficence). The effect is to generate conflicting duties. When considering the ethics of accepting organ donations from strangers, hospitals must consider not only duties to sick children, but also duties to themselves as institutions, to the donors, and to vulnerable third parties.

The duties of nonmaleficence and patient benefit bear on donations by strangers in a fundamental way. Consider one connection, producing a basic rule in medical ethics: Physicians are not to harm patients without the prospect of patient benefit. As Sharon Johnston, codirector of Baylin's Office of Ethics, remarks, "Doctors can't operate on an individual simply because that person asks them to. There has to be patient benefit to justify harming them in the first place."[13]

Stated in more traditional terms, Johnston's comments gesture toward the principle of totality. In Catholic moral theology, where that principle finds its pedigree, the principle of totality "means that all parts of the human body, as parts, are meant to exist and function for the good of the whole, and are thus naturally subordinated to the good of the whole body."[14] The principle of totality thus allows for the mutilation of part of the body for the good of the whole, but it does not obviously allow for the mutilation of one body in order to benefit another because, in the words of Gerald Kelly, S.J., "no human being is subordinated to another as part to whole."[15] Interpreted in this way, the principle of totality would not justify organ donations from living donors.[16]

Kelly subsequently revised this idea, arguing that considerations of "totality" could be expanded to allow for nonmedical benefits because *human* well-being surely involves more than physical benefit alone.[17] "Totality" could include prospective psychological and moral benefits to the donor that might justify performing surgery on that person so that he or she could benefit another. On this logic, the "moral wholeness" of the donor would allow for the sacrifice of a physical part. Summarizing this idea, Warren Reich writes, "Perhaps the principle of 'helping thy neighbor' is not so distinct from, but is an amplification of the principle of totality—of the totality of all the dimensions and not just the physical requirements" of a person. On this description, donors subordinate their physical welfare not to the physical welfare of another, but to their "own perfection of grace and charity."[18]

Although the ethics of mutilation as governed by the principle of totality derives from Catholic sources, in my view, it does not depend exclusively on the Catholic tradition. Two basic values are relevant: equality and human dignity. The first idea prevents using some persons as a means only to benefit others; the second understands our humanity to be enhanced by morally and socially responsible acts. This latter idea in particular provides a rationale for *nonmedical* benefits of living organ donations—namely, the moral and psychological benefits of doing good for another.

A moral or psychological benefit to organ donation is easy to understand when the donor and recipient are bound by ties of familiarity. Relatives may feel a sense of domestic obligation or may wish to redeem a tragic set of circumstances bearing on family life. Parents can derive nonmedical benefit from the survival of a child because the family would be diminished by the loss. Teresa Grabcek, a mother who donated her kidney to her adolescent son at Baylin, put the point this way: "I wanted to be a part of him because he's a part of me. I'm happy when he's happy. When he's not well, I'm not well. . . . Yes, there is a loss. But I don't want to dwell on that. The other part is the reward. It's like giving birth again."[19] The family acts for its own preservation as a unit when one member contributes to the survival of another. Analogously, donating an organ to a needy child, friend, student, or neighbor contributes to the benefit of the local common good.[20] In cases of relatives or community members, benefits can be understood as "a part contributing to the whole," and such contributions can bring great psychological and moral benefits to donors.

In general, fellow-feeling for the near neighbor is more understandable than fellow-feeling for the distant neighbor. Liberal cosmopolitans or inveterate Stoics might see their donations as adding to the good of humanity, but it is difficult to ascertain in concrete terms "the whole" to which that potentially life-saving decision contributes. In the argot of theology and philosophy, preferential loves are easier to understand than nonpreferential loves.[21] Benefits to donors are harder to conceive when they are total strangers, especially given the pain and medical risks that surgery can entail. Altruism in its standard form is unconditional and unmotivated, and unmotivated actions by definition defy explanation.[22] Can doctors be expected to inflict harm on individuals whose motivations are opaque or incongruous? Without some clear indication of benefit to the donor—even psychological benefit—the answer seems to be no. Stated differently, benevolence that is *beneficial to the donor* must be connected to real human associations.

Herein lies the first obstacle: Without some idea of benefit to the donor, the sacrifice seems inordinate—indeed, inconceivable. George Thomas of Baylin's renal transplantation service put the point graphically to the ethics consult: "I don't consider volunteers seriously unless they've had something like a gallbladder operation. Not the new way [with a small incision]. They should come in, lift up the shirt, and show me a scar that runs across the abdomen. Then I know that they know the kind of pain involved in this kind of operation."[23] Voluntarily taking on bodily risks and undergoing great discomfort to benefit a complete stranger is, for the vast majority of people, simply unimaginable. Friends can more plausibly make the case that their generosity includes outcomes that are psychologically beneficial to themselves. Given the absence of compensatory benefit in cases involving strangers, however, the duty not to harm may not be overridden by donors' benevolence. Hospitals may thus justifiably discriminate between friends and strangers in the pool of biologically unrelated donors.

Yet this conclusion appears to frustrate some prospects of doing good for others. Altruistic efforts are trumped by the code of medical professionals, which appears so stringent that it leaves suffering patients in need. Indeed, as I have described this issue, resolving on the negative side leaves no room for the possibility of heroics. Are we unable to conceive of radically self-sacrificial choices?

Approaching this answer in the context of organ transplantation engages issues that are in part philosophical. Altruistic offers, as unconditional offers, do not suffice to explain why an individual would voluntarily suffer. That is, pure altruism fails to include reasons for taking on grave risks;

the altruist seeks no reciprocity or return. Without knowing what benefit donors might enjoy in return for their risks, it is difficult to honor their willingness to take on those risks. Accordingly, the obstacle to granting permission to strangers as donors lies in the nature of the offer itself.

Second, there are grounds for suspicion about strangers as donors if we consider the likelihood that some donations will be compensated under the table. Here the problem shifts from the incongruity of motives to an all-too-familiar incentive: financial reward. Many ethicists and policy makers in the United States view such acts as degrading to the body, a form of self-instrumentalism according to which the ends justify the means. William F. May writes, "We debase the meaning of some goods when we put them up for sale. When we bribe judges, buy babies, or purchase prizes intended to honor excellence, we corrupt the meaning of the good so purchased." A society that allows the merchandising of bodies or organs "demeans itself and its members and fails to solve its problems fittingly. The desperately ill ought not to solve their health care needs through the desperately poor."[24] James F. Childress argues that selling bodily organs is not intrinsically immoral, but adds that commerce in organs is counterproductive and that more feasible and morally preferable means are available for procuring organs.[25] Apart from these moral considerations, the 1984 National Organ Transplant Act bans the selling of bodily organs (but not blood or semen). Hence the second obstacle: In the United States, there is a legal ban and an arguable moral position against selling body parts. Hospitals that accept such donations use legally tainted sources; they are correct to screen for counterfeit virtue and to protect themselves from its effects.

Parenthetically it should be noted that the issue of accepting legally damaged goods is *not* a matter of illicit cooperation. As defined by Edwin F. Healy, S.J., *cooperation* refers to "acting together with another in doing something that is morally wrong or . . . supplying another with what is helpful to him in doing something that is morally wrong."[26] Hospitals that accept tainted sources are not guilty of immoral cooperation because they are not assisting in the commercial arrangements between vendors and families who promise to pay them. Those arrangements may be foreseen, but not intended by hospital personnel.

In this respect, accepting legally tainted sources is different from, say, investments in the tobacco industry, or investments in corporations that did business in South Africa during apartheid. Such investments materially facilitate morally questionable practices and thus can be classified as cooperation. Accepting organs from paid donors, in contrast, does not put the hospital in a causal chain by "supplying another with what is helpful . . . in doing something that is morally wrong." Accepting legally damaged goods does not operate in the same kind of nexus in which dirty money does its work.

Nor is the problem of using tainted sources, strictly speaking, one of direct scandal. In Catholic moral theology, where this issue has been paradigmatically formulated, *scandal* refers to acts or failures of action that induce another to commit wrongdoing. In scandal, one person directly or indirectly corrupts the character of another. Direct scandal is a malicious action in which one tries to induce another to sin; indirect scandal, in Healy's words, "is that in which another's sin is foreseen but not wished."[27] According to Healy, the latter is morally acceptable if great goods would be gained through the practice. One might argue that creating a black market of body parts is "foreseen but not wished" by hospitals, and that the merits of helping suffering children outweigh moral qualms about hospitals using legally damaged goods.

It is rather the case that the prospect of a hospital using tainted sources creates an occasion of wrongdoing, and is thus morally suspect. In Catholic casuistry, an "occasion of sin" refers to circumstances in which the temptation to wrongdoing arises; in accepting tainted sources, hospitals create occasions for individuals to exploit themselves or others. Policies that allow the use of commercialized body parts create opportunities that are morally undesirable. Moreover, although such opportunities might not be directly scandalous as Healy defines the term, such practices doubtless tarnish a hospital's reputation and compromise public expectations about medical practice. Hence the need for hospitals to be vigilant about whether policies regarding organ transplantation encourage the commercialization of the body.[28]

A third obstacle arises in cases when altruistic individuals increase risks to their dependents, compounding incongruous motives with dangerous ones. Consider the fact that one of the volunteers at Baylin was a father of six children and that Joyce Roush was the mother of five. Assume for the sake of argument that these volunteers were motivated by their communal values, religious ideals, or cultural heroes, and that they were financially well-off. They thus could overcome the first obstacle by making sense of their actions, and they could overcome the second by virtue of their economic situation. In fact, Roush met both of these criteria. She came from firm, familiar religious ideals and was financially secure. A middle-class health care professional, she believed that "God has a purpose for us. We say, 'Show me the way. Okay, I'll go. You lead me.' I'm open, I'm a vessel for God's direction." But convincing hospital personnel was not easy; she had to expend considerable effort to persuade doctors in Baltimore that she was psychologically fit. "They finally realized that I was sane. I was persistent without being obnoxious."[29]

Yet in cases like Roush's, considerations of others' welfare seem warranted, for donors are not the only individuals whose well-being is at risk. When donations touch on relationships with vulnerable third parties, donors' altruism is socialized, imposed their dependents. In these instances, hospital personnel seem justified when barring a donation. Volunteers may convince a hospital that they need no protection from themselves, but they are not the only relevant individuals in the case. Hence the third obstacle: Hospitals must consider risks to vulnerable third parties.

PARAMETERS

We have, then, three problems with donations by strangers: incongruous motives, tainted sources, and risks to donors' dependents. Together, they seem to prohibit virtually every possible source because they cast doubt on unmotivated actions as well as motivated actions of an obvious and frequent sort. Yet we should not forget that young patients need organs and that there is a vast shortage of available organs in the United States. Is it not possible for a hospital to construct parameters for screening donations from strangers that avoid these difficulties?

The first obstacle—the incongruity of motives—is considerable but not insuperable. The fact that altruism is incongruous may say something about our social expectations; as I shall indicate below, it stands on the margins of our moral intuitions and practices. In any event, not all candidates for altruism should be eliminated from the pool of unrelated donors. The problem of incongruous motives can be resolved by learning more about the donor's cultural, religious, or social background, features of which might allow us to conceive of an action that combines self-sacrificial risk with (some) motivations. The donor might reveal that he is motivated by the values of his religious and ethnic community, which places a premium on service to others. He might cite the example of a sister, an Army sergeant in 1992 who risked her life in Somalia for an effort widely described as a humanitarian intervention. Or he might refer to the example of religious dissidents, civil disobedients, or community activists, arguing that social progress typically does not occur until individuals or groups consciously depart from centers of power or mainstream values.

Benefits to the donor—connections to family heritage, the esteem of the community, participation in a narrative of heroism—may be less tangible than benefits to those in more familiar relationships to the recipient, but they are nonetheless real. Let us call this offer to donate a quasialtruistic act. The effect is to understand some behavior as "motivated altruistically" and to diminish the incongruity that surrounds some "selfless" actions.

Indeed, when compared with circumstances in which a family must decide whether one of its members should donate an organ to a relative, motivated altruism offers some advantages. Consider, for example, a parent of an adolescent in acute renal distress. She finds herself in a situation of having to donate an organ or watch her son die. Her choice is tragic: She must immediately agree to the risks of surgery, organ removal, and recovery, or watch physicians detach her son from life support. To say that an individual autonomously chooses to donate an organ in such circumstances strains credulity. Limited resources, physiological matching, emotional agony, family pressures, and tangible suffering conspire to compromise autonomy. In these circumstances, isn't the hospital being asked to accept a donation from a tainted source? By comparison, the motivated altruist can claim to act more autonomously.

Given the possibility of a quasialtruistic donation, professional obligations justify inquiry into a potential donor's motives. Yet on its face, such an inquiry would seem to compromise a donor's autonomy and to run counter to the general ethos of tolerance in physician–patient relationships. Noting the difficulties involved in such inquiries, Childress points to the fact that donors typically act with mixed motives, suggesting that those who wish to query motivations must risk wading through a veritable swamp of human dispositions.[30] Rather than involve hospital personnel in such murky and indeterminate matters, it would thus be morally preferable (and more feasible) to construct mechanisms that protect the donor's autonomy and leave it at that.

But Childress's counsel pertains to donations arranged near the time of death, and live donors pose problems that go beyond respect for autonomy. As I have said, the duty not to harm is likewise relevant, and it cannot be overcome without compensatory benefit. Inquiry into motivations, although surely difficult, is neither an abuse of a hospital's institutional power nor an act of moralistic intolerance. Rather, it is a function of professional responsibility, driven by the need to justify harming individuals to benefit others.

Each of the other two obstacles is sufficient to prohibit donation. Using tainted sources implicates health care practitioners in immoral conduct; it is prohibited by considerations that surround the occasions of wrongdoing and concern for the public trust. Protecting dependent third parties is a reasonable principle on which health care professionals should act; it is implied as a general feature of medical responsibility for human welfare. As I argued in the previous chapter, persons do not have the right to demand certain forms of treatment from medical professionals: Autonomy is a negative right, not a positive one, in patient-professional relationships. The ethics of accepting organs from strangers is morally complex, requiring hospitals to weigh duties to themselves and vulnerable third parties. How can these considerations be enshrined in a policy to screen potential donors?

GUIDELINES AND RATIONALES

Baylin's ethics consult proposed guidelines that function to honor these and other considerations. Creating a high but not insuperable bar for accepting donations, they embody impartial principles that are widely shared in the medical profession and American society. They are as follows.

1. *No medically unacceptable risks.* This guideline is justified by the norm of nonmaleficence and the duty to protect the donor's well-being.

2. *No mental illness or psychological instability.* This criterion, like the first, is designed to ensure the donor's well-being. It is also justified by the norm of autonomy, seeking to ensure that the donor is providing informed consent.

3. *No financial or commercial benefit.*

4. *No other clandestine incentives, such as occupational or personal favors.* The third and fourth criteria protect donors from exploitation, and they protect the hospital from implication in the use of tainted sources and the occasioning of wrongdoing. However, these criteria should not rule out the removal of disincentives to donate—for example, compensation for time or work lost, or payment of hospital expenses.

5. *No appreciable risks to third-party dependents.* The norm of beneficence prohibits health care providers from cooperating with donors whose voluntary choices render their dependents vulnerable. Here the idea is to protect third parties from having their parents' altruism socialized. (St. Louis Children's Hospital, where Fondie Foster awaited donation, bars women of childbearing age who have not yet had children.[31] Presumably the idea is to protect future third parties from their mother's altruism. However, in order to avoid the charge of discriminating against women of childbearing years, this policy would have to indicate why it is not applied to men as well.[32])

6. *Comprehensible social relationship.* Donors should be able to show that their actions stand within an intelligible religious, social, or cultural framework, that their decision to donate is voluntary, and that they understand the risks.

If hospitals are to accept organs from strangers, they are justified in screening carefully against counterfeit or imprudent virtue. When screening against the former, hospitals rightly protect themselves. When screening against the latter, they protect vulnerable third parties. Guidelines 3 to 5 function in accord with such obligations, and Guideline 6 functions to protect patients from themselves. In cases presenting the prospect of altruism, no simple response will do. Donations by strangers involve hospitals in a conflict of duties, which can be resolved only by clear policies and procedures that aim to address the moral complexity of the case.

The effect of these guidelines is to shift moral presumptions. I began by suggesting that various ethical considerations—virtue, casuistry, and fairness—suggest a strong presumption in favor of accepting organ donations from strangers. But questions about incongruous, counterfeit, and imprudent motives are too weighty to let that presumption stand. Rather, the potential donor should assume the burden of proof in establishing a case for donation; the hospital should not be required to make the case for refusing donations. The unusual nature of the offer, the potential for abuse, and the risks to third parties all suggest caution as a matter of policy. The fact that an individual has the right to volunteer an organ does not establish a duty for professionals committed to medical welfare to accede to that individual's desire. Owing to the special role responsibilities of medical providers (especially responsibilities informed by the duty of nonmaleficence), patients' rights and professionals' duties are not always symmetrical.

Shifting presumptions in this way appears to produce a policy of medical paternalism because it seems to restrict a person's liberty in order to produce a good or prevent a harm to that person. But such an appearance is mistaken because in the case of organ donation the volunteers are not, strictly speaking, patients. The idea of screening potential donors is to determine whether they *qualify* to enter into a relationship with a medical provider. To deny volunteers that chance is to limit their access to medical treatment. That denial is different from the paternalistic practice of refusing to comply with the wishes of a someone who has *become* a patient. As I noted above, the value of autonomy in medical care—however poorly it may be understood—does not permit persons to demand certain kinds of actions from a medical provider. As a side constraint on professionals' conduct, autonomy functions to limit what a medical professional may presume to do for a patient. As we saw when discussing the asymmetry between autonomy and beneficence in Chapter 5, viewing that limit as a positive claim on the professional misunderstands the meaning of freedom in relationships between patients and medical professionals.

TWO CONCEPTS OF LOVE

I noted in my references to Ramsey at the outset of this chapter that motivational issues are vexing in this case, and I want to turn our attention directly to those issues by drawing on resources in religious ethics. Readers familiar with religion and ethics know that motivational issues surrounding altruism and the potential for self-sacrifice follow well-worn paths. The first cluster of problems to which I referred—incongruous motives and nonpreferential loves—echoes Kierkegaard's normative account of Christian *agape*. Love is a duty, Kierkegaard insists, that is rigorously unconditional, disinterested, and egalitarian. No qualities or features of the neighbor merit our care; love is an obligation that binds the Christian regardless of any features that render the neighbor attractive. In this respect, Kierkegaard understands *agape* to be unmotivated and nonpreferential: Nothing about the beneficiary ought to prompt one to love him or her; one's love should be spontaneous, self-generated, undiscriminating, and unchanging. Christian love involves no reciprocity or return; it cannot entail what Kierkegaard calls a "bookkeeping-relationship."[33] Actions based on conditional terms flow from "double-mindedness," producing a mixture of motives that are impure and insincere.[34] In contrast, love as uncalculating remains unshakable in the face of contingencies that would otherwise disappoint. In Christian *agape,* the right is prior to the good. In this way, *agape* is both free and bound: free from considerations of mutuality and desire; bound by the demands of duty. The effect, in Kierkegaard's mind, is to produce a concept of love as eternal, outside time, requiring ongoing self-renunciation.[35]

Kierkegaard recognizes that such an account is counterintuitive—that unmotivated duties are incongruous given the natural tendency to expect our love to be returned. *Agape* requires the kind of commitment he describes as absurd in his masterpiece, *Fear and Trembling.* On account of this absurdity, he argues, Christian love is forever countercultural. *Agape* is an "offense" to the masses (including standard accounts of Christianity itself). Kierkegaard writes, "Christianly understood," the inwardness and perseverance required by *agape* "is sacrifice, and it is also, humanly understood, madness."[36]

If Kierkegaard provides the definitive word on altruistic conduct, then the problem of incongruous motives when screening for altruism might be insuperable, for it is difficult to extract a motivational rationale from love characterized as ongoing self-renunciation. But there is a more nuanced position, perhaps unacceptable to Kierkegaard but considerably more plausible given the issues under review. I have called it an account of quasialtruistic behavior, and its progenitor is Augustine.

Like Kierkegaard, Augustine argues on behalf of charitable motivations that are not premised on securing some benefit or reward as a foreseeable outcome. For theological reasons that go beyond our present discussion, Augustine crafts his views against the Pelagian notion that individuals can perform loving deeds under the assumption that God will reward meritorious action. For Augustine, such notions bind the deity to a contractual relationship and compromise the sovereignty of God. So Augustine, like Kierkegaard, wants to construct an understanding of loving action that is uncalculating and nonreciprocal.

Yet Augustine refuses to sharply separate the right from the good, thereby opening the door to actions that are altruistic and motivated in a broad sense. The challenge is to describe such actions in a way that avoids the double-mindedness of Pelagius and the apparent madness of Kierkegaard's *agape.*

For Augustine, the key lies in the distinction between instrumental actions and enjoyment, what he calls *amor uti* and *amor frui*.[37] Calculating actions of the kind Kierkegaard criticizes are *amor uti*, using some good merely as a means to one's own end. *Amor uti* is a love that instrumentalizes, but *amor frui* is different and more subtle.[38] For Augustine, to do a loving deed for its own sake is to participate in the Good, to be framed by a horizon that is larger and more expansive than the self. Participation in larger, more encompassing goods satisfies the heart's quest to attach itself to increasingly stable objects, objects that will be faithful to the heart's desire for truth and beauty. The pinnacle in that quest is the Supreme Good, the sole good that is eternal and thus the source of ceaseless enjoyment.

The main point for Augustine is that the right joins the good: Noninstrumentalizing conduct enables the agent to partake in the enjoyment of the expansive, encompassing Good as a by-product of virtuous action. In this way an altruistic action can be understood as motivated in a broad sense. The agent who acts out of virtue has responded to the bidding of the Good, itself a source of desire's satisfaction, and in the process experiences the good of enjoyment.

Augustine's theocentric eudaimonism provides the kind of theory that enables us to see how screening for altruism can overcome the problem of incongruous motives. The suggestion is not to ascertain whether potential donors are potential Augustinians or neo-Platonists. It is rather that we can make sense of motivations by learning more about the horizons in which potential donors situate their conduct, the range of goods according to which such individuals frame their self-interpretations. Such "frameworks," writes Charles Taylor, provide the basis for an individual to make "strong evaluations," that is, "discriminations of right or wrong, better or worse, higher or lower, which are not rendered valid by our desires, inclinations, or choices, but rather stand independent of these and offer standards by which they can be judged."[39] Frameworks articulate an ensemble of largely unarticulated understandings about what it means to be an agent and what is important in the exercise of that agency.

A policy that interrogates donors' cultural, religious, or social contexts seeks to uncover the enjoyments that derive from frameworks or horizonal understandings. It requires administrators to ascertain whether the donor's act is narratively intelligible. The goal is to understand donor agency as combining self-sacrificial risk with (some) motivations and, in this way, to ascertain how the agent's altruism joins the right with the good. The horizonal values I have mentioned—family heritage, the esteem of the community, participation in a narrative of heroism—point to the love of enjoyment rather than to that of instrumentalization. Proceeding in this way, medical professionals can understand some behavior as "motivated altruistically" and eliminate the incongruity that surrounds self-sacrificial conduct.

AT THE LIMITS OF POLICY AND CUSTOM

Yet even if we follow Augustine rather than Kierkegaard when screening for altruism, it remains true that the guidelines developed by Baylin's ethics consult situate the generosity of strangers on the margins of what is customarily presumed in organ donation. The guidelines both reflect and reinforce that marginality, making it difficult but not impossible for strangers to donate organs. My conclusion, echoing the epigraph from Aquinas with which I began this chapter, is that sacrificing the body, or part of the body, for a stranger marks the perfection of charity, one of its highest expressions. More important, the pursuit of charity's perfection shoulders a burden of proof when it obligates health care practitioners to harm an individual as a means to an end. I want to conclude by identifying practical and theoretical components to that marginality.

Practically speaking, we should not expect that allowing donations from strangers will change much in the overall delivery system. Robert Hamilton, a pulmonologist and member of Baylin's Ethics Advisory Committee, rightly observes, "Such donations are unlikely to have much impact on the current shortage of organs."[40] In order to remedy that shortage, we need nationwide attention to structural improvements in the procurement system as a whole. One alternative to current practice would be to develop policies based on presumed consent, which would allow hospitals to take organs from the dead unless potential donors or families explicitly refuse. Another proposal is to make express donation easier, by asking individuals not whether they would agree to donate, but whether they would agree to let their families or a designated individual make the decision about donation at time of death.[41] I mention these alternatives not to argue for them, but to identify plausible proposals that rely on structural changes rather than on private initiative. My point is that issues of availability and distribution are unlikely to vanish if hospitals widen their pool of prospective donors to include organs from strangers. The ethical issues surrounding donations from strangers, as a practical matter, are marginal to the larger problem of organ availability.

One corollary of this practical point concerns the potential consequences of allowing a marginal practice. A policy that accepts donations from strangers could do more harm than good. If public knowledge of the policy of accepting donations from strangers appears to contribute to an overall downturn in donations, then it may be better to establish a wholesale ban on the practice of accepting strangers' offers to donate. Benevolence must be beneficial, as I have indicated in various ways throughout this book. Individual altruism is no solution to the problem of limited resources, and in fact may impede the solution.

The fact that a policy makes it difficult but not impossible for a stranger to donate an organ has a theoretical component as well. Screening for altruism as I have proposed seems intuitively correct, at least when we consider the rightful place of "the perfection of charity" among our moral practices. Given the extraordinary nature of the offer, individuals who wish to volunteer an organ should be expected to make the case that harm to them is justified. The presumption against donations by strangers both reflects and reinforces the difficulty of the act. Theologians like Augustine and philosophers like Taylor conceive of distinctions that render altruistic actions unusual but intelligible. Altruistic behavior is strenuous; it taxes our moral strengths and brings us near the dark void of unconditional action. Potential donors and health care professionals are wise to approach that realm, as Kierkegaard would surely advise them, in fear and trembling.

TEN

The Politics and Ethics
of a Hospital Ethics Committee

DELIBERATIVE AND NONDELIBERATIVE PROCEDURES

Discussions at Baylin about whether to accept organ donations from strangers involved a case consult that never expanded into a proposal for a formal policy requiring the hospital administration's approval. Guidelines for screening donors were circulated to a working group of ethicists and surgeons for feedback, but nothing official came of those conversations. That process contrasts with the work of crafting ethical policy, for which the Ethics Advisory Committee (EAC) served as the hospital's main deliberative body. To fulfill the goal of forming policy, the EAC met monthly to discuss case consults and broader issues that were relevant to the hospital as a whole, and it is to that work that I want to direct attention here.[1]

Composed of physicians and nurses from different services, chaplains, family members, legal counsel, ethicists, and outside observers, Baylin's EAC—like other hospital ethics committees—served several functions:

1. *To educate hospital staff about moral and legal standards in medicine.* Hospitals must learn to be ethical—not once, but on an ongoing basis. Staff turnover, new cases, and changes in biomedicine all contribute to the need for continuing education.

2. *To review case consults brought to their attention by the hospital's staff to determine whether formal policy is needed.* Committees must serve as the hospital's casuists, settling cases of conscience and representing the moral voice of the institution.

3. *To informally advise and support health care providers who confront moral issues in the treatment of patients and families.* Individuals have crises of conscience even (perhaps especially) when institutions do not.

4. *To craft official hospital policy regarding the provision of care.* Such policy may include do not resuscitate (DNR) orders, futility policy, or in-

formed consent, drawing on developments and arguments in contemporary bioethics.

5. *To institutionalize a hospital's commitment to moral standards by providing an official venue for the discussion of ethical issues.* In that capacity, ethics committees serve to dispose members of the institution to deliberate about ethical issues and to seek reasonable and workable solutions. Committees are thus facilitators of virtue—the virtue of practical reasoning—producing occasions for moral deliberation about health care policy and practice.

In this chapter, I want to focus on the last two items here—forming official policy and disposing institutional members to deliberate about policy—keeping in mind that these two functions might be distinct in theory but not in practice. Specifically, I am concerned with how a hospital committee monitors itself in its attempt to craft ethical policy. I want to consider ethical questions that surround the *procedures* of committee decision making. When forming policy, is it possible for ethics committees to behave ethically? Are there standards of practice that should govern how a committee comports itself?

Note that we are *not* focusing on the professional norms that characterize the goods of medical practice, norms that should infuse the ethos of hospitals and the first-order, day-by-day deliberations of personnel and committees: beneficence, nonmaleficence, autonomy, or fairness in resource allocation.[2] Instead, I want to inquire in a second-order way into the ethics of crafting ethical policy in an institutional setting, drawing on ideas that might ground those first-order norms but exceed them in their implications for administrators who must fashion policy in institutional contexts. It is tempting to think that the process of crafting policy is problem-free, that orchestrating policy deliberations is either morally neutral or that those responsible for orchestrating such deliberations are agents of virtue, needing no moral standards. But we know that neither of these assumptions is true: There are better and worse ways of producing policy, and those who can be trusted as virtuous leaders are trustworthy in part because they satisfy moral norms such as respect for persons. Those whom we do not trust we suspect of acting "politically"; they rely on procedures that may be effective and prudential, but they fail to respect persons by providing reasons to justify their actions.

Proceeding in this second-order way, I will assume that forming official policy and disposing institutional members to deliberate about policy cannot avoid certain practices that we call "political." That is, forming policy may require an ethics committee not only to respect persons by providing reasons for their actions, but also to negotiate, caucus, vote, and compromise for the sake of producing a workable consensus—even if this means putting aside the best reasons for a policy in order to "make things work."

Ethics and politics—or justice and efficiency—are frequent partners in the formation of hospital policy, and their alliance is not surprising. We need to examine that partnership with some care in order to determine which of its aspects are acceptable in principle. Hence my questions: What is the ethics of forming hospital policy? How should we evaluate the various practices that bring those policies about? Are some political practices more ethically acceptable than others? Can hospitals form policies that are both just and justly achieved?

In exploring these questions, I will borrow from recent discussions in political philosophy about deliberative democracy. When thinking about hospital ethics committees, we must consider norms by which to measure good government. Deliberative democrats argue—rightly, I believe—that good government rests in part on the disposition to provide substantive moral justifications for decisions or policies. The core idea is that by providing shareable reasons we respect each other as moral equals. The goal of this vision is principled social cooperation, in which decisions or policies grow out of a deliberative process structured by reciprocity, openness, and accountability.[3]

Yet describing good government in this way emphasizes the *deliberative* features of democracy, potentially obscuring *nondeliberative* practices that are nonetheless democratic. I have mentioned a few nondeliberative procedures—caucusing, negotiating, voting, and compromising[4]—because they were very much alive in a case at Baylin, about which I will say more below. In nondeliberative processes, people express their interests or convictions, but not through rational argumentation premised on mutual respect. When we vote, we are not asked to provide reasons for our decision; when we strike a compromise, we concede some of the conclusions to which our reasons have led us. Democratic politics, in a hospital no less than in other institutional contexts, frequently requires us to depart from deliberative ideals because deliberation can become interminable, repetitive, or both. Striking the proper balance between deliberative and nondeliberative procedures defines an ethical challenge for individuals who direct hospital ethics committees (and other groups as well).

Most readers of this book likely serve on committees—at work, in civic and religious activities, in professional organizations, or in other volunteer work. "Life is in meeting," we might say, expressing the ideas of Martin Buber with self-reflexive irony. Yet however ubiquitous committee work might be, little attention has been devoted to how committees ought to operate—how there might be duties and virtues in administrative life. Like the norms of parenting, the norms of committee work are assumed to be obvious or self-explanatory. At the same time, service on a committee is often met with dread. With a clearer sense of the challenges and trade-offs that committee work involves, perhaps that need not always be the case.

To anticipate my conclusion, I will argue that there is a strong presumption but not an absolute prohibition against nondeliberative practices in a committee's procedures. Nondeliberative practices are regrettable because they can be manipulative or coercive rather than respectful of persons. They can be justified on one of two counts: first, insofar as they might dispose members to deliberate; second, insofar as they function as a last resort, when mechanisms of deliberation reach an impasse. The politics of policy making is not to be regretted when it satisfies one of these two conditions. In addition, the decision to abandon deliberative procedures should itself be deliberated about; choosing not to deliberate ought to be a decision for which reasons are given. In any event, we should not overlook the fact that reason and ethics have a material life, that principle and prudence must coexist. *How* they rightly coexist is a (second-order) question for us to consider.

THE AUTOPSY THAT WOULD NOT DIE

During the summer months before I began my stint as a participant-observer, Baylin's EAC began a comprehensive review of the hospital's procedure for securing parents' informed consent for an autopsy on their child when he or she dies in the hospital. That review was prompted by a family's complaint that they received inaccurate information from a physician after their child died at Baylin, and that they subsequently gave permission for an autopsy without adequate information. At issue were differing accounts about what the doctors conveyed when the parents were approached for an autopsy regarding the ultimate disposition of the body's organs. The family believed that the child's organs would be returned to the body; the physician believed that the hospital's consent form stated that organs were to be retained by the hospital. In fact, the consent form allowed for unspecified restrictions on the autopsy and stated that organs would otherwise be retained. Autopsies might be limited by restricting the procedure to a specific organ, by obtaining tissue samples for biopsy with a needle, or by limiting the incisions to specific areas of the body. Because the family did not indicate any limits on postmortem procedures, the pathology service thought it acceptable to retain some of the child's organs. Believing that the organs (partially) represented their dead child, the parents became upset once they learned that the organs had not been returned. Acting on the parents' wishes, the hospital arranged to have the child's organs transported for a ceremony in which the organs were buried with the rest of the child's body. The mother was subsequently treated for depression brought on by her child's death, autopsy, and burial; the family threatened a lawsuit. Believing that the sensitivity of the issue and the mother's disposition rendered the case unwinnable, Baylin's general counsel agreed to settle out of court.

The EAC's policy review began with the formation of a subcommittee headed by Michael DeVries, the associate director of the intensive care unit (ICU); the hospital chaplain; a community representative who is also a legal expert in health care law; and a medical resident. The subcommittee first sought to determine the policies and practices of other hospitals by researching 165 teaching hospitals across the United States. Their specific aim was to learn how many of those institutions provide the option of a limited autopsy, and what they regard as adequate informed consent. DeVries submitted a questionnaire about autopsy consent forms to these hospitals and followed up with queries about what the chief residents knew about autopsy procedures and autopsy consent. His questionnaire generated a response rate of 68 percent (82 of 119) from internal medicine programs and 98 percent (45 of 46) from pediatric programs. DeVries learned that 92 percent of the forms describe the option of a restricted postmortem examination, but that only 7 percent of those forms provide an clear, explicit place for families to authorize the procedure.[5]

The general wording of existing consent forms, DeVries observed, is "sparse and ambiguous."[6] Virtually all of the chief residents who were surveyed admitted that they knew little about autopsy procedures and autopsy consent. Together with the subcommittee's medical resident, DeVries set out to craft a document that would function within the hospital as well as provide a standard for other hospitals, and he conferred with the hospital's pathology service to learn about existing protocols for postmortem examinations.

In the fall, DeVries presented an initial draft of a consent form at the monthly meeting of the EAC. This draft, which aimed to inform parents fully, provided a wide array of options by listing organs, bodily areas, procedures, and instructions, and allotted additional space for parents to identify items that were not listed. The document was, in effect, a "designer form," allowing parents to tailor a postmortem examination to their specific wishes.

The EAC quickly decided that this document was too informative, that its details were too harsh for a grieving parent. Moreover, pathologists on the committee argued that providing options *endorsed* the idea of a limited autopsy, an endorsement that failed to represent their disagreement with the very premise of restricted examinations. Among other things, the pathologists noted, recent studies demonstrate that 25 to 30 percent of standard autopsies produce clinically significant findings that were unknown before death.[7] That information could have a substantial impact on understanding the patient's course of disease and physiological decline. Some of that information, moreover, has the potential to revise the physician's diagnosis of the cause of death and to provide significant information for surviving relatives. The pathology service generally agreed to accept a request for restrictions, and agreed in particular about the importance of returning the eyes to the body. But they argued that proposing further limits would lend official backing to procedures that are antithetical to the purpose of an autopsy, are contrary to the research and teaching mission of the hospital, and may provide incomplete or inaccurate information.

On the advice of the committee, DeVries agreed to develop another draft in consultation with one of the hospital's pathologists. Seeking to work out an acceptable document, DeVries conferred over the next two months with Tom McDowell of the pathology service. In the revised document, DeVries retained the option of restricted examinations, but deleted the list of specific organs, bodily areas, procedures, and instructions. The revised document simply mentioned the option of limited autopsy and left a line for parents to specify what they would want done (or not done). In return for those changes, DeVries added new material to compensate for reducing the information from the initial draft. The new material sought to capture some of the reasons that parents might have for restricting a post-mortem examination, the most important of which stated,

> Many religions and cultures have specific views about autopsies. For example, some families have decided in the past to exclude an organ or organs from the autopsy. Other families have requested that the organs be returned to the body after samples have been obtained. I understand that I have the option to limit the autopsy or to make a specific request about the autopsy. However, limiting the autopsy may reduce the chance of obtaining information or answers to the questions being asked. I also understand that I have the option to speak with others who share my spiritual beliefs, hospital chaplains, or with physicians, regarding limiting the autopsy.

In effect, DeVries decided to inform parents by including reasons rather than choices involving restricted autopsies.

In January, DeVries presented his new draft at the meeting of the EAC; six members of the pathology service attended that meeting to present an alternative proposal. In preparation for the meeting, the chair of the EAC, Sharon Johnston, conferred briefly with the hospital's legal counsel, Robert Dugan, to arrange the sequence of presentations. The strategy was to begin with Dugan presenting information regarding the lawsuit implicating the hospital, which resulted from parents alleging that they were provided inaccurate information by the hospital before giving consent. The plan was to reveal the legal stakes of the existing consent form to those in the pathology service who were reluctant to revise it.

The pathologists' alternative permission form mentioned limited autopsies in one brief sentence, omitted reference to religious or cultural practices, and directed parents to pathologists for advice (but not to chaplains or others who might share the parents' beliefs). The pathologists' draft placed the burden of proof for securing a restricted autopsy on the parents by leaving a line that asked parents to confirm that "our questions have been answered." Moreover, the pathologists vigorously argued against the presence of the clause in DeVries's draft that stated, "limiting the autopsy may reduce the chance of obtaining information or answers to the questions being asked." In their view, that clause was an insufficient deterrent (although the alternative, which mentioned limited autopsy, did not mention its disadvantages).

At the end of a very tense meeting, their objections did not prevail. Committee members argued that DeVries's draft more adequately informed parents about reasons for and against limited autopsies, and various committee members proposed ways of strengthening the clause about the drawbacks of restricted examinations—in keeping with the substance of the pathologists' concerns. But the pathologists experienced the outcome as defeat, not dialogue, and in a strategy of retreat proposed that the hospital revert to the original form. Recognizing that they had not achieved consensus, the committee agreed to endorse DeVries's form as the basis for further negotiations between DeVries and the pathology service.

Before the meeting fully adjourned, the pathologists won a brief, concluding skirmish. Protesting the presence of the clause about religious and cultural beliefs, the pathologists claimed that such a clause suggested that standard autopsies are irreligious. That idea, the pathologists noted, slanted the information negatively by implying a religious presumption against autopsy. In effect, the pathologists were asking the committee not to draft a document that stigmatized their practice. Moreover, the pathologists believed that the information was gratuitous. In their view, adherents of religions that have specific rules about handling dead bodies can generally be relied on to possess that knowledge in advance of a family member's death; they do not need the hospital to instruct them about religious doctrine.

In response, the committee decided to vote over electronic mail about whether the "religion clause" should remain on the form. The choice was whether to keep the clause, against the pathologists' objections, or to include it on a supplementary information page that would have less authority than the consent form. The information sheet would help to inform parents, but there would be no guarantee that house staff would use it consistently, and it included no mechanism to secure consent. It might not be read or considered by all families, especially given the circumstances of grief. Despite these obvious limits, the EAC acceded to the pathologists' wishes by voting over E-mail to place the "religion clause" on the information page.

Between January and April, DeVries worked with the pathology service in the hope of producing a final document. DeVries and McDowell shared information about the flexibility of their respective groups (the EAC and the pathology service) on specific points. More frequently, however, their discussions turned on political procedure. The pathologists were unhappy about playing a subordinate role in the hospital's review of a research practice in which they were obviously and directly involved. They questioned the standing and legitimacy of the EAC as the proper agency for crafting a new form. DeVries negotiated with McDowell and his colleagues to secure their participation in the process. DeVries thus worked at two levels: first, with regard to what information should be included in the revised document; and second, with regard to the EAC's authority to establish hospital policy.

DELIBERATIVE CIRCUMSTANCES

In seeking to craft a reasonable and acceptable permission form for pediatric autopsies, the EAC engaged in practices that were ethical and political. We might clarify that partnership by considering the circumstances in which such a committee deliberates, circumstances including moral uncertainty, plurality of participants, and the need to produce a justifiable outcome. As I hope to make clear, the latter two circumstances help us understand what is at stake when we inquire into the ethics of committees and sharpen the challenge of directing administrative committees in an ethical way.

Moral Uncertainty

Ethics committees convene in order to answer moral questions or to resolve moral disputes. Typically, uncertainty turns on the need to *specify* the implications of a general norm or prior policy, *settle an apparent conflict* between rival values by weighing or balancing them, or determine a service's *degree of moral accountability* for carrying out a procedure or practice.[8] A committee asks, for example, whether a DNR order properly specifies how to honor patients' autonomy given their implied wishes when express statements are lacking, or whether triage practices fairly allocate resources.

In developing an informed consent form for pediatric autopsies, the EAC faced the question of how to balance the family's needs with the hospital's legitimate therapeutic and research interests. The committee confronted uncertainty about how best to specify each value and how to assign relative weight to each. Providing detailed information about autopsies—including a list of organs and procedures—might lead parents to make choices that are properly informed. By choosing to limit an autopsy, however, parents might compromise the effectiveness of the autopsy and of hospital research. Moreover, the facts about autopsies are harsh details for a grieving parent. Yet giving hospital pathologists carte blanche to perform standard autopsies seems to fail to respect the legitimate interests of family members who grieve the loss of a child. Various religions (e.g., Islam, Conservative and Orthodox Judaism, Christian Science, Jehovah's Witnesses) ban or limit autopsies except when legally or medically indicated. Denying the option of a limited autopsy can be insensitive to the demands of a family's cultural and religious identity.

Hospital ethics committees address moral uncertainty that is practical, not theoretical. Committee members do not debate foundational issues about the nature of rationality, deontology versus utilitarianism, correspondence versus coherentist theories of truth, or whether moral dilemmas exist. Their mission is concrete and directive: They are to eliminate uncertainty about how individuals or services are rightly to carry out their respective practices. Hence discussions about one or another policy must eventually find resolution. Moral uncertainty is thus a function, in part at least, not of theoretical quandaries, but the need to relate norms and virtues to actual practice within a complex institutional setting.

Institutional Pluralism

Committees that set out to eliminate uncertainty do so, of course, as a group. At Baylin, the EAC comprises about twenty-five individuals who come from various services and specialties: intensive care, chaplaincy, pulmonology, surgery, respiratory therapy, urology, psychiatry, law, and extended care. Adding to the mix of specialists are parents and occasional outside visitors.

Over the past decade, observers of ethics committees have lauded this kind of pluralism. Diversity provides a check on the power of any one service or role by representing the moral claims of others. Having doctors and nurses deliberate in an open forum diminishes advantages that might otherwise accrue to physicians in a professional culture that privileges their rank. Participation in ethics committees can be contagious, affecting the ethos of specific services or departments. (One member of the EAC at Baylin regularly orchestrates ethics rounds for nurses and house staff in the ICU.) Diversity also promises to broaden imaginative horizons. By including outsiders (e.g., parents and visitors), committees reduce the possibility of "groupthink," the tendency of individuals within an institution to think and feel within well-worn grooves. Moreover, the committee's outside members connect the hospital to its "moral constituency,"[9] the larger moral community to which the hospital is accountable as a member of civil society.

Accompanying these advantages are practical challenges. As a collective entity, an ethics committee illustrates what Dennis F. Thompson aptly calls "the moral responsibility of many hands," the fact that numerous individuals contribute in different ways to the decisions and policies of an institution.[10] One challenge is that policy must be acceptable across a spectrum of interests. More specifically, the moral responsibility of many hands points to the fact that policy making must not only aim at justice and good reasons, but that it must also produce consensus, something that "everyone can live with."

In terms of political philosophy, the responsibility of many hands alerts us to the fact that policy must be democratically legitimate. If policy is going to coerce the consciences of hospital personnel, it will be tyrannical if it lacks popular consent. Consensus is a practical as well as moral requirement, for it honors others as equals by attempting to take their claims into account. Failure to consult a diverse range of services and specialties will produce policy that is disrespectful and unrepresentative. Without a wide consultation, an ethics committee might function despotically.

One of the greatest benefits of a diverse committee is that it minimizes the disadvantages that some groups might experience as a result of their place in the hospital hierarchy. Diversity functions in part as a check on rank; it can have a (commendable) leveling effect on decision-making procedures. But that potential can be realized only if deliberation is morally constrained. Diversity brings with it the potential for special pleading, filibustering, or strategizing to promote self-interest. Without some moral norms, deliberation in circumstances of diversity can do more harm than good.

In *Democracy and Disagreement,* Amy Gutmann and Dennis F. Thompson propose three norms to constrain democratic deliberation, all of which bear on how hospital ethics committees might assess themselves in a second-order way: *reciprocity, publicity,* and *accountability.*[11] These norms can function to keep deliberative parties respectful of each other as persons, regardless of their substantive moral positions or their places in the hospital hierarchy.

Reciprocity expresses a sense of mutuality in deliberative forums. The goal is to offer "reasons that can be accepted by others who are similarly motivated to find reasons that can be accepted by others."[12] Underlying the norm of reciprocity is an ethics of coercion, or a theory of justified coercion: Insofar as policies or decisions are mutually binding, deliberators "should aspire to a kind of political reasoning that is mutually justifiable."[13] The idea of reciprocity is to constrain discussion so that each contributor is treated as a moral equal rather than as an instrument of another party's interests or calculations. In that way, deliberators can take collective ownership of the policy that they produce; policy is the product of shared reasons, not the interests of a particular group.

Publicity helps the norm of reciprocity to achieve its full potential. It expresses the idea that deliberation should not occur in private. Failing that condition, publicity requires that private meetings should be subsequently disclosed. Deliberating in the open protects against procedures that jeopardize the moral equality that reciprocity is meant to enshrine. Secret deliberations communicate the idea that some are worthier than others in the formation of policy. Secrecy disadvantages some individuals or groups, (re)creating asymmetries of power. With these concerns in mind, Kant constructed the publicity principle to hold that "all actions which relate to the right of other [persons] are contrary to right and law [if their] maxim does not permit publicity."[14] Accordingly, the Kantian understanding of publicity holds that a policy is unacceptable if exposing it would render it self-defeating.[15]

Moreover, publicity can have the salutary effect of improving the quality of argument. When committees convene openly, they express the conviction that deliberators are capable of good reasoning. That conviction can be as much a duty as a compliment: Publicity requires that committee members be ready to argue in ways that are substantive and strong. Deliberating openly thus has the merit of producing conditions that obligate individuals to put their best foot forward. As Mill observes, "People will give dishonest or mean votes . . . more readily in secret than in public."[16]

Accountability, Gutmann and Thompson argue, is a norm that requires deliberators to justify their decisions to those who will be bound by them.[17] Obviously implied by reciprocity, accountability expresses the idea that when committees deliberate well, their members are morally responsible to themselves and to the larger hospital constituency. Committees must answer questions about the merits of their decisions or policies; they exercise accountability insofar as they take moral ownership for the results of their debates. They express their own dignity as moral subjects to the extent that they are willing to accept praise or blame for their deliberations.

Policy Formation

So obvious as to be easily overlooked, there is a goal to deliberation: the formation of an ethically sound policy, one that is secured by the balance of good reasons. That circumstance alerts us not to issues of legitimation, but to justification. Committees seek to solicit a variety of voices not only as an end in itself, but as a means to the end of producing a morally superior policy. Like collaborative learning, deliberation involves (or can involve) a synergistic process in which reasons are strengthened by dialogue and debate. A committee's ideal, of course, is to overcome moral uncertainty with a policy that is morally justified and democratically legitimate. But results, not process, are the goal. Failing to achieve that goal, a committee can find only partial solace in the fact that it used commendable procedures.

APPLIED ETHICS, NARRATIVE, AND CASUISTRY

The goal-oriented aspect of deliberation focuses our attention on the need for ethically sound results—a policy that is backed by good reasons. I call attention to that goal here in part to distinguish my views from those of Margaret Urban Walker, who argues that hospital ethicists are architects of moral space within the health care setting, as well as mediators who are responsible in part for the quality of the conversations taking place within that space.[18] Walker connects that mode of ethics consultation with a narrative-based approach to moral deliberation. For Walker (and others), narrative ethics thinks "about morality as a medium of progressive acknowledgment and adjustment among people in (or in search of) a common and habitable moral world."[19] Walker contrasts such an approach with what she and Arthur Caplan call the engineering model of consultation, with its "top-down application of code-like theories."[20] According to Walker, we ought to envision ethicists' contributions to hospital deliberations less in terms of mastering the technique of specifying principles, weighing rival values, or relating norms to cases, and more in terms of keeping "open, accessible, and active (and if necessary to create and design with others) those moral-reflective spaces in institutional life where a sound and shared process of deliberation and negotiation can go on."[21]

Walker echoes the current tendency to view options in practical moral reasoning in terms of either applied ethics or narrative ethics.[22] I share her dissatisfaction with top-down, mechanical moral reasoning, aspects of which I discussed in the case of Ericka's sepsis in Chapter 8. Walker is correct in calling for an approach to ethical consultation that is sensitive to the richness, complexity, and densely textured quality of ethical problems in hospital settings, for such accounts more truthfully represent a hospital case's moral properties than do brief, streamlined accounts. But her model of ethicist as architect—"someone who designs a structure to fulfill a function at a given site"[23]—fails to capture hospital ethics committees' responsibility to produce policies that can boast the merit of sound reasons. A good resolution to a disagreement is not merely one that "might come from stakes being clearly assessed, parties becoming clear on their own and others' legitimate positions, compromises being achieved that will stand up satisfactorily to later review because of the care with which they were constructed."[24] All of those conditions can be met by a committee that fails to produce a substantively sound decision or policy. Walker does not adequately distinguish between the importance of sound *process,* on the one hand, and the importance of *substantive reasons,* on the other. As a result, her recommendations fail to provide sufficient guidance at a second-order level about the ethics of directing ethics committees.

In the context of Baylin's autopsy dispute, deliberative procedures had less to do with keeping reflective spaces open than with settling a question about how to weigh competing norms in the resolution of a practical issue. Casuistry, not narrative ethics, was operative, for the hospital committee set out to resolve an institutional case of conscience by employing standard features of case-based reasoning: paradigms, presumptions, analogical reasoning, and attention to circumstances.[25]

The committee began by perceiving the case of securing informed consent for autopsies through the paradigm of securing informed consent from parents who are deciding whether to begin or continue medical treatment for their child. Acting on that paradigm and a presumptive respect for parental autonomy, a physician is to inform parents about risks and benefits of treating or not treating their child. Specifically, physicians must describe the risks and benefits of a proposed procedure, the risks and benefits of alternative procedures (when relevant), and the risks and benefits of doing nothing. The overall task is to help parents evaluate treatment within a therapeutic alliance.

The challenge to the EAC was to reason analogically from this paradigm to the case of autopsies, in which actions performed on the child have no therapeutic dimension. Risks and benefits are to be weighed not in relation to the child's well-being, but in relation to the family's well-being and social customs. *Patient benefit, a key assumption in the standard paradigm, is moot in securing consent for pediatric autopsies.*

With patient benefit moot, competing values such as medical training and research interests acquire greater importance. True, in the standard paradigm, it is possible for parents justifiably to consent to nontherapeutic research on their child. As I will argue in Chapter 11, there are principled reasons for parents to volunteer their children for nontherapeutic research if the risks are minimal. In the case of dead patients, the risks to the individual are obviously nonexistent, allowing countervailing concerns such as research benefits to rise to the fore. Informed consent thus turns on instructing parents to weigh those benefits in tandem with other considerations that bear on *their own* well-being.

Hence the task of weighing competing norms that emerge in the process of reasoning analogically from the standard paradigm of informed consent to consent for pediatric autopsies: Informing parents of risks and burdens is an attempt to honor their autonomy as decision makers, but considerations of "benefit" are different from those that operate within the standard paradigm. When considering pediatric autopsies, we need not balance risks and therapeutic benefits to the patient, or weigh risks to the patient against other social needs. But that does not mean that "benefit" is irrelevant or uncomplicated. Rather, considerations of beneficence remain relevant and generate tensions with autonomy at two levels.

Consider the need to inform parents adequately about what an autopsy does. One goal is to clarify the risks that they may endure as parents who have a legitimate interest in respecting their dead child. Worries about bodily integrity, funeral arrangements, and disfigurement need to be addressed. Out of respect for families respecting (and mourning) their dead, the ethics committee drafted a form that described the basic features of postmortem examination, leaving open the option of restricting the autopsy and returning organs to the body. In that way the EAC worked to honor parental autonomy and, more specifically, a family's right to refuse recommended action when that refusal does not harm their child.

Yet there are benefits to a full autopsy that even well-informed parents might deny themselves. Herein lies one tension between autonomy and beneficence: Parents may choose to limit the autopsy out of a concern for bodily integrity and thus deny themselves important (and desirable) information. As I noted, 10 to 15 percent of standard autopsies produce clinically significant data, which might bear on the child's cause of death. That information might be helpful to surviving blood relatives, and it is not possible to acquire it with limited autopsies.

Moreover, medical and research benefits follow from standard autopsies. Herein lies the second tension between autonomy and beneficence: Clinicians are trained in the practice of postmortem examination, and science gains information that is compromised or lost when autopsies are limited.

Hence the problem about which the ethics committee deliberated: Providing information and allowing for limited autopsy seems to honor parental autonomy and negative liberty, but it does so at the expense of the benefit to the parents, the hospital, and society. Given that conflict, the ethics committee sought to frame a consent form that allowed for limited autopsies and yet clearly stated the benefits of standard autopsies. To the pathologists, this approach either surrendered too much to autonomy or misinterpreted its meaning. On their account, a family's choice should be a rational choice, and a limited autopsy, in their view, is irrational. Thus they preferred phrasing the form to avoid encouraging limited autopsies. Their goal was to ensure that the form did not lead to a state of affairs that was harmful to parents and the hospital alike.

DELIBERATIVE LIABILITIES

So much for the EAC's casuistry. What about the moral quality of their deliberations? Given what we have learned from Gutmann and Thompson, what can we say about the EAC as deliberative democrats?

The last two features of policy making that I mentioned—the need for consensus and the need for sound policy—point to a potential tension between *legitimation* and *justification* in deliberative processes. Legitimation and the need for consensus do not guarantee that a morally sound policy has been crafted; sound policy, which must be justified by a balance of strong arguments, does not require consensus. We can see the appeal of a theory of deliberative democracy, for it appears to resolve what might become a dilemma. By allowing for widespread participation, deliberative procedures satisfy the need for representation and popular consent. By drawing on different moral voices, moreover, deliberative procedures attempt to increase the likelihood that the best reasons are stated in the crafting of policy. Seeking to strike a balance between process and substance, deliberative democrats appear to provide the best of both worlds.

Of course, a convergence of legitimation and justification is easier to conceive in theory than reality, for it is not uncommon for their respective aims to pull apart. The need to produce consensus may require policies whose reasons are weaker than is morally desirable; uncontroversial reasons are not necessarily the strongest. Conversely, seeking the strongest moral policy might not secure the approval of all interested parties.

The causes of these tensions are familiar: self-interest, intractable moral disagreement, or incomplete understanding. When these forces hold sway, deliberative processes become repetitive, circling around familiar arguments. Like other democratic practices that seek consent, deliberation can be inefficient and regressive, relying on the will of the people. Deliberation in the real world is not without its problems, and their solution lies outside deliberative procedures themselves.

Baylin's attempt to deal with such liabilities came in the form of four nondeliberative practices: caucusing, negotiating, voting, and compromising, both within the ethics committee and between committee members and the pathology service. Caucusing and negotiating occurred, rightly in my view, in the effort to keep deliberative procedures moving on the right track. Voting and compromising occurred once those procedures reached an impasse; they can be justified as a last resort. Nondeliberative procedures, then, are generally warranted when they are instrumental to deliberation itself, or when they function as an alternative to deliberative mechanisms that have exhausted themselves.

More specifically, the principles and advantages of deliberative measures generate a strong presumption on their behalf. Deliberation aims to respect persons, secure consent, and solicit the strongest possible reasons. Nondeliberative procedures may be efficient and effective for producing results, but they do less to respect persons and cannot ensure that good reasons will rise to the fore. Their moral merits lie in their ability to keep deliberation going, or as an alternative when deliberation lamentably ceases.

Even when presumptions are overridden, however, they leave what Robert Nozick calls "moral traces."[26] That is, they continue to exert pressure on the moral quality of action. Once one departs from a presumption, one does not abandon it; it continues to cast a moral shadow over the subsequent course of action. The goal is to restrict the departure from the presumption as much as possible, conceiving that restriction in terms of duration, importance, and number of people affected. Ideally, that means that nondeliberative procedures should be brief, provide a reasonable hope of success, affect or involve few individuals, and approximate the goods enshrined in deliberative practices. Moreover, a departure is best when it aims to serve the ends of deliberation itself. In that respect, justification for nondeliberative action is strongest when it is carried out on behalf of ethical ends.

On these terms, each of the nondeliberative practices at Baylin fares well. Private caucusing occurred between members who conferred behind the scenes to orchestrate the pivotal committee meeting in January. Seeking to reveal the legal stakes of the original form to those in the pathology service who were reluctant to revise current policy, Johnston (the chair of the EAC) conferred with Dugan (the hospital's legal counsel) before the meeting to arrange the sequence of presentations. The aim was to begin the meeting with the hospital's general counsel presenting information about a lawsuit implicating the hospital. With the stakes clear from the outset, it was hoped, the committee would be in a better position to deliberate about an alternative.

Those caucusing arrangements were brief, limited to one strategic conversation. Caucusing aimed solely at staging the initial sequence of events at the January meeting. Without a clear and concrete set of issues to be addressed, it was feared, the pathologists might prevail in the attempt to preserve the status quo. Moreover, Johnston began that meeting by revealing that she and Dugan had caucused about arranging the sequence of presentations, thereby honoring the presumption of publicity that she had previously overridden.

Johnston's and Dugan's caucusing was prudent. The fact that the pathologists were willing to propose the original form once their alternative was defeated reveals the extent of their conservatism. Had they not been required to shoulder the burden of proof from the outset of the meeting, they might have easily turned the tables and placed the burden of proof on DeVries's efforts, thereby returning the debate to its earliest phase. Revealing the inadequacy of the original form and the legal state of play, Johnston and Dugan were able to prevent deliberation from regressing. Private caucusing was justified, in short, because it was an effective attempt to improve the conditions of deliberation and because its relevant details were disclosed to the committee as a whole.

Negotiating can be seen in similar terms. During the heat of the controversy, DeVries conferred twelve times with the pathology service about how to construct a new informed consent form. Although it might seem that these discussions were deliberative, only occasionally did they involve questions about how much information the pathology service considered appropriate to include on the revised form. DeVries and McDowell discussed substantive points, especially how much weight each group (the EAC and the pathology service) assigned to specific items of information on the revised document, seeking to ascertain which items each group considered nonnegotiable. More frequently, however, they debated political process and the proper jurisdiction of the EAC. DeVries regularly confronted the tasks of defending the ethics committee's role in the hospital's review of postmortem examinations, and of persuading the pathology service to continue in respectful dialogue with the committee. The pathologists challenged him to account for the committee's authority and the pathology service's subordinate role in the review process.

Doing so required DeVries to make a case for the committee's administrative authority. Negotiation was justified to the extent that it sought to sustain conditions for deliberative procedures, thereby maintaining dialogue between the ethics committee and the pathology service. DeVries's task was political, having less to do with the ethics of informed consent than with the need to smooth over tensions among committed individuals with strong personalities. He worked to ensure that ideas were transmitted between groups, that a spirit of good faith and mutual effort could prevail as long as possible.

Although compromising and voting might be justified as a last resort in many deliberative arrangements, that condition was not met in this case. As a result, the compromise vote seems the least commendable of the committee's nondeliberative acts. At the January meeting, the pathologists adamantly insisted on removing the clause referring to religious or cultural reasons for limiting autopsies. They complained that this clause stigmatized their practice by suggesting a religious presumption against standard autopsies, and that it included unnecessary information because the relevant population would be likely to know their religious beliefs about postmortem treatment. The effect of the pathologists' protest was to create an impasse, to which the EAC decided to respond in a nondeliberative way. Rather than holding to the position that the religion clause must remain in the document (or discussing it further), the committee compromised its position by voting on whether the clause ought to remain on the form. By placing the clause on a supplementary information page, it was hoped, the policy could maintain its goal of producing an informed consent form while mollifying the beleaguered pathology service.

The committee's decision was hasty and unfortunate. However correct the pathologists might have been about the form stigmatizing their practice or functioning gratuitously, they were wrong to insist that reference to religion be deleted. Removing that clause denies some families a vital piece of relevant information about autopsies and cultural beliefs. The clause did not assert that autopsies are wrong. It pointed to the hospital's spiritual resources for families in difficult emotional circumstances who may have questions about the acceptability of standard autopsies. To delete this reference—as if death, the body, cultural norms, and religion were not appropriate matters for families to consider at the time of their child's death—is not properly to inform them. It might lead them to choose a course of action that they would regard in retrospect as undignified or religiously harmful. The pathologists' complaint thus failed to appreciate not only autonomy, but the full range of issues that beneficence bids us to consider. It is notable that the hospital chaplain was absent from the meeting during which this compromise resolution occurred. The committee did not sufficiently deliberate the decision to abandon deliberative procedures; it thus departed from deliberative measures in a twofold way.

FIRST- AND SECOND-ORDER TRADE-OFFS

The case of "the autopsy that would not die" illustrates two sets of moral trade-offs in the administrative life of a hospital. At a first-order level, the committee deliberated about how to interpret, weigh, and balance the meaning of autonomy and beneficence when constructing an informed consent form for pediatric autopsies. That task was generated by issues that emerged as the committee reasoned analogically from the standard paradigm of informed consent to circumstances in which risks and benefits to the patient are moot. That task of casuistical reasoning shaped the moral tensions between the ethics committee and the pathology service. At a second-order level, the moral trade-offs bear on the operation of the committee itself, involving the choice between deliberative and nondeliberative procedures. Hospital ethics committees behave ethically when they institutionalize a strong presumption in favor of deliberative methods. Those methods attempt to overcome moral uncertainty, produce sound policy, and secure consent. When committees depart from that presumption, they should do so in ways that nonetheless honor its force. They should thus deliberate about the reasons for their departures, thereby honoring the presumption in favor of deliberation in a self-reflexive way. And they should limit their departures to those that serve the interests of deliberative practices, or to those circumstances that materialize when deliberation fails to secure the goods it is meant to serve.

ELEVEN

Ethical Issues in Pediatric Research

I do consider children vulnerable. We have to limit the
amount of risk that we expose children to.[1]
—*Marilyn Waters, Director of Research Compliance,
Baylin's Institutional Review Board*

There is a moral imperative to formally study drugs
in children so that they can enjoy equal access to
existing as well as new therapeutic agents.[2]
—*American Academy of Pediatrics*

THERAPEUTIC ORPHANS

I noted in the last chapter that one function of an ethics committee is to
educate hospital staff about moral and legal standards in biomedicine—
to function as a school of sorts—especially in response to new developments in science, culture, and technology. To that end, Baylin's Ethics Advisory Committee (EAC) convenes a retreat each spring to orient new
members, to thank members who are rotating off their three-year term,
and to present educational materials for discussion and review. The day-
long meeting occurs at a large retreat center, away from the rhythms and
routines of the hospital, and offers a precious commodity for busy medical
professionals: time to reflect about the moral challenges of their work. Typically, members of the EAC's core group—Sharon Johnston, Michael De-
Vries, Robert Hamilton, and Christopher Martin—give presentations and
guide discussion on a select topic.

One spring, while I was completing a draft of this book, the EAC con-
vened a special retreat to discuss the ethics of pediatric research. The goal of
that meeting was to bring together members of the hospital's Institutional
Review Board (IRB) and members of the hospital's ethics committee to dis-

cuss federal regulations, moral arguments, and concrete cases regarding the use of children in scientific research. Baylin's IRB (like all IRBs) is responsible for screening research proposals involving human subjects to ensure soundness of research design and proper protection of individuals who are enlisted in investigative studies. The EAC has little direct influence over the workings of the IRB; they are two relatively independent groups. The general feeling at Baylin was that matters were becoming more complex because the IRB was being presented with an increasing number of research protocols that posed risks to patients and offered financial incentives to researchers and families. In Johnston's mind, "It was important to bring together people who knew something about ethics with people who new something about research."[3] A retreat that generated discussion between members of the EAC and members of the IRB, it was hoped, would enable each group to educate the other. In a research hospital such as Baylin, the tensions between medicine and science are not insignificant—aspects of which we have already considered in the cases of Billy Richardson and pediatric autopsies. Here, as before, we are reminded that in biomedicine ethical norms and virtues are often mediated by different groups in institutional settings. Given the complexity of issues in medicine and research, moreover, bioethics sometimes requires a division of labor.

Retreat participants included members of Baylin's EAC and IRB, workers at a local extended care center, employees of the drug industry, and myself. All of those who attended were provided a folder of reading materials in advance of the retreat to help focus the day's discussions. Among those readings were the following real-life cases, drafted by Marilyn Waters, the Director of Research Compliance on Baylin's IRB.

- An investigator is looking at the relationship between a pediatric urological condition and fertility. If the condition threatens fertility, early surgery might prevent problems later in life. The investigator would like to collect semen samples from adolescent boys age thirteen and up. Who should be approached first, the adolescent or the parent?
- An investigator proposes to conduct a focus group of adolescent girls with Down syndrome and their mothers to explore the special needs of these girls as they start menstruating. Two focus groups are proposed, one with the mothers and the one with the girls. Many of these adolescents are capable of providing some level of assent. Are there special considerations for enrolling these subjects onto the trial? How should the investigator recruit participants and obtain permission/assent?
- An investigator is testing the hypothesis that in patients with attention deficit hyperactivity disorder (ADHD), behavior can be modulated by a special diet. The study involves a total of two days on a general clinical research unit—two one-day visits at least one day apart. While in

the hospital, the children are fed a specific diet, wear an electronic activity monitor, and take a computerized attention test. No ADHD medications are allowed during the admission. The IRB has approved the protocol as well as approving a $50 gift certificate for Tower Records or Barnes and Noble for the child and reimbursement expenses for the parent to cover parking, food, and transportation costs. Yet the investigator had trouble recruiting subjects. The investigator has approached the IRB at least three times and requested permission to raise the amount of compensation offered. The most recent request is for $200 for KayBee Toys or Toys R Us. He advises the IRB the following: "Most of the people we interviewed lost interest because the study provided little direct benefit to their child and there is an extensive time requirement. Drug trials seem to have less difficulty because the children are at least exposed to a treatment arm for a period of time."

• Dr. Cobb is interested in studying arginine metabolism and requirements in children with sepsis. The goal of the study is to gain information that will eventually help in providing the best nutritional and metabolic support for these patients. Arginine, an amino acid that is found in proteins such as eggs, meat, vegetables, and dairy products, is important because it is a precursor to nitric oxide. Nitric oxide is a gas normally produced by the body. However, during severe infection, the production of nitric oxide increases and may be responsible for some of the problems seen in patients with severe infections (e.g., low blood pressure).

One arm of Dr. Cobb's study will involve sixteen patients, aged two to six, who are diagnosed with sepsis and who are admitted to the intensive care unit. Patients with anemia will be excluded from the study. All children will already have intravenous and arterial lines and a nasojejunal tube in place, and all will be receiving enteral nutrition as part of their medical treatment. Each patient will receive two eight-hour infusions of intravenous and intragastric stable isotope tracers of arginine, citrulline, and leucine. The tracers have been used safely with children. Subsequent blood samples will be obtained from the arterial line; breath samples will be obtained from the endotracheal tube, the consumption of energy will be calculated from the respirator; and all urine excreted during the twenty-four-hour period will be collected and studied. The tracer will be administered in minuscule doses, and the proposed dose of tracer will not affect the stability of patients. Subjects will not be compensated and will receive no direct medical benefit. However, the results will lead to a better understanding of the metabolic pathway under septic conditions with the final goal of providing adequate nutritional and metabolic support to these patients.

When she submitted her proposal to NIH for funding, Dr. Cobb was advised to include data from healthy, normal controls. Control data are thought to be essential in collecting complete relevant information. Dr. Cobb thus submitted a second protocol to study arginine metabolism in healthy children. Her plan was as follows: Thirty children aged two to six who are scheduled for elective surgery (orthopedic, urologic, and ophthalmologic) but who are otherwise healthy will be approached for the study. No information is available on normal metabolic rates for this age group. The child's attending physician will give authorization to approach the families. Patients will be admitted to the General Clinical Research Center the evening before their scheduled surgery. These children would normally not come into the hospital until the day of their surgery. Two intravenous lines will be placed after a local anesthetic and EMLA cream. The lines will then later be used in surgery. An eight-hour tracer infusion study with stable isotopes as listed above will be performed. Blood samples, breath analysis, and urine collection will occur at the same time points as the experimental group in the intensive care unit. Compensation will be provided in the form of a $100 gift certificate for toys or clothes.

These cases enabled retreat members to gain a sense of the type and range of issues comprised by the ethics of pediatric research. But looming large in the background of the retreat was a recent twofold development that these cases fail to capture. First, the problem of insufficient data on pediatric medications has become increasingly acute. As noted by a recent policy statement by the American Academy of Pediatrics, "a survey of the 1991 *Physicians Desk Reference* showed that 81% of listed drugs contained language disclaiming use in children or restricting use to certain age groups. A survey of new molecular entities approved by the Food and Drug Administration from 1984 through 1989 revealed that 80% were approved without labeling for children."[4] In 1997, the U.S. Food and Drug Administration (FDA) listed ten drugs widely used for children that contained no or inadequate labeling for use with young people. Included in the FDA's list were the following statistics about drugs prescribed in 1994: Albuterol, an inhalant, was prescribed over 1.5 million times for children with asthma under the age of twelve; Zoloft, an antidepressant, was prescribed 248,000 times for children under the age of sixteen; Ritalin, a treatment for attention deficit disorders, was prescribed 226,000 times for children under the age of six; and Prozac, a treatment for obsessive-compulsive disorder and depression, was prescribed 349,000 times for children under the age of sixteen and 3,000 times for children under the age of one.[5]

It is thus necessary for drugs to be studied in children to determine their safety and effectiveness. Growth, differentiation, and maturation can alter the kinetics, end organ responses, and toxicities of drugs in newborns, infants, children, and adolescents. Drug studies in adult humans may not adequately predict the effects or properties of drugs in children. Given the lack of information about the safety and efficacy of drugs, Loretta Kopelman observes, "clinicians face a dilemma. If they use untested interventions, they may endanger their patients. . . . Yet if clinicians only use tested interventions, they are severely limited in their treatment options."[6] Our culture appears to discriminate against children, leaving them more at risk than adults when it comes to drug safety and efficacy. In the words of one commentator, lack of information and proper labeling about the safety and efficacy of drugs have left children as "therapeutic orphans."[7]

The second development is related to the first. In 1997, Congress passed the Food and Drug Modernization Act, which provides economic incentives to drug companies (six-month extension of patent or market exclusivity) for conducting pediatric clinical trials. In 1998, the FDA proposed a regulation—the "pediatric rule"—requiring data supporting safety and efficacy for pediatric age groups for all new molecular entities and supplemental new drug applications after December 2, 2000.[8] FDA regulations now require drug manufacturers to test new drugs on children, thereby increasing the need for children to serve as research subjects. As a result of these regulations, the FDA has asked the pharmaceutical industry for 332 "postmarketing studies"—to be conducted after a drug has been approved for adults—that could involve more than 20,000 children.[9] In 1998, the National Institutes of Health (NIH) adopted a policy and guidelines that require researchers to include children as research subjects or to explain why they have decided not to do so.[10] Hence IRBs across the country have recently received an increase in research proposals involving children. As a result of these developments, policy and practice have shifted from a protectionist to an inclusionist approach to enrolling children onto medical research trials.[11]

In this chapter, I want to comment on federal regulations and new developments in pediatric research, drawing on cases, comments, and questions from the EAC-IRB retreat as a springboard for reflection about federal rules, the use of money to recruit research subjects, and a legal case involving the use of children in research.[12] To prepare for that discussion, I want first to examine an argument that serves as a benchmark for ethical reflection about pediatric research: Paul Ramsey's trenchant critique of research with children in *The Patient as Person*. Ramsey develops a conservative position regarding pediatric research, and no intelligent treatment of the topic can ignore his argument. Aware of the vulnerability of children, their inability to provide valid consent, and the need to protect them from the interests of others, Ramsey insisted that only therapeutic research with children is permissible. Though there are problems with his position, it lays out paradigmatic terms for approaching the topic of children as research subjects—terms that, properly critiqued, refined, and amended, can instruct us at the levels of theory and practice.

THE ARGUMENT OF PAUL RAMSEY

Ramsey takes up the issue of research with children as the "prismatic case" for the new ethics of medicine in general and the meaning of informed consent in particular.[13] If we accept Albert R. Jonsen's judgment that *The Patient as Person* is "the first truly modern study of the new ethics of science and medicine,"[14] then the case of pediatric research is foundational to bioethics, for it is the first case that Ramsey takes up.

Focusing on the importance of securing informed consent in research and medicine, Ramsey argues restrictively: Children who are unable to consent should not be volunteered for nontherapeutic studies. Ramsey's position captured much of the initial spirit about the ethics of pediatric research, which tended to be protectionist in response to scandals and abuses regarding children in research settings.[15] At the heart of his argument is the following statement:

> Any human being is more than a patient or experimental subject; he is a *personal* subject—every bit as much a man as the physician-investigator. Fidelity is between man and man in these procedures. Consent expresses or establishes this relationship, and the requirement of consent sustains it. Fidelity is the bond between consenting man and consenting man in these procedures. The principle of an informed consent is the cardinal *canon of loyalty* joining men together in medical practice and investigation. In this requirement, faithfulness among men—the faithfulness that is normative for all the covenants or moral bonds of life with life—gains specification for the primary relations peculiar to medical practice.[16]

Coordinating ideas of humane treatment, fidelity, respect for persons, and informed consent, Ramsey sets an absolute limit on all medical experimentation: Experiments may not violate a research subject's autonomy. Without reasonably free and informed consent, "experimentation and medicine itself would speedily become inhumane."[17]

For Ramsey, all nontherapeutic research with children is impermissible because they are unable to provide consent. Equally important, he maintains that *proxies* are eligible to consent for children only when treatment promises to be therapeutic. Ramsey's prose leaves readers with little doubt about his raw feelings: "To experiment on children in ways that are not related to them as patients is already a sanitized form of barbarism."[18] Parents or guardians who agree to volunteer their children reveal a basic failure to care. Ramsey remarks, "No *parent is morally competent* to consent that his child shall be submitted to hazardous or other experiments having no diagnostic or therapeutic significance for this child himself."[19] Ramsey thus rejected the idea of proxy consent to nontherapeutic research as right or good. Recognizing that banning children from nontherapeutic research would leave them without adequate medications and available therapies, he exhorted researchers to "sin bravely": the ethically trustworthy investigator would be one who did not "deny the moral force of the imperative he violates."[20]

By focusing attention on the issue of proxy consent, however, Ramsey confuses two norms that need to be distinguished. His core concern has less to do with respect for autonomy—the principal value grounding informed consent—than with beneficence as a basic principle of pediatric care. On this view, parents are ineligible as proxies if their decisions do not promise to benefit their children. Respect for their autonomy is secondary to a more fundamental test—namely, patient benefit.

Failing to see this point, Ramsey argues at length that nontherapeutic experimentation on children is wrong because it cannot meet the standards of true and informed consent. He writes, "No child or adult incompetent can choose to become a participating member of medical undertakings, and no one else on earth should decide to subject these people to investigations having no relation to their own treatment."[21] But in stating that children cannot choose to become participants in nontherapeutic medical trials, Ramsey proves too much, for children (or at least very young children) cannot competently choose to become participants in *any* medical trials, beneficial or nonbeneficial. Children's incompetency would exclude them from medical research *tout court.*

Ramsey in effect conflates two sets of foundational regulations, those of the Nuremberg Code, drafted in 1945, and the Helsinki Declaration, first drafted in 1964. The Nuremberg Code bans all forms of experimentation with patients who cannot consent. Ramsey prefaces his chapter on pediatric research by citing the Nuremberg Code, which begins by stating, "the voluntary consent of the human subject is absolutely essential."[22] Yet Ramsey adopts a more permissive position, allowing for proxy consent for therapeutic research with nonconsenting human subjects, echoing the principles of the Helsinki Declaration.[23] For Ramsey, there is no problem with parents consenting to experimentation with their child in cases that might prove medically beneficial for that child.[24] His claim that "no parent is morally competent to consent that his child shall be submitted to hazardous or other experiments having no diagnostic or therapeutic significance for this child himself"[25] leaves open the moral possibility of proxies consenting to potentially therapeutic experimentation on children.

Nonetheless, Ramsey's canon of loyalty for protecting noncompetent patients is too broad, for it excludes all young children from any experimentation, which is not his aim or final position. His argument turns on a basic confusion: The fact that he allows parents to permit therapeutic research with children indicates that beneficence, not autonomy, defines the basis for protecting children from being instrumentalized in medical and research contexts. That is to say, beneficence and the corresponding requirement to provide therapeutic treatment specifies the first criterion or canon of loyalty in Ramsey's pediatric ethic, not the criterion of informed consent. *Consent may be secured only for research that has passed a prior test, namely, that it is potentially therapeutic.* On his logic, parental permission is a relevant consideration *after* the treatment's aims are evaluated. His argument on behalf of protecting children is internally gnarled because it presumes that respect for autonomy rather than beneficence can provide a discriminating basis for protecting a young person's basic interests.

Had Ramsey seen matters more clearly, he would have argued that canons of loyalty to a child in research settings must begin not by focusing on criteria for validating parental consent, but with determining whether the proposed intervention is in that child's basic medical interest. Beneficence is a norm that can stand independently of autonomy; each norm is subject to different tests. Ramsey thus stumbled when thinking about pediatric research ethics, seeking to squeeze concerns about care and beneficence into the mold provided by the norm of autonomy and its corresponding requirement, informed consent. One result of his confusion is to invoke substantive concerns to determine the merits of proper procedure. Stated differently, Ramsey mistakenly uses the criterion of *patient benefit* as a test for determining the *competence* of parents or guardians who are asked to provide proxy consent for pediatric experimentation.

Ramsey erred in ways that I have generally sought to correct in this book because he failed adequately to think about basic differences between the ethics of adult and pediatric care. He reasons as if he could extend the adult model of informed consent to the case of research with children. Better instead to distinguish between pediatric and adult paradigms of care in research and medical settings. In the former paradigm, as I indicated at the outset of this work, beneficence is generally prior to the value of autonomy. In its (first) revised form, the pediatric paradigm respects parental autonomy on the condition that such autonomy is constrained by the duty to care. The pediatric paradigm (and its first revision) actually shapes how Ramsey tackles the issue of research with children: Once the beneficent aims of the research have been established, researchers may consider whether the conditions of proxy consent have been satisfied.

The concrete implications of this problem bear directly on how (and to whom) canons of loyalty ought to apply when assessing protocols for pediatric research. Ramsey's theory is designed to assess the competence of parents or guardians as proxies: They are ineligible to grant permission to enroll their child if they agree to nontherapeutic investigations. But that line of argument places the onus on parents without first examining the moral merits of an investigator's proposal. If Ramsey had properly understood his own argument about pediatric ethics, with beneficence as the prior norm, moral responsibility would have been placed first on researchers and those who oversee them rather than on parents.[26] On his terms, researchers who propose nontherapeutic experimentation commit a moral wrong. That is not to say that parents are free of moral responsibility in considering the interests of their child, only that the first line of normative inquiry should target the research proposals of scientific investigators rather than the decisions of parents or guardians. Understanding how to order the values in pediatric research enables us to see that the first line of moral responsibility falls on investigators and IRBs—those who are to review research protocols—not on parents or guardians who may agree to enroll their children.

The pediatric paradigm as it pertains to research with human subjects would help straighten out Ramsey's views, for it would clarify how he actually wanted to rank basic values in pediatric research and it would point us in the right direction when thinking about how to institutionalize screening procedures. Ramsey's restrictions mean that pediatric research should occur within a therapeutic alliance among investigators, proxies, and children, limiting the freedom of parents or guardians in the recruitment of young persons for scientific investigations. As I will argue in the concluding chapter, there are good reasons for supporting some of his reservations about respecting parental autonomy and family privacy given the main lines of a (liberal) ethic of care. But Ramsey's "therapeutic" position does not adequately resolve the specific case of pediatric research, for it bars all forms of nontherapeutic research which, as I have indicated above, is vitally necessary to generate important and beneficial knowledge about (among other things) the effects of drugs on children of different age groups. Ramsey's restrictive position may ironically leave countless children at medical risk, contrary to the spirit if not the letter of the duty to care. Thus the question: Is it possible to allow some nontherapeutic research without sacrificing Ramsey's core concern, namely, the desire to protect children from being unduly instrumentalized, from being treated as things rather than as persons? Assuming the need to produce effective therapies for children *and* the need to protect children from callous utilitarianism, is it permissible to enroll children onto some forms of research without exhorting researchers to "sin bravely?"

One nonutilitarian way to justify some nontherapeutic research on children would be to draw on the ethics of fair play and turn-taking, building on a modified version of the Golden Rule. Given that current children benefit from research performed on previous children, it seems fair to expect current children to shoulder the burden of assisting in further research. The guiding maxim is, "Do unto current and future generations of children as prior generations of children have done unto you." Underlying that maxim is the value of fairness, according to which society is to distribute burdens not only contemporaneously but across time. We all are "thrown" into societies that possess opportunities and benefits that are the result of sacrifices assumed by earlier generations. Our current quality of life is a function in part of discoveries and initiatives for which previous groups are responsible. Those who benefit now from such risks and sacrifices but who refuse altogether to assume some comparable burdens make exceptions of themselves; they are "free riders." Children's medical welfare is a product in part of risks that previous children have assumed, and expecting them to shoulder some burdens of medical research is a function of the need for them to take their turn in the process of improving therapeutic opportunities.[27]

Some nontherapeutic pediatric research may thus be justified on principled rather than utilitarian grounds. The core idea is intergenerational reciprocity, giving in ways that are comparable to the "gifts" that have been received. Here the focus is on children's debts to others who have assumed risks to advance researchers' investigations into therapies that are focused on children's metabolic and psychological peculiarities, knowledge about which cannot be acquired from research on adults or animals. Unlike a utilitarian justification, mine does not look ahead to future benefits to justify burdening current generations. Rather, my justification looks back to prior risks that have helped produce current benefits and opportunities, and asks members of the current generation to assume commensurate burdens. Instead of saying "the ends justify the means," a reciprocity-based rationale for nontherapeutic pediatric research says that it is fair to expect current members of society to assume some of the risks that have helped to produce the benefits that they now enjoy. In that way, we share in our common finitude in the quest to advance human health and well-being.

This rationale should be distinguished not only from a utilitarian rationale, but also from a rationale premised on respect for parental autonomy. Approaching the issue of nontherapeutic pediatric research according to an intergenerational version of the Golden Rule first asks whether imposing risks on children is appropriate. It does not ask whether parents who accept or reject the rule are competent to guard their children's interests. Questions of parental competence would be relevant *after* determining whether the risks of the research are justified. It is not necessary, *pace* Ramsey, to squeeze concerns about pediatric care and the protection from harm into the mold provided by informed consent and its underlying value, autonomy. Following the general contours of the pediatric paradigm, my view is that risks should be evaluated prior to and independent of considerations of parental autonomy and family privacy.

Yet this justification does not open up the door to any and all forms of nontherapeutic pediatric research. Proper limits must be honored. Given children's lack of power, they deserve special protections to safeguard against the possibility of exploitation or abuse. Hence the need to place limits on the risks expected of children—to minimize the risks to which they are subject and to ensure that only minor risks are imposed. Nor is it fair to ask members of one generation to assume unjust burdens on the argument that prior generations have had such burdens imposed on them. Sharing in our common finitude does not entail continuing a legacy of neglect or exploitation. The requirement to constrict nontherapeutic experimental procedures to those involving minimal risks aims appropriately to ensure that the burdens of risk-sharing do not exploit the voiceless and vulnerable.[28]

Over the course of the past thirty years, national policy has developed with an eye toward permitting some forms of nontherapeutic pediatric research. Those permissions are premised on the need to generate potentially valuable knowledge while protecting children from undue burdens or exploitation. Current federal guidelines identify several classes of research with children, each with specific, albeit vague restrictions about how IRBs should screen investigative protocols.

FEDERAL REGULATIONS AND PEDIATRIC RESEARCH

Federal regulations identify four categories of permissible pediatric research, the first three of which I want to analyze carefully.[29] All of these permissions are constrained by the obligation to minimize risks to human subjects in research. Federal regulation 45 CRF46.111 requires investigators to use "procedures which are consistent with sound research design and which do not unnecessarily expose subjects to risk" and, whenever appropriate, to use "procedures already being performed on the subjects for diagnostic or treatment purposes."

The first category permits research with *no greater than "minimal risk"* if it provides for informed parental permission and children's assent (45 CFR46.404). (Throughout the federal guidelines, children's *assent* refers to "a child's affirmative agreement to participate in research." It differs from the idea of assent that I described in Chapter 3 in that it provides children over the age of seven with veto power in research settings.) The second category permits research with *greater than minimal risk* if the risk is justified by the anticipated direct benefit to the child, if the risk/benefit ratio is at least as favorable to each subject as available alternatives, and if adequate provision is made to secure parental permission and the child's assent (45 CFR46.405). These first two categories, respectively, allow minimal risks in all pediatric research, and allow proportionate increases to minimal risks in research that promises to benefit the child directly.

The third category pertains to nontherapeutic research that may go beyond the minimal risk standard (45 CFR46.406). It permits studies with a "minor increase" over minimal risk where the overall risk resembles the child's "actual or expected medical, dental, psychological, or educational situation," the research is likely to yield generalizable knowledge about the subject's disorder which is of vital importance for understanding or ameliorating that disorder, and when provisions are made for parental permission and the child's assent. A researcher may thus enlist children who suffer from a condition that needs to be studied but who may not benefit from the study, if the research involves only a small increase over minimal risk and provides for informed consent.

The fourth category refers to research that cannot fall within the first three categories—for example, nontherapeutic research that exposes a child to more than a minor increase over minimal risk (45 CFR46.408). Such research might be approved if it presents a reasonable opportunity to further the understanding, prevention, or alleviation of a serious pediatric health problem and the study is approved by the secretary of the Department of Health and Human Services after consulting with a panel of experts about the study's ethical aspects, and if adequate provision is made for parental permission and the child's assent.

The first three federal regulations thus allow pediatric research that involves *minimal risk,* research "above" minimal risk in which there is a *proportionate balance* of risk and benefit, and nontherapeutic research that involves a *minor increase* over minimal risk to learn more about a condition from which a child suffers. Note that these regulations follow the main lines of the pediatric paradigm in that they establish a floor of acceptable risk before considerations of parental permission. Federal regulations presume the need to protect research subjects independently of whether their parents or guardians will volunteer their children for research. That is to say, *parental permission may be secured only for treatment that has passed a prior test, namely, that it poses an acceptable level of risk.* Owing to the priority of beneficence (and nonmaleficence) to autonomy, representation and parental "consent" are relevant considerations *after* the treatment's risks and benefits are evaluated.

That is not to say that the regulations are problem-free, however. "Minimal risk" and "minor increase over minimal risk" are subject to widely different interpretations by IRBs. That problem is compounded by the fact that federal regulations' definitions of these categories are vague and confusing.

The *first* permission focuses attention on research that imposes less than "minimal risk." In fact "minimal risk" serves as a guideline in all four regulations. According to U.S. 45 CFR46.102.i, "*Minimal risk* means that the probability and magnitude of harm or discomfort anticipated in the research are not greater in and of themselves than those ordinarily encountered in daily life or during the performance of routine physical and psychological examinations or tests." The initial part of this definition calibrates minimal risk on the standard of risks encountered in ordinary life. The latter part of this definition calibrates minimal risk to risks encountered in routine medical examinations. An immediate difficulty presents itself: These two calibrations are quite different because the risks of ordinary life typically exceed those encountered in routine medical examinations. Hence one question: How "risky" may "minimal risk" be?

Further difficulties appear when we consider this unclear standard of risk in light of the federal regulations' specific permissions for pediatric research. The first permission (45 CFR46.404), as I have noted, allows for pediatric research in which there is less than minimal risk and if the investigator makes adequate provision for parental permission and children's assent. The problem here, as several participants in Baylin's retreat noted, lies in interpreting and applying the "minimal risk" standard. Take the initial part of the definition, which implies a wide range of acceptably risky activity: People encounter different degrees of risk in everyday life, including high-risk activity; many people (firefighters, police, soldiers, emergency medical teams) routinely take on danger in their everyday occupations. If "minimal risk" is seen in light of those facts, then investigators may impose considerable risks on research subjects.

If federal regulations presume that the definition of minimal risk would refer to risks that *children* face in everyday life, matters are no clearer. Children ordinarily encounter a wide range of risks: psychological pressures in school and play; physically demanding practice regimens in the performance arts or sports; personal setbacks in relationships with parents, siblings, and friends; crime and drugs at school or in the neighborhood; high-risk sexual activity during adolescence. Moreover, our culture tolerates widespread neglect of children's welfare. At the retreat, one participant put the point: "Our society tolerates huge risks to children: abuse, poverty, undereducation, vulnerability to disease through underinsurance. In everyday life, children suffer and we as a society do nothing about it."[30] Measuring "minimal risk" on the standard of "risks in everyday life" will provide children with few real protections as research subjects.

The *second* permission (45 CFR46.405), allowing for a proportionate balance of risk and benefit in research that involves greater than minimal risk, adopts a standard from medical practice to regulate research: Risks are justified by prospective benefits. As we saw in Chapter 9, harm to individuals is justified in medical settings on the condition that it is offset by the pursuit of patient benefit. I see no difficulty with this idea as it applies to research with sick children.

However, this regulation bans the use of healthy children as a control group in research that aims to benefit (some) sick children because the healthy children do not stand to benefit from the proposed study. For reasons that I will cite below, this regulation raises questions of distributive justice. Moreover, this regulation is premised on the distinction between interventions that are beneficial to a child-subject, and interventions that aim to benefit children generally. However, only the latter is truly "research," and such research may need to enroll sick and healthy children.

The *third* permission (45 CFR46.406), allowing for a *minor increase* over minimal risks in nontherapeutic research, sets the baseline of permissible risks according to a different standard than the risks of everyday life that all people or children might encounter, or that people typically encounter in routine medical examinations. According to this regulation, permissible risks in nontherapeutic research must be "commensurate with those inherent in [the subject's] actual or expected medical, dental, psychological, social, or educational situations."

Once again we're met with the fact that some situations—school, for example—allow a fair amount of high-risk activity, such as field hockey or football practice. Moreover, and more problematically, this permission allows for unequal levels of risk, depending on the sickness of the child or the child's familiarity with and tolerance of various procedures given his or her medical history. The sicker children are or have been, the more they may experience interventions imposed for purposes of research, because sick children encounter many more invasive procedures in the course of their medical treatment. By allowing risks with some children that would be prohibited in other children, the regulation appears to produce a double standard of protection.

One prong of this regulation would forbid nontherapeutic research on healthy children altogether, and herein lies another problem with the federal regulations. According to 45 CFR46.406(c), nontherapeutic research should aim to "yield generalizable knowledge about the subjects' disorder or condition which is of vital importance for the understanding or amelioration of the subjects' disorder or condition." That requirement allows investigators to recruit children who suffer from a general condition but who would not benefit from the research. Children who are healthy are ineligible from this research, removing them as a control group in investigative studies. Thus another double standard exists, one that allows researchers to recruit from only one pool of children—namely, sick ones, thereby distributing the overall burdens of research inequitably.

Federal regulations were promulgated in 1983 and need to be reconsidered. At that time, few studies included children as research subjects, and the general ethos was protectionist rather than inclusionist. Given recent incentives to enroll children onto medical research trials, and given the increase in complex and sophisticated research methods, federal regulations need to be revisited. To that end, I recommend consideration of the following issues, perhaps by a special bioethics commission that convenes a national forum on the ethics of pediatric research. Composed of pediatricians, researchers, ethicists, parents, and children of different ages, the commission should seek to ascertain how medical professionals have interpreted and applied the ideas of "minimal risk" and "minor increase over minimal risk" in investigative settings. The commission should solicit information in a national forum and through a questionnaire that is widely distributed to medical researchers and families, with sections for children to complete when possible. That attempt should seek to gather information about and resolve the following issues.

1. *The categories of "minimal risk" and "minor increase over minimal risk" need to be reviewed, with concrete cases and practices in mind.* Do multiple venipunctures exceed "minimal risk"? If so, how many? Similar questions about whether specific interventions are acceptable as either minimally risky or only a minor increase over minimal risk should be discussed: lumbar punctures, aspirating bone marrow, pricking an ear drum, administering a placebo, to name a few. Consider Waters's third case above: Is withdrawing prescribed medications from children with ADHD a "minimal risk"? Is it justified because the prospective benefits outweigh the risks to those research subjects? Why should children who already have access to safe and effective medications be made ill with, for example, the use of placebos rather than medication, in order to promote medical research?[31] Data about these and related matters indicate that researchers' views of "minimal risk" vary widely across the United States.[32]

2. *New regulations must incorporate developmental factors.* Current federal regulations show no attention to differences in childhood development and maturity.[33] Some interventions may be experienced as more stressful by children who are younger or developmentally delayed than by "normal" adolescents. The second case I describe above should call attention to special challenges posed by developmental differences. No less than in medical care, the ethics of calibration should inform pediatric research. Having fixed notions of risk and acceptable increases to risk that do not account for levels of development or maturity among children will likely prove exasper-

ating to investigators. Marilyn Waters, the mother of a preadolescent boy and the Director of Research Compliance on Baylin's IRB, observes, "At different ages they'll be different levels. Some places have separate forms for different levels."[34]

My recommendation would be to abandon the distinction between "minimal risk" and "minor increase over minimal risk" in pediatric research. In its place, I would recommend maintaining a standard of "minimal risk" calibrated in two ways. For preadolescents, I would recommend a standard of minimal risk that is calibrated to the inconveniences that may be intentionally imposed by standard physical and psychological examinations. The core idea would be to use standards in the medical world to set expectations for what can be allowed in research. For adolescents, I would propose maintaining the standard of minimal risk for research that would be calibrated in light of risks that teenagers take on voluntarily in high-quality school or work environments, or that may be intentionally imposed on them in those environments for educational and developmental purposes.[35] That is to say, for adolescents, we would calibrate risks not according to the risks that they must endure in socially impoverished contexts, but according to what we know characterizes workplaces and schools that meet the gold standard for childhood safety and welfare. For research that enrolls children younger than seven, parental permission would be required. For research involving children seven and older, the assent of the child and parental permission would both be required.

The advantage to these changes would be to eliminate the confusions and contradictions that surround the idea of a "minor increase over minimal risk" for pediatric research, the different expectations of risk in research that seeks direct benefit for the child as opposed to information about, for example, the child's condition. At the same time, we may allow increases that are indexed to the child's age and maturity. The background idea is that society allows for increasing risks in school and play as children mature. It seems commonsensical to draw from those habits and patterns of changing expectations in the world of childhood education and development to guide standards of risk in research settings. Having a simpler and more straightforward standard to apply to pediatric research is necessary. Hence my suggestion: Pediatric research must impose no more than minimal risks in nontherapeutic research. The older the research subject, the more risks researchers and IRBs might reasonably consider, premised on standards that pertain to school and play. (Enrolling children for nontherapeutic research is justified according to the idea of turn-taking and fair play, as I argued above.[36]) For studies that promise to benefit the subject, then (as with current federal regulations), risks must be proportionate to benefits.

The rationale for allowing nontherapeutic research that includes a minor increase over minimal risk cannot be justified. According to the federal regulations, studies may impose a "minor increase over minimal risk" when the research is likely to yield generalizable knowledge about the subject's disorder which is of vital importance for understanding or ameliorating that disorder. This permission allows adults to enroll children if the costs to the research subject are outweighed by the potential benefits to society and medicine. Justifying pediatric research in this way instrumentalizes children. It allows the ends to justify the means and increases risks to a vulnerable population.

3. *Cultural factors should be considered.* Recall from the story of Lia Lee that a lumbar puncture, a procedure that is considered routine by some medical professionals, raises enormous worries among the Hmong, who fear that such a puncture will lead to a flight of a person's soul. New regulations must be crafted with the awareness that biomedicine has its own culture, and that medical investigators must learn how nonmainstream cultures and traditions view others' conceptions of high- and low-risk activity.

4. *The issue of equity in distributing research risks needs to be discussed.* As I noted above, current regulations prohibit researchers to recruit healthy children but permit them to recruit sick children (45 CFR46.406[c]) onto some protocols.[37]

REIMBURSEMENT, RECOGNITION, RECRUITMENT, AND INDUCEMENT

The most animated discussion at the EAC-IRB retreat focused on the increasing role of money in pediatric research. Federal regulations make no reference to the appropriateness of financial payments in research with human subjects, but recent developments have rendered the problem acute in pediatrics. Waters expressed her concerns: "The FDA's exclusivity law . . . allows drug companies 6 extra months for their patent if they do pediatric trials. This is a good idea; we can't avoid pediatrics anymore. However, now there is a financial incentive for drug companies to do this. I sense this pressure. There are not huge cohorts of kids who are sick. So companies are willing to pay children for their participation."[38] The FDA's provision has proven lucrative to pharmaceutical companies. Eli Lilly received a six-month extension for Prozac, its antidepressant, enabling the company to reap an additional $1 billion in sales, $700 million of it in profits.[39]

In addition, Waters observed, "there are financial issues between drug companies and investigators. There are extra bonuses offered if investigators succeed in increasing the pool of research subjects. Research nurses, too. They can get $50 if they recruit someone."[40] A report in the *New York Times* indicates that researchers can earn $2,000 for each child they recruit in a pediatric drug trial.[41]

Recall that the pediatric paradigm sets a baseline of acceptable risk prior to and independent of parental permission. As it pertains to pediatric research, the pediatric paradigm generally presumes a priority of beneficence (and its minimal standard, nonmaleficence) to autonomy. But even with a baseline of acceptable risk in place, children remain vulnerable to having risks imposed on them, for researchers' conduct or parents' judgments can be unduly affected in ways that render children less than adequately protected. In a capitalist society, offering money or material goods provides one obvious way to reward sacrifices and provide incentives for people to act in one or another way. Whether that is a good thing in pediatric research—whether it compromises an investigator's or a parent's integrity—is an important matter to consider. Although Waters's comments reverse the priority of beneficence to autonomy in the care of children, her remarks summarize the problem: "The element of coercion is so much a part of the informed consent process. To respect autonomy, the decision has to be removed from coercive processes. Then there is the idea of children as a vulnerable population. How do we protect them? We like to think of parents as making decisions in their [children's] best interests. That may be true. Are they likely if there's a large sum of money attached?"[42]

Exactly how we are to understand the problems that surround money in pediatric research requires some important distinctions. Helena Kramer, a fellow in Baylin's Office of Ethics, put the question provocatively: "Why are parents and kids expected to be 'pure' of money while researchers and companies can be motivated by money?"[43]

To Kramer, we can say that money can operate in legitimate and illegitimate ways; hence the need for moral categories and limits. Moreover, money's illegitimacy needs to be understood properly, requiring additional distinctions that reflect some of the special challenges of working with children. Money can operate legitimately when it functions to repay families for time, inconvenience, and their out-of-the-pocket expenses. It may also function appropriately as an expression of gratitude for a child's contribution to medical research. It operates inappropriately when it serves as an incentive for adults to volunteer or recruit children. The key distinction is between money as a form of reciprocity and money as a form of inducement. Providing a set of restrictions that permit the limited role of money in pediatric research is of utmost necessity.

As *reimbursement* for inconvenience and out-of-the-pocket expenses, money serves an appropriate function. Families who volunteer children for research incur expenses for travel, parking, meals, child care, and loss of work time, to name the most obvious costs. Research protocols that assign funds to compensate families for their inconvenience and out-of-pocket expenses are justified by reciprocity. One mechanism for maintaining limits on such compensations would be to set a per diem rate that is sufficient to accommodate a reasonable range of expenses, following the model of universities' reimbursements to professors for travel and research expenses. Families whose expenses exceed the per diem rate could be compensated after they complete a request for supplemental compensation, providing a rationale, receipts, and the like to support their claims.

As an *expression of gratitude,* small gifts can fulfill the norm of reciprocity, returning the kindness of a child's time and generosity. Moreover, small gifts can function as a means of *recognition,* acknowledging (and positively reinforcing) a child's volunteerism in a public way. As I noted in Chapter 9, civic agapism is an important virtue for civil society, and hospitals have a stake in fostering it, providing one avenue for connecting with their "moral constituency."[44] In order to reduce the chance that these expressions might become inducements to volunteer, however, it may be wise to exclude this feature of the research protocol from the consent process. As a policy statement of the American Academy of Pediatrics observes, "If remuneration is to be provided to the child, it is best if it is not discussed before the study's completion. This will help assure that the remuneration is not part of the reasons that a child volunteered or is volunteered for the study."[45] On that account, the third case above is problematical. Offering $200 to research subjects is a clear inducement to volunteer. The offer should have been excluded from the research protocol.

As an *incentive for researchers to recruit research subjects,* money functions perniciously. The danger of a conflict of interest is obvious. Although no researcher is free of bias, money only adds to the problem of self-interest. IRBs that nonetheless allow researchers to be rewarded for enlisting subjects should require them to disclose that fact in the informed consent process. Baylin's policy on this matter is admirably strict: In no circumstances may medical staff, hospital staff, or house officers accept any type of recruitment incentive provided by a sponsor above and beyond the actual costs associated with enrolling and evaluating a research subject.

Similarly, money functions perniciously when it is offered as a *reward to parents or guardians,* above the per diem reimbursement they rightly deserve for their time, inconvenience, and out-of-pocket expenses. Providing financial incentives for parents or guardians generates an obvious temptation to overlook the basic interests of their children.

These concerns about the role of money as reimbursement, recognition, inducement, and reward provide only broad parameters for evaluating possible conflicts of interest in pediatric research. My comments are deliberately sketchy and overlook important variables in childhood development. For example, paying adolescents for their time in research studies may be a fair expression of reciprocity given the fact that adolescents understand that their time has monetary worth. For some adolescents, payment may be justified to compensate for loss of comparable work time. In any event, the role of money in pediatric research calls out for more fine-grained analysis. Hence another topic for a national commission on pediatric research:

5. *The proper and improper role of money as an incentive for research and recruitment in pediatric trials, (again) with appropriate attention to research subjects' differences in development and maturity.*

Why money operates inappropriately as an inducement needs to be considered. The standard idea—repeated several times at the EAC-IRB retreat—is that money functions coercively, attenuating the parent's autonomy or corrupting the investigator's integrity. On that account, the core value at stake is freedom and self-determination: Money poisons the consent and research situation by introducing factors that naturally lead to mixed motives. A parent or guardian's decision is no longer "purely" free and disinterested, but is bound by self-interest. So, too, with the researcher's incentives: A researcher motivated by profit does not seek knowledge disinterestedly, but out of financial interest. Hence researchers may devise efforts to coerce parents or children into participating in a study.

This understanding of money's dangers can confuse us, for it proceeds from basic intuitions that inform the adult paradigm of informed consent in medical and research settings. That is not to say that we should ignore the issue of freedom and consent altogether, but attention to differences in pediatric contexts is necessary here. In adult medicine, patients should not be coerced or unduly influenced by a medical professional; adult decision making begins from a presumption against professional power and paternalism. Out of respect for patient freedom and equality, professionals are to respect their adult patients' informed decisions to accept or refuse treatment. But in pediatric research, autonomy is not always or obviously the chief value to be honored, and worrying about its demands can mislead.

In Chapter 4, I argued that issues of permission or "consent" in pediatric settings can be informed by distinctions drawn from political philosophy. I argued that, generally speaking, proxies function in pediatric contexts as *guardians* on behalf of young children, and as *delegates* or as *representatives* with adolescents. One idea is that guardians cannot rely on the (precompetent) wishes of persons whose interests they are to defend. They are to *care for,* not *speak for,* others.

In pediatric research contexts, it is not a parent or guardian's *autonomy* that is chiefly at stake when material inducements are introduced, but their resolve to act on the duty to care. If we were to assign respect to parental decisions owing to the value of autonomy, we would say that such decisions "are 'worthy of respect' . . . in virtue of being 'the product of free and voluntary choice,' in virtue of being beliefs of a self unencumbered by convictions antecedent to choice."[46] The core principle would be respect for the dignity that inheres in the capacity to choose freely. Given the general priority of beneficence to autonomy in pediatrics, however, we must remember that proxies are responsible for *protecting* precompetent children as research subjects. Herein lies the basic reason for limiting the place of money as a means of recruitment: It may weaken the responsibility of parents or guardians to care for those who cannot defend their basic interests in investigative settings. Stated differently, money puts virtue at risk.

We thus come full circle to issues that are central to the world of pediatrics. Money should be limited owing not to the value of self-determination for free and equal persons, but owing to the demands of moral responsibility in the care of children. Given the need to triangulate care in pediatric settings, money poses a different danger than in adult settings. With adults, money can weaken the capacities of patients to deliberate freely about whether they want to take on risks in research. With children, the influence of money is socialized; it can produce a conflict of interest between parents and children.

If money or material reward has a place beyond reimbursing families for their time, inconvenience, and out-of-the pocket expenses, it should be limited to expressions of gratitude for the sacrifices or risks that the research subjects endure. The basic virtue is reciprocity, the disposition to return in kind. Limited in that way, studies will have fewer incentives for others to recruit or volunteer research subjects for reasons that may conflict with children's basic interests.

Such limits pertain to matters of parental permission and research integrity. The reach of money is more extensive, however. In drug research, money can intrude into larger, "macro"-level aspects of pediatric research because it generates incentives for companies to test only patented drugs, allowing drugs whose patents have expired to remain untested. Again we see the danger of an asymmetry, this time between cohorts of drugs rather than between cohorts of patients. The FDA's exclusivity law did not spur testing of some drugs that are widely used for children, including albuterol (for asthma), and ampicillin (an antibiotic), because they lack patent protection.[47] Waters recognized the issue: "One problem concerns off-patent drugs that we are using that have not been tested. These remain."[48] Hence another issue for policy and practice:

6. *Determining which drugs, especially off-patent drugs, need to be tested for their effects on children.*[49]

TESTING CHILDREN FOR ENVIRONMENTAL HAZARDS

Though not dealing with children and drug research, two cases brought before the Maryland Court of Appeals (Maryland's highest court) illumine important moral issues surrounding pediatric research: *Grimes v. Kennedy*

Krieger Institute, Inc., and *Myron Higgins, a minor, etc., et al., v. Kennedy Krieger Institute, Inc.* Taken up in one decision by the court,[50] these cases concern alleged negligence involving children who developed elevated levels of lead dust in their blood while participating in a research study by the Kennedy Krieger Institute (KKI), a research outfit associated with Johns Hopkins University. Between 1993 and 1996, researchers at KKI tested children who were residing in homes undergoing different degrees of lead paint abatement in Baltimore. At the time the study was planned, investigators estimated that 95 percent of low-income housing in Baltimore had lead hazards, and that 40 to 50 percent of the children living in these homes had elevated lead levels in their blood.[51] Landlords in Baltimore's low-income housing were eligible to receive subvention from the state of Maryland for lead abatement modifications. Aware of this state program, KKI enrolled children from families living in the low-income housing to test the effectiveness of different levels of lead abatement modifications. Before embarking on the experiment, Dr. Mark Farfel and his associates at KKI submitted their proposal to the Johns Hopkins University Joint Committee on Clinical Investigation—the Hopkins IRB—for review.[52]

The specific aim of the research was to find the cost of the minimal level of effective lead paint or lead dust abatement procedures in order to help landlords assess the commercial feasibility of attempting to abate lead dust in low rent urban housing. The goal was *not* to remove all lead paint and dust, but to find a less than complete level of abatement that would be safe and economical, enabling Baltimore landlords with lower socioeconomic rental units to retain their properties. (The cost of full abatement far exceeded with value of the properties themselves.) Children living in five groups of homes of twenty-five homes each were to have their blood tested six times over a two-year period. Homes in Groups I, II, and III were all known to have lead and received different degrees of repair. The amount of renovation increased from Group I to Group II to Group III. Homes in Groups IV and V were assumed to be safe, either because they had been previously abated of all lead paint and dust (Group IV), or because they were built after lead paint had been banned in the United States (Group V). Children in homes I, II, and III would have their contamination levels compared with each other and with children who resided in Groups IV and V. Children in Groups IV and V thus functioned as a control group.

Two cases were brought to the Maryland Court of Appeals by families who lost their civil suits against KKI in lower court rulings. The Court of Appeals sent the cases back to the Circuit Court of Baltimore City for trial, but not before making sweepingly condemnatory statements about the research. The court's dictum is restrictive: "In our view, otherwise healthy children should not be the subjects of nontherapeutic experimentation or research that has the potential to be harmful to the child."[53] The court thus limits parental authority: "In nontherapeutic research using children, we hold that the consent of the parent alone cannot make appropriate that which is innately inappropriate."[54] Because there are few state court cases involving research with children, this decision by the Maryland Court of Appeals will be closely watched and will likely have a chilling effect on pediatric research.

According to the first case, *Grimes v. Kennedy Krieger Institute, Inc.*, KKI recruited Viola Hughes in March 1993 to conduct research on her home and her daughter, Ericka Grimes. Hughes had lived on Monroe Street in Baltimore since 1990. Although her home was part of Group IV, and presumably safe from contamination, researchers immediately found several "hot spots" where the level of lead was "higher than might be found in a completely renovated house."[55] This information was not furnished to Hughes until December 1993, nine months after it had been discovered, and three months after Ericka's blood was found to contain highly elevated levels of lead.

Hughes sued KKI for failing to warn of or abate lead paint hazards that researchers found in her home. As a result of KKI's negligence, Hughes argued, she and her daughter were unaware of the dangers to which the daughter was being exposed. Hughes alleged that KKI's consent form did not adequately disclose the fact that the child might accumulate lead in her blood, or that in order for the research to succeed, it was necessary for the child to remain in the house for two years.

According to the second case, *Myron Higgins, a minor, etc., et al., v. Kennedy Krieger Institute, Inc.*, Mr. Polakoff, a landlord, volunteered some of his property for KKI's lead abatement study. Polakoff owned property on Federal Street in Baltimore that had documented levels of lead based paint in the unit. Once accepted into the state program, that property was assigned to Group II of partial abatement, which was completed in April 1994.

Catina Higgins began renting the Federal Street property in May 1994. Later that month, Ms. Higgins agreed to enroll her home and her son, Myron Higgins, in KKI's study, enabling researchers to collect dust samples from Higgins's home and to obtain blood samples from Myron. According to her suit, KKI's consent form did not clearly disclose that children would accumulate some level of blood contamination and that obtaining children's blood would be one way to determine the effectiveness of various abatement procedures.

In May 1994, researchers collected dust in two ways: using an experimental cyclone dust vacuum, and wiping dust from surfaces in the home. Higgins was only given information derived from the latter, less sophisticated method. Although the cyclone vacuum samples showed high levels of dust concentration, the dust wipe samples indicated that no area in her house had concentrations higher than a newly renovated house, and KKI only reported this second, "safer" set of data. Results from Myron's blood tests in July, August, and December 1994 showed that he had concentrations ranging from moderately elevated to highly elevated. When she learned this fact, Higgins sued, arguing that KKI was negligent for not arranging a full abatement of lead dust in her home and claiming that researchers misled her about the hazards in her home by only informing her of the dust samples taken from the less sophisticated, dust-wipe method.

In each case, KKI provided material incentives to participants. In return for enrolling in KKI's study, families were given $5 for answering questions and for allowing researchers to sketch their homes, and $15 for completing a questionnaire. Researchers also promised to provide parents with specific blood-lead results, and to contact families to discuss house test results and how to reduce risks of exposure. In addition, the court found a "stream of compensation flowing to the research subjects and the parents."[56] The researchers' application to the Environmental Protection Agency for funding approval stated that

> a number of incentives are planned both in the clinic and in the home of the type that were well received in the recently completed Maryland Lead in Soil Project, i.e., (1) coupons for things ranging from skating trips to groceries; (2) gifts for the children such as T-shirts in the summer, and hats and gloves during winter clinic appointments; (3) ongoing incentives for parents such as $10 to $20 food coupons provided at each clinic visit for blood collection.[57]

According to the court,

> otherwise healthy children . . . should not be enticed into living in, or remaining in, potentially lead-tainted housing and intentionally subjected to a research program, which contemplates the probability, or even the possibility, of lead poisoning or even the accumulation of lower levels of lead in the blood, in order for the extent of the contamination of the children's blood to be used by scientific researchers to assess the success of lead paint or lead dust abatement measures.[58]

In its lengthy discussion of these cases, the court raised numerous legal and ethical points; I will comment on the latter here.[59] The court's position that "otherwise healthy children should not be the subjects of nontherapeutic experimentation or research that has the potential to be harmful to the child"[60] imposes a stricter limit on pediatric research than we find in the federal regulations because those regulations allow for a minor increase over minimal risk in research that examines a general medical condition but that does not promise direct benefit to research subjects if they agree to participate in the study and their parents permit them to do so. Indeed, the court appears to rule out the imposition of *any* risk, thereby voiding the possibility of any form of nontherapeutic research. That position would ban virtually all forms of pediatric research in the state of Maryland.

Beyond this problem, four specific issues present themselves: How to understand (1) the risks and benefits proposed by KKI's research, (2) parental authority and consent (3) the responsibilities of researchers and IRBs in human subjects research, and (4) the matter of material incentives offered to parents and children.

The first issue concerns how to understand the risks and benefits imposed by KKI's research. Note that some of the children enrolled onto the study were already residing in low-income housing with high levels of lead. It is not the case that KKI imposed those risks onto the research subjects; as residents of old homes, the children were subject to such risks regardless of the research. An analogy would be research on persons who live near Superfund sites to monitor the effects of toxic waste on their health. The research does not place the subjects at risk, but aims to measure environmental risks of subjects who reside in unhealthy areas. On this description, the risks that researchers intentionally imposed were confined to drawing blood and asking questions. The investigative procedures did not expose the children to more than minimal risk, even if their environment did.

For this reason, it may well be that the research on the children in homes with lead hazards abided by the federal guidelines. Recall that federal regulations in pediatric research allow research that involves *minimal risk,* research with risks "above" minimal risk in which there is a *proportionate balance* of risk and benefit, and nontherapeutic research that involves a *minor increase* over minimal risk in order to study a child's condition. Research that imposes further increases in risk must be submitted for review at the federal level. Given the data available at this writing, the venipunctures and survey appear to fall within the category of minimal risk.

The court devotes scant attention to this vital issue of the appropriate level of risk and the distinction between risks imposed by the investigation and risks imposed by the environment. Granting the difficulties in interpreting and applying this standard of minimal risk, the court should have asked KKI's researchers how they viewed risks to the children in their investigations. Unfortunately, the court speaks only once—and vaguely—to this issue, stating that "there was clearly more than minimal risk involved."[61]

The research's benefits also seem to have been misunderstood. The court recurrently referred to the research as "nontherapeutic," understood as research that "generally utilizes subjects who are not known to have the condition the objectives of the research are designed to address, and/or is not designed to directly benefit the subjects utilized in the research."[62] But enrolling healthy children onto pediatric trials does not necessarily mean that the research is nontherapeutic. For example, healthy children can be vaccinated and thereby benefit from a medical intervention. The key factor is not whether the research subject is ill, but whether he or she can benefit from the research. On that account, KKI's research might be labeled "therapeutic" because its results could inform the parents about the need to lower their children's blood levels.

Still, there is some uncertainty as to KKI's moral and perhaps legal liability regarding the risks to which the children were exposed. The court alleges that "in return for permitting the properties to be used and for limiting their tenants to families with young children, KKI assisted the landlords in applying for grants or loans of money to be used to perform the levels of abatement required by KKI for each class of home."[63] Whether this is true will be determined by the trials remanded to the Circuit Court of Baltimore City. If the allegation is true, then KKI may have been complicit in exposing children to hazards that obviously go well beyond the risks of venipunctures and survey questions.

The second issue turns on matters of consent. The court approached the cases within the broad contours of the pediatric paradigm, in which considerations of appropriate risk are prior to the matter of informed consent. "If the research methods . . . are inappropriate . . . then the consent of the parents, or of any consent surrogates, in our view, cannot make the research appropriate or the actions of the researchers and the Institutional Review Board proper."[64] On the matter of foreseeable risks and informed consent, the court correctly understood that the task of assessing risks stands independently of the ethics of informed consent. Parents' consent is not sufficient to authorize research on children. Indeed, according to the court, parental rights are no stronger than researchers' rights; both are subject to the same measure: "Parents . . . have no more right to intentionally and unnecessarily place children in potentially hazardous nontherapeutic research surroundings than do researchers. In such cases, parental consent, no matter how informed, is insufficient."[65]

In my view, the court is correct in framing the consent requirements in this way: risks should be assessed prior to and independent of parental consent to pediatric research. More controversial is the requirement to provide informed consent *during* the study itself. In the court's mind, researchers have the duty to ensure that consent is truly informed—that full disclosure of risks is essential, before *and* during the study. The key of informed consent is to provide information for subjects "to freely choose whether to participate, and continue to participate, and receive promptly any information that might bear on their willingness to continue to participate in the study."[66] The court calls for a dynamic, ongoing duty to seek informed consent when new information becomes available that bears on the interests and welfare of research subjects. For KKI to presume that consent is valid when not all the risks are known is to turn the informed consent process into an empty formality. The core idea, as the Nuremberg Code makes clear, is that proper consent must include information about *all* the risks that subjects might encounter from their participation in the experiment, not just those imposed by the researchers' interventions (venipunctures and questionnaires).[67]

In the care of children, beneficence constrains respect for parental autonomy. That idea shapes how we are to understand adults' responsibilities in pediatric research. As I noted when discussing Ramsey, moral responsibility should first be placed on researchers and those who oversee them rather than on parents. That is not to say that parents have no moral responsibilities when enrolling their children onto research trials, only that the first line of normative inquiry should target the proposals of scientific investigators.

On this count the court hammered home a criticism of the Hopkins IRB, and herein lies the third aspect of the case to which I want to draw attention. An initial draft of the KKI research protocol received the following response from the IRB:

> *Federal guidelines are really quite specific regarding using children as controls in property in which there is no potential benefits.* To call a control a normal control is to indicate that there is no benefit to be received. . . . So we think it would be much more acceptable to indicate that the "control group" is being studied to determine what exposure outside the home may play in total lead exposure[,] thereby indicating that these control individuals are gaining some benefit, namely, learning whether safe housing alone is sufficient to keep the blood levels in acceptable bounds. We suggest that you modify the consent forms . . . accordingly.[68]

In the court's view, the Hopkins IRB "encouraged the researchers to misrepresent the purpose of the research in order to bring the study under the label of 'therapeutic' and thus under a lower safety standard of regulation."[69] More generally, the IRB abdicated its role as watchdog and advocate for the interests of research subjects, and sought to help researchers instead. In this the IRB failed in its duty: "An IRB's primary role is to assure the safety of human research subjects—not help researchers avoid safety or health-related requirements."[70]

As I noted above, however, there are plausible reasons to describe KKI's research as therapeutic in that it promised to provide information that would directly benefit the families in the study. Consider the presence of the control group—the most difficult cohort to describe as benefiting from the research. The control group was not deliberately exposed to unabated lead poisoning in order to compare their blood levels with the blood levels of the children residing in the modified housing. Because lead was likely to exist in the soil around the housing of the new and fully abated housing, the children in those homes would likely register increased levels of lead and would benefit from knowing that fact; so too with the children in housing that had lead paint. Calling such research "therapeutic" for these groups was not a ruse.

Fourth is the court's discussion of compensation and incentives. Legal defense in *Grimes* admitted that "there was some remuneration involved as incentive [in KKI's research] to get the participants to enroll and continue to follow through."[71] The court described the families as "improperly enticed by trinkets, food stamps, money or other items"[72] and worried that such incentives compromised parents' ability to provide free and informed consent. Although this worry is generally on target, we do well to remember the core value that ought to inform the court's concerns. Given the general priority of beneficence to autonomy in pediatrics, parents or guardians should *protect* precompetent children as research subjects. Herein lies the basic reason for limiting money or other material incentives as a means of recruitment: It may weaken the responsibility of parents to care for those who cannot defend their basic interests in investigative settings. Unfortunately, the court failed to probe either the problems around KKI's recruitment efforts or the underlying values at stake.

Throughout its discussion of both cases, the court claims that there are various kinds of "special relationships" that give rise to a "duty of care." One question the court puts to itself is whether research situations create special relationships that imply a corresponding duty of care, including the duty to warn research participants about risks they are experiencing in the course of an investigation. The court all but answered that question in the affirmative as it remanded the *Grimes* and *Higgins* cases to the lower court.

The court's dictum that "otherwise healthy children should not be the subjects of nontherapeutic experimentation or research that has the potential to be harmful to the child."[73] returns matters in Maryland to Ramsey's argument. One hears echoes of his claim that "to experiment on children in ways that are not related to them as patients is already a sanitized form of barbarism."[74] The court should be commended for its attention to the duties of researchers and IRBs, for its understanding of the structure and demands of parental permission regarding pediatric research, and for its concerns about the potential collusion between researchers and landlords who had a financial interest in recruiting or retaining tenants. The court should be faulted for imposing a standard of protection that exceeds that required by federal regulations, for failing to distinguish the risks imposed by KKI's research from the environmental risks, for overlooking how research subjects might benefit from participating in the study, and for failing to indicate why incentives were a problem in KKI's research.

DISTINGUISHING BETWEEN
UTILITARIANISM AND PATERNALISM

Pediatric research covers a broad range of scientific questions, medical and social needs, and investigative practices. But whatever the specifics, in pediatric research adults are responsible for trying to avoid a potential danger that differs from potential dangers in pediatric medicine. Up to this chapter, our main focus has been on the duties and virtues of medical professionals and parents or guardians, and their need to form a therapeutic alliance in medical contexts. Accordingly, the main idea is to craft how we are to conceive of professional and parental responsibilities in relation to patients who are young and sick. One danger is *paternalism,* the idea that "doctors know best." Medicine tempts professionals to infantalize patients or parents, treating them "below" their capacities and competencies. My arguments on behalf of a presumption in favor of parental autonomy and the idea of a child's basic interests develop with an eye toward limiting professional power without completely barring the possibility of intervention and rescue.

In research contexts, other dangers loom. Here the challenge is to protect research subjects from *utilitarianism*—from being instrumentalized in researchers' quests for scientific knowledge. Ramsey was rightly concerned about this problem, however much he might have overreached in his efforts to protect against it. More generally, Ramsey might mislead if we take research with human subjects as the "prismatic case" for modern bioethics. Rather than posing the danger of infantalizing patients, research poses the danger of unduly sacrificing their interests for the collective good. In paternalistic contexts, I must subordinate my freedom to another person's account of *my* overall welfare. In utilitarian contexts, I must subordinate my freedom to the demands of *others'* overall welfare.

Paternalism and utilitarianism are twin dangers in bioethics, but they rear their ugly heads in different institutional settings. Physicians must be guarded against the former, researchers the latter. No less than virtue, vice sometimes involves a division of labor. In research hospitals such as Baylin, the same person may occupy both roles. That said, it is important to keep those roles and their corresponding temptations distinct.

In the quest for safer and more effective pediatric care, it is vitally necessary to learn more about how children at different stages are affected by various illnesses, drug treatments, and other interventions. It is no less imperative to protect children as research subjects in the investigative process. Thus it is necessary to balance children's interest in access to safe and effective treatments with their interest in bodily and psychological welfare in research settings. At least six issues shape how children's needs must be considered, and how we must guard against situating children within adults' conflicts of interest.[75]

In my view, pediatric research is justified on principled terms, as an expression of turn-taking, reciprocity, and fair play. But that justification includes limits that aim to protect children from exploitation and abuse. Potentially therapeutic research should be limited by proportionality; the burdens may not outweigh prospective benefits. Nontherapeutic research should be confined to studies that impose minimal risk, where risk is calibrated according to age and maturity. In all research investigations, children seven and older must provide consent, and parents of all children must provide permission. Allocating money is justified to reimburse families and express gratitude to children for taking their turn in assuming risks to benefit current and future generations of young and ill patients.

Conclusion:
On Liberal Care

In Parts I and II of this book, I sought to draw broad contours of pediatric bioethics (*Moralität*) as a framework for considering specific issues and experiences in the medical culture of pediatric care (*Sittlichkeit*). Although Part I emphasized an ethics-distant orientation and Part II an ethics-near orientation to medical ethics, I sought to keep both orientations in focus in proceeding from theory to culture, from contours to cases. I want to conclude by isolating and commenting on a topic that is fundamental to both parts, namely, the family in private and public life. As we saw in Part I, there are strong, albeit qualified, reasons for respecting parental autonomy and family privacy. As we saw in Part II, there are good reasons for outsiders sometimes to intrude into a family's internal affairs. Both of these facts remind us that parental autonomy has presumptive, but not absolute, weight in cases regarding a child's welfare. Many parents make decisions for their children in fear and trembling, but what do we make of those who don't?

In Chapter 2, we saw why, and to what extent, parental autonomy ought to be respected, and now I want to identify reasons why the shield of family privacy should not be impenetrable. My reasons are moral, political, or a combination of both. Not all of them warrant intervention in the domestic lives of others, but each of them points to reasons why families are not immune from moral criticism, either from within or from without.[1] Whether a child is raised by a married couple, a single parent, a divorced couple sharing custody rights, a gay or lesbian couple, an unmarried heterosexual couple, or grandparents, or in a women's collective or a kibbutz, they have certain basic claims to protection and care.

My ideas draw largely from liberal philosophy, especially the ideas of John Rawls, which is sometimes associated with promoting a high level of freedom and tolerance in nonpublic affairs—thereby making it difficult to evaluate or intrude in the domestic lives of families. Contrary to that impression, Rawls includes the family in the "basic structure" to which the principles of justice ought to apply.[2] To be sure, Rawls does little to develop those ideas systematically, leaving untouched some obvious questions about whether and on what terms family privacy is to be respected. But liberal doctrine offers resources to prevent families from becoming small tyrannies, aspects of which I want to develop now.

Here I will isolate several of Rawls's claims and briefly develop their positive implications for an ethics and politics of the family, focusing on the rearing of children.[3] The liberal understanding of care that I developed in Chapter 2 suggests how that might be possible, and why family privacy is not an absolute value in liberal social thought. There, I indicated that respect for parental autonomy must be understood within a framework defined by adult responsibilities and the duty to care. I argued, among other things, that respect for parental autonomy must be constrained by virtues and norms, especially benevolence and beneficence. Family privacy is not an incorrigible principle, and liberal social critics have reasons to insist that it be qualified. Viewed normatively in liberal terms, the family is (1) a school of personal moral development, (2) an equitable, intimate social grouping, (3) a source of personal self-worth, (4) an aid to opportunity, and (5) a school for political citizenship. Each of these ideas merits comment.

First, the family is expected to facilitate the moral development and education of children, and in that regard it is a central institution in any society.[4] Amending Rawls's language, let us say that families should impart a "sense of care," a strong desire to act on virtues that dispose us to attend to others' needs. We acquire such virtues, Rawls observes, as we develop moral sentiments that are first nurtured in family settings. Although Rawls's attention to moral development in the much-neglected third section of *A Theory of Justice* focuses on acquiring a "sense of justice," much of what he says also explains how we develop the virtues and duties of care.[5] Those ideas, in turn, shed light on the role of the family in imparting civic virtues, blurring the boundaries between public and private life. Given that the family can nurture sentiments of justice and care, so important to our common life, family practices and institutions cannot be entirely shielded by considerations of privacy.

Echoing Piaget, Rawls argues that we develop moral sentiments in three stages.[6] Pivotal is the experience of care and the subsequent desire to reciprocate caring practices and affections in the first developmental stage, "the morality of authority." The love of parents for a child "is expressed in their evident intention to care for him. . . . Their love is displayed by their taking pleasure in his presence and supporting his competence and self-esteem."[7] Generally, Rawls observes, "to love another means not only to be concerned with his wants and needs, but to affirm his sense of the worth of his own person."[8] Parents' love for a child arouses "in him a sense of his own value and the desire to become the sort of person that they are."[9] In that way, "the love of the parents for the child gives rise to his love in return."[10]

At the subsequent stage of development, the "morality of association," the family also figures importantly in the development of moral sentiments.[11] By filling various roles and positions in the family, we increase our moral affections and capacities for care. Crucial here is our ability to take up different points of view and to learn from others, seeing things from their perspectives. As daughters or sons, sisters or brothers, children learn behavior that is appropriate to their roles in the family, along with corresponding expectations and responsibilities. Without such experiences, Rawls notes, "we cannot put ourselves into another's place and find out what we would do in his position."[12] On the basis of family relationships and corresponding role responsibilities, we are able to develop empathy—a "capacity for fellow feeling"[13]—vital for social interactions as we assume nonfamilial roles and relationships. Empathetically understanding another's situation, we can "regulate our own conduct in the appropriate way by reference to it."[14] Such skills enable us to move into various associations with the capacity to perceive others' needs and perspectives apart from our own immediate interests. "As we assume a succession of more demanding roles with their more complex schemes of rights and duties," Rawls observes, we acquire the ability "to view things from a greater multiplicity of perspectives."[15]

At the final stage, "the morality of principles," Rawls claims that persons are supposed to attach themselves to moral principles that can rise above their immediate heritages and traditions.[16] But rather than arguing on behalf of impartial, impersonal principles of justice so often associated with liberal theory, he notes that at this stage our moral sentiments are "continuous with the love of mankind."[17] Moral principles are to display an independence from our backgrounds and attachments, but not entirely: "Our natural attachments to particular persons and groups still have an appropriate place."[18] An empathetic imagination is crucial to this stage of moral development, for we are expected to see ourselves in the circumstances of others. Summarizing what he calls the laws of moral development, corresponding to the morality of authority, association, and principle, Rawls states that these laws

> are not merely principles of association or of reinforcement. . . . They assert that the active sentiments of love and friendship, and even the sense of justice, arise from the manifest intention of other persons to act for our good. Because we recognize that they wish us well, we care for their well-being in return. Thus we acquire attachments to persons and institutions according to how we perceive our good to be affected by them. The basic idea is one of reciprocity, a tendency to answer in kind.[19]

In each stage of moral development, our experiences of warmth, trust, and care are psychologically foundational to developing the capacity to empathize for others. Rawls thus writes, "Certain natural attitudes underlie the corresponding moral feelings: a lack of these feelings would manifest the absence of these attitudes."[20]

Yet affection in the family is a finite resource, and for that reason, too, it is subject to ethical analysis. Herein lies the second reason that we must open the family to moral evaluation: Parents and families operate within conditions of finitude and must think about how fairly to distribute the good of care. In many ways, what appear to be loving families can enshrine injustice, privileging some members' needs to the neglect of other members' needs, or privileging some members' needs for morally arbitrary reasons.

This view of family life and human finitude runs against the idea that justice is an inappropriate virtue for families. According to Michael Sandel, the family is a social group characterized by "more or less clearly defined common identities and shared purposes," unlike social groupings characterized by the "circumstances of justice," understood to be a moderate scarcity of resources to be distributed among persons with different ends and purposes and who make conflicting claims on those resources.[21] For Sandel, the family is where we develop "enlarged affections," a set of dispositions to act generously and lovingly.[22] Seeing the family in this light seems to refute Rawls's claim that justice is the first virtue of social institutions,[23] for in a "more or less ideal family situation," solidarity and spontaneous affection will prevail, thereby reducing the problems posed by scarcity and diversity as these constraints characterize the circumstances of justice.[24]

Given that fact, Sandel argues, the arrival of justice in an intimate group may mean not a gain but an overall loss of virtue. Justice on Sandel's account would repair morally compromised conditions of discord and disagreement. If that is so, then the *absence* of these conditions "must embody a rival virtue of at least commensurate priority, the one that is engaged in so far as justice is not engaged."[25] That is to say, the absence of justice can mean the prevalence of good will and benevolence. As Aristotle remarks, justice is unnecessary between friends.[26] For Sandel, a gain in justice can come about "where before there was neither justice nor injustice but a measure of benevolence and fraternity such that the virtue of justice had not been extensively engaged."[27] In those cases, "when an increase of justice reflects some transformation in the quality of pre-existing motivations and dispositions, the overall moral balance might well be diminished."[28]

Sandel's view of benevolence in intimate groups fails to account for challenges to families that operate in even the best of natural and social circumstances, for it fails to note that benevolence itself is a finite resource, not merely a fund of virtue that enables us generously to allocate (or receive) other scarce resources. Among humans, love is not infinite, however much we might wish that it were. A child has just claims to parental affection, and those claims are among many that parents must consider when they weigh their attachments to their other children, to themselves, to their own parents, to friends, to vocational and avocational ideals, and to civic and recreational associations. Love requires justice and practical reasoning so that children are cared for fairly.[29] Even if benevolence entails self-sacrifice—an arguable idea, to be sure—it does not entail having infinite resources. That is to say, even if love is self-sacrificial, it needs to be informed by justice, for the question would otherwise remain: *To whom* is the sacrifice properly owed? Hence the need for practical guidance and a list of priorities when allocating care to vulnerable persons in need. Benevolence cries out for general principles of equity in order to ensure that parents aspire to meet each of their children's basic interests.

A third reason for liberal social critics to scrutinize the family derives from the link between a person's family experience and self-esteem. The experience of love and care in the family imparts a sense of self-worth to individuals, a crucial psychological feature in all persons' lives. From parental love comes the child's "sense of his own value and the desire to become the sort of person that they are."[30] A sense of self-worth, perhaps the most important primary good in Rawlsian liberalism,[31]

> includes a person's sense of his own value, [the] secure conviction that this conception of his good, his plan of life, is worth carrying out. . . . [Moreover], self-respect implies a confidence in one's ability, so far as it is within one's power, to fulfill one's intentions. When we feel that our plans are of little value, we cannot pursue them with pleasure or take delight in their execution.[32]

Without self-worth, nothing may seem worth doing. On this description, self-worth is not so much a particular plan of life as it is a sense that one's plans are worth pursuing.[33] A young person's agency is thus critically dependent on relationships with others. We admire ourselves when we are admired by others around us, and the development of reflexive admiration is especially vulnerable during our formative years. Self-worth is relational, for we rely on others' esteem to develop our own sense of self-worth. Families that deny their children this vital good can leave permanent, ineradicable scars.

Self-worth is a primary good in Rawlsian liberalism, a good that we need whatever else we want. Without it, we would lack the confidence to pursue our other goods; we would be psychologically handicapped. As a primary good, self-worth is an attribute to which all children have a rightful claim. For that reason it is an important *political* value, not merely a private one, for it comprises a good that requires proper allocation. That is to say, liberal doctrine has an interest in the quality of family life, given the role that families play in providing or denying an important primary good.

The idea that the family can strengthen or weaken a young person's sense of self-worth is a commonplace that I will not pursue further, except to note the gendered dimensions of self-worth and family experience.[34] Liberal social critics have due cause to worry about gender relations in the family insofar as such relations in societies with a history of patriarchy can foster the idea that women are second-class citizens. Girls in families likely suffer greater barriers to self-worth in domestic arrangements that privilege male authority, impose inequitable distribution of domestic responsibilities on women, or bar their access to public culture. That families can be a barrier to gender justice and the equitable distribution of self-worth cries out for social criticism and demands efforts to correct patterns that privilege male power. That such reforms would directly or indirectly affect the shape of the family should be important to Rawls, for Rawlsian liberalism rejects the idea that the family is a prepolitical unit that is unaffected by state action. According to Rawls, a domain such as the family "is not . . . something already given apart from the principles of justice. A domain . . . is simply the result, or upshot, of how the principles of political justice are applied, directly to the basic structure and indirectly to the associations within it."[35] Because the family is an association made up, in part, of future citizens, its patterns of allocating the good of self-worth are obviously eligible for liberal social criticism and reform. For that reason, the family sits on the boundary between the public and private realms, subject to moral and political criticism.

Related to this third claim is a fourth: Our experience of love and self-worth, or lack thereof, can seriously affect our life chances. Doubtless this is a crucial reason for liberal social critics to scrutinize family life: Families can directly affect individuals' future prospects, their opportunities.[36] Liberal societies are committed to the equality of opportunity; they enshrine a vision of social conditions in which persons are not handicapped from pursing their intimations of the good for reasons that are morally arbitrary. If, as Rawls argues, one goal of liberal justice is to nullify "the accidents of natural endowment and the contingencies of social circumstance,"[37] then we must assess how life chances are enhanced or attenuated by family experiences. One's family background is among "the contingencies of social circumstance" that affect an individual's freedom and well-being. Whether that experience is for good or ill is an important question for liberal social criticism.

Fifth, as Rawls observes, the family is a school of political virtue and citizenship. A "sense of care" and a "sense of justice" are foundational to a fair, well-ordered society, for without them, citizens would have few psychological resources to sustain just social institutions. In this respect, the four aspects of family experience that I have mentioned help to focus our attention on the idea of civic virtue. Empathy and reciprocity that derive from the experience of care and justice; the intimate experience of fairness; the primary good of self-worth and its implications for moral and political motivation; and experience of hope as it derives from the assurance of opportunity—these experiences empower children to acquire dispositions necessary to treat others benevolently and equitably in public affairs. The experience of injustice, in contrast, tends "to undermine children's capacity to acquire the political virtues required of future citizens in a viable democratic society."[38] As *future* citizens, children need to develop civic virtues, the excellences of character that dispose them to care for others and the common good.

For these reasons, families must be caring and just. Children who will develop into socially responsible adults must spend their early, formative years in social groupings that are loving and equitable, and persons who treat young people well must exhibit "primary virtues"—dispositions to care for children's needs, whatever those children may eventually want. Although liberal, Western societies assign a wide latitude to families in matters of child rearing, that liberty must be constrained by considerations of basic rights and civic virtue. The idea that children are objects of property or instruments for others' use, like the idea that women are naturally inferior to men, is (or ought to be) a relic of the past.

The young persons we have met in the course of this book—Jean St. Jacques, Martin Seiferth, the infant in *Custody*, Henry Gucci, Aaron Wolfe, Kevin Sampson, Ahmet Ali, Billy Richardson, Jackson Bales, Ericka, and Lia Lee—all came from relatively good families. None of them was "abused" in any obvious sense, and some of them enjoyed medical outcomes that resulted from a therapeutic alliance between their care providers and their families—however awkward it might have been to form such an alliance in some instances. These children's medical fates were not uncomplicated, and sometimes respect for their parents' wishes was insufficient to address their basic needs. The welfare of children and adolescents is a social responsibility, and their claims cry out for advocacy and protection. Liberal societies that care about their youth have due cause to evaluate family life, situated as it is on the boundary between private and public affairs.

NOTES

INTRODUCTION

1. Over the course of this development, patients' rights have taken on different functions. In response to early abuses in research in the 1960s, the defense of individual rights functioned to protect research subjects from *utilitarianism,* that is, from being instrumentalized in researchers' quests for scientific knowledge. Soon thereafter, those rights assumed a different role in medical as opposed to research contexts. In medical situations, the language of rights was invoked to protect patients from *paternalism.* Rather than posing the danger of instrumentalizing patients, paternalism poses the danger of infantalizing patients. Rights are meant to protect individuals' dignity and equality, but the implications of those values differ, depending on the context. I am grateful to Heather McConnell for enabling me to see this point.

2. I borrow the idea of a basic moral paradigm and subsequent revisions from Michael Walzer's approach to war in *Just and Unjust Wars: A Moral Argument with Historical Illustrations* (New York: Basic Books, 1977), chaps. 4–6.

3. Brian Clark, *Whose Life Is It, Anyway?* (New York: Dodd, Mead, 1978).

4. The idea of "first" and "second" languages comes from Robert Bellah et al., *Habits of the Heart: Individualism and Commitment in American Life* (Berkeley: University of California Press, 1985). According to Bellah et al., the first language of individualism often mutes the second language of communal action and social responsibility, on which Americans often, if unconsciously, rely.

5. Philippe Aires, *Centuries of Childhood: A Social History* (New York: Random House, 1965), 38.

6. See Angel Ballabriga, "One Century of Pediatrics in Europe," in *History of Pediatrics, 1985–1950,* ed. B. L. Nichols, A. Ballabriga, and N. Krechner (New York: Vevey/ Raven Press, 1991), 1–21.

7. Children's rights have developed in American law, unevenly to be sure, either by extending adults' rights, e.g., the right to some medical care without parents' consent, or by recognizing children's unique needs and interests, e.g., the right to an education up to a certain age. In Chapter 2, my argument for children's moral rights will follow these two developments in their main lines. For a discussion of children's rights and American law, see Hillary Rodham, "Children under the Law," *Harvard Educational Review* 43 (November 1973): 487–514.

8. The language of ideal and nonideal theory draws from John Rawls, *A Theory of Justice* (Cambridge, Mass.: Belknap Press, 1971), 8–9, 245–46.

9. David J. Rothman, *Strangers at the Bedside: A History of How Law and Bioethics Transformed Medical Decision-Making* (New York: Basic Books, 1991), 9.

10. Ibid. Although not a product of the era about which Rothman writes, Edwin N. Forman and Rosalind Ekman Ladd draw extensively on cases in their contribution to pediatric ethics. See Edwin N. Forman and Rosalind Ekman Ladd, *Ethical Dilemmas in Pediatrics: A Case Study Approach* (Lanham, Md.: University Press of America, 1995).

11. Clifford Geertz, *Local Knowledge: Further Essays in Interpretive Anthropology* (New York: Basic Books, 1983), 57.

12. Daniel F. Chambliss, *Beyond Caring: Hospitals, Nurses, and the Social Organization of Ethics* (Chicago: University of Chicago Press, 1996), 6.

13. Arthur Kleinman, *Writing at the Margin: Discourse between Anthropology and Medicine* (Berkeley: University of California Press, 1995), 49–50. See also Kleinman, *The Illness Narratives: Suffering, Healing, and the Human Condition* (New York: Basic Books, 1988).

14. Kleinman, *Writing at the Margin,* 51.

15. That is not to accept Chambliss's and Kleinman's characterizations of bioethics as entirely accurate. I critically address their claims in "Religion, Ethics, and Clinical Immersion: An Appraisal of Three Pioneers," in *Caring Well: Religion, Narrative, and Health Care Ethics,* ed. David H. Smith (Louisville: Westminster/John Knox Press, 2000), 17–42.

16. Geertz, *Local Knowledge,* 57.

17. Rawls, *Theory of Justice,* 20.

18. Richard B. Miller, "Love and Death in a Pediatric Intensive Care Unit," *Annual of the Society of Christian Ethics* 14 (1994): 21–39.

19. My remarks here are informed by Michael Walzer's view of social criticism in *The Company of Critics: Social Criticism and Political Commitment in the Twentieth Century* (New York: Basic Books, 1988), 3–28.

20. These parallels grow out of the work by Carol Gilligan, *In a Different Voice: Psychological Theory and Women's Development* (Cambridge, Mass.: Harvard University Press, 1982). For recent discussions that challenge these parallels, see the essays in *Feminism and Bioethics: Beyond Reproduction,* ed. Susan M. Wolf (New York: Oxford University Press, 1996).

1. PARENTAL RESPONSIBILITY IN FEAR AND TREMBLING

1. Personal interview, January 1998.

2. For a discussion of illness and identity, see William F. May, *The Patient's Ordeal* (Bloomington: Indiana University Press, 1991).

3. Søren Kierkegaard, *Fear and Trembling,* trans. with an introduction by Alastair Hannay (New York: Penguin Books, 1985).

4. Ibid., 65.

5. Ibid., 71.

6. Readers alert to distinctions in moral theory might retort that Abraham is asked to kill Isaac—that the story begins as a tale about divinely authorized infanticide—and that decisions about infanticide are morally off-limits to health care providers and parents. According to American law and medical morality, the most that care providers and parents may do is withhold or withdraw treatment, thereby allowing a child to die, when that treatment is futile or imposes burdens that are disproportionate to medical benefit. Those facts seem to render our biblical tale irrelevant to pediatric contexts in general and Adrienne in particular.

Yet in an important essay by James Rachels, the distinction between killing and letting die has been critically revisited, yielding important conclusions. Rachels rightly argues that allowing an individual to die may be just as heinous as killing, that no *moral* distinction rests on the distinction between omissions and commissions. Accordingly, a parent would be just as guilty of wrongdoing for allowing her son to drown as she would be if she deliberately poisoned his meal. Thinking that omitting treatment is more easily justified than killing can lead parents and health care providers into self-deceptive practices that are morally negligent. Rachels reminds us that acts of commission and acts of omission must be justified according to second-order evaluations. Indeed, actively killing someone (e.g., an unjust assailant) is prima facie more acceptable than allowing a person to drown who could easily be saved.

Rachels's article has led moral theorists to reconsider the ethics of killing and letting die, leading to refinements in action theory, discussions of moral responsibility, and debates about euthanasia and physician-assisted suicide. His argument is also relevant to the broader background features of the healer's art that I am seeking to highlight here. When combined with our biblical story, Rachels's analysis reminds us that some decisions that parents must make are no less trying than the one that Abraham faced, even if those decisions are "only" about omitting treatment. Not only do acts of commission and omission cry out for moral justification, decisions about them tax the souls of parents who must confront the fact that their child is suffering. Decisions about whether to authorize or omit action can be equally challenging, equally Abrahamic, for (in either case) parents are summoned by the trial of relinquishing a child to powers that seem mysterious and sometimes untrustworthy. See James Rachels, "Active and Passive Euthanasia," *New England Journal of Medicine* 292 (1975): 78–79.

7. This point about responsive agency is made most notably by H. Richard Niebuhr, *The Responsible Self: An Essay in Christian Moral Philosophy,* with an introduction by James M. Gustafson (New York: Harper and Row, 1963).

2. THE DUTY TO CARE

1. Personal interview, June 1998.

2. Personal interview, March 1998.

3. Personal interview, June 1998.

4. For a discussion of several of these issues, see Gene Outka, *Agape: An Ethical Analysis* (New Haven, Conn.: Yale University Press, 1971).

5. See Peter Harvey, *An Introduction to Buddhist Ethics* (Cambridge: Cambridge University Press, 2000).

6. See K. R. Srikanta Murthy, "Professional Ethics in Ancient Indian Medicine" in *Cross Cultural Perspectives in Medical Ethics: Readings,* ed. Robert M. Veatch (Boston: Jones and Bartlett Publishers, 1989), 126–30; "Hinduism (Thought and Ethics)," s.v. in *The HarperCollins Dictionary of Religion,* ed. Jonathan Z. Smith and William Scott Green (San Francisco: HarperCollins, 1995).

7. Fazlur Rahman, *Health and Medicine in the Islamic Tradition* (Chicago: ABC International Group, 1998), 29–30.

8. "The Hippocratic Oath," in *Cross Cultural Perspectives,* ed. Veatch, 6–7.

9. American Medical Association, "Principles of Medical Ethics" (1957), in *Cross Cultural Perspectives,* ed. Veatch, 37.

10. Moral norms for the role morality of health care professionals, as I am developing them here, are a special case of general morality, not a set of exceptions to or excuses for departing from that morality. For an example of the former, see Robert M. Veatch, "Medical Ethics: Professional or Universal?" *Harvard Theological Review* 4 (October 1972): 531–59. For an example of the latter, within the context of law, see David Luban, *Lawyers and Justice: An Ethical Study* (Princeton, N.J.: Princeton University Press, 1988), chap. 7.

11. Aristotle, *Nicomachean Ethics,* 1094b21.

12. Onora O'Neill, *Towards Justice and Virtue: A Constructive Account of Practical Reasoning* (Cambridge: Cambridge University Press, 1996), 194.

13. Ibid., 148.

14. Lainie Friedman Ross rejects the language of children's rights on the assumption that rights language and the authority they assign to children endanger the value of family

intimacy, in which the child has an interest and over which parents rightly presume authority. Ross agrees that children are owed primary goods and have basic interests, but she inexplicably eschews rights language as a way of indicating that children have a claim to the protection of basic interests and the provision of primary goods. Her view of surrogate decision making for children "is based on parental autonomy constrained by the principle of respect for persons modified to apply to children" (50). Developing a model of "constrained parental autonomy," Ross assigns wide latitude to parents in medical decision making for their children. But she ignores the fact that respect for parental authority may not cohere with the value of family intimacy because parents can insist on decisions that wear down a family's sense of solidarity—even when those decisions honor the baseline needs of their offspring in keeping with "the principle of respect for persons modified to apply to children." Parents who routinely exercise their authority in impersonal or imperious ways might exercise autonomy at the expense of family intimacy. Ross would do well to develop an account of the virtues on which the cultivation of family intimacy would presumably rely and according to which the exercise of parental authority should be evaluated. In my view, the language of care and responsibility provides the proper starting point for considering the moral challenges of treating children in medical and research settings. That is not to gainsay the value of parental autonomy, only to situate it within moral contours wider than one finds in Ross's argument. See Lainie Friedman Ross, *Children, Families, and Health Care Decision-Making* (Oxford: Clarendon Press, 1998), chap. 3 and passim.

15. John Rawls, *A Theory of Justice* (Cambridge, Mass.: Belknap Press, 1971), 249. As will become clearer in the next chapter, Rawls's terminology is not entirely precise. The principles he develops do not entail paternalism, strictly speaking, because they do not enjoin ignoring the wishes of a person in order to prevent a harm or produce a good for that person. Still, I will follow his language here.

16. For a critical discussion, see Eva Feder Kittay, *Love's Labor: Essays on Women, Equality, and Dependency* (New York: Routledge, 1999).

17. Rawls, *Theory of Justice*, 249.

18. Rawls's principles of paternalism and its implications for the duty to care are overlooked in Eva Feder Kittay's critique of Rawls. See Kittay, *Love's Labor*, chaps. 3, 4.

19. Rawls, *Theory of Justice*, 504–12; Rawls, *Justice as Fairness: A Restatement*, ed. Erin Kelly (Cambridge, Mass.: Harvard University Press, 2001), 18–19.

20. Donald VanDeVeer, *Paternalistic Intervention: The Moral Bounds of Benevolence* (Princeton, N.J.: Princeton University Press, 1986), 375–90.

21. Rawls, *Theory of Justice*, 509. These ideas about the capacity for moral personality and the principles of paternalism receive insufficient attention in the critique of Rawls's theory by Samantha Brennan and Robert Noggle, "Rawls's Neglected Childhood: Reflections on the Original Position, Stability, and the Child's Sense of Justice," in *The Idea of a Political Liberalism: Essays on Rawls,* ed. Victoria Davion and Clark Wolf (Lanham, Md.: Rowman and Littlefield, 2000), 46–72.

22. See Michael J. Sandel, *Liberalism and the Limits of Justice*, 2d ed. (Cambridge: Cambridge University Press, 1998); and "The Procedural Republic and the Unencumbered Self," *Political Theory* 12 (February 1984): 81–96.

23. Rawls may weaken his case by emphasizing the importance of seeking terms of "mutual advantage" behind the veil of ignorance. The principles of paternalism suggest the need for arrangements that are not mutually advantageous for adults and those in their care.

24. See, e.g., Onora O'Neill, "Begetting, Bearing, and Rearing," in *Having Children: Philosophical and Legal Reflections on Parenthood,* ed. Onora O'Neill and William Ruddick (New York: Oxford University Press, 1979), 31.

25. Rawls, *Theory of Justice,* 11–17.

26. Ibid., 15. This is not to say that I aim to provide an argument regarding the justice of access to health care institutions and related provisions. The duty to care grounds adults'

social responsibilities to protect the welfare of children, but it is not sufficient to provide principles for determining just procedures for distributing the good of health care. In short, arguments on behalf of *social responsibility* differ in important ways from arguments regarding principles of *distributive justice*. In many modern societies, it is doubtless necessary to construct such principles premised on the absence of any shared vision of the good. At the same time, the value of equal opportunity may provide a widely shared, noncontroversial basis for beginning such a discussion. Balancing the need to provide health care in light of other pressing social demands is not an endeavor I am equipped to undertake. Suffice it to say that commitment to protect a child's primary goods with an eye to their connection to children's fair share of opportunity suggests a viable starting point for thinking about the design of social institutions that allocate the good of health care in pluralistic societies. For an important discussion, see Norman Daniels, *Just Health Care* (Cambridge: Cambridge University Press, 1985).

Daniels might take issue with my concentration on primary goods and the rights they generate as a baseline for thinking about medical ethics. Despite my appeal to the distinction between the grounds for *social responsibility* and principles of *distributive justice*, Daniels might worry that appeals to baseline goods and rights are nonetheless misguided for theoretical and practical reasons, and these bear directly on important distributive issues.

At a theoretical level, Daniels, following one line of Rawlsian liberalism, claims that "rights are not moral fruits that spring up from bare earth, fully ripened, without cultivation. Rather we are justified in claiming a right to health care only if it can be harvested from an acceptable, general theory of distributive justice, or, more particularly, from a theory of justice for health care" (*Just Health Care*, 5). On that account, rights are not pretheoretical but rather depend on a broader theory for their justification. Without a prior, grander theory, their grounds are question-begging. For Daniels, such a theory would proceed by assuming the social obligation to protect fair equality of opportunity and then set terms for the design of social institutions, including health care institutions, to meet that obligation (79).

At a practical level, the point of denying the force of pretheoretical rights in the context of health care is to prevent appeal to rights from establishing a bottomless pit of demand for health care needs. Apart from a theory to ground and order rights, claims to health care are potentially expensive and may deplete resources that are needed for other goods and services.

Despite these theoretical and practical concerns, it is clear that Rawlsian liberalism cannot eschew the language of pretheoretical rights altogether, as evidenced by the importance of primary goods, and the claims they generate, in Rawls's theory. Daniels's theory concedes that fact, proceeding from the principle of fair equality of opportunity to the right to health care that aims to protect "species-typical normal functioning" (26–28, 42, 55).

27. I prefer the phrase *parental autonomy* to *family autonomy* The former is narrower than the latter, focusing on parental authority and discretion. As Margaret Steinfels rightly notes, family autonomy involves the effects and influences of children's behavior on the parents. Parental autonomy, in contrast, refers to parents' or guardians' ability to control and channel a set of commitments into the domestic sphere. *Family privacy* refers to the rights of families to be left alone. See Margaret O'Brien Steinfels, "Children's Rights, Parental Rights, Family Privacy, and Family Autonomy," in *Who Speaks for the Child? The Problems of Proxy Consent,* ed. Willard Gaylin and Ruth Macklin (New York: Plenum Press, 1982), 223–63.

28. See James F. Childress, *Who Should Decide? Paternalism in Health Care* (New York: Oxford University Press, 1981).

29. Ibid., 55–74, and passim.

30. Ibid., chap. 5.

31. Tom L. Beauchamp and Laurence B. McCullough, *Medical Ethics: The Moral Responsibilities of Physicians* (Englewood Cliffs, N.J.: Prentice-Hall, 1984), 98–101. In the 5th edition of their jointly authored work, Beauchamp and Childress allow for some forms of strong paternalism, arguing in defense of acts "that prevent major harms or provide major

benefits while only trivially disrespecting autonomy." See Tom L. Beauchamp and James F. Childress, *Principles of Biomedical Ethics*, 5th ed. (New York: Oxford University Press, 2001), 185. I will address issues of paternalism in the next chapter.

32. Will Kymlicka, *Multicultural Citizenship: A Liberal Theory of Minority Rights* (New York: Oxford University Press, 1995), 89, citing Avishai Margalit and Joseph Raz, "National Self-Determination," *Journal of Philosophy* 87 (1990): 449.

33. For this reason, liberal political philosophy can provide a basis for protecting the family as a social institution. The family provides, among other things, a context in which individuals develop the capacity for self-determination. This fact, along with the implications of Rawls's principles of paternalism, are overlooked in Ezekiel J. Emanuel's judgment that liberalism provides no basis for affirming the family or providing a basis for protecting patient medical interests. I shall delineate flaws in Emanuel's depiction of liberalism more directly in Chapter 5. See Ezekiel J. Emmanuel, *The Ends of Human Life: Medical Ethics in a Liberal Polity* (Cambridge, Mass.: Harvard University Press, 1991), chap. 3.

34. See Michael Walzer, *Just and Unjust Wars: A Moral Argument with Historical Illustrations,* 2d ed. (New York: Basic Books, 1992), chap. 6.

35. Allen E. Buchanan and Dan W. Brock, *Deciding for Others: The Ethics of Surrogate Decision-Making* (Cambridge: Cambridge University Press, 1989), 88, 236; Ferdinand Shoeman, "Parental Discretion and Children's Rights: Background and Implications for Medical Decision-Making," *Journal of Medicine and Philosophy* 10 (1985): 45–61.

36. Joel Feinberg, "The Child's Right to an Open Future," in *Whose Child? Children's Rights, Parental Authority, and State Power,* ed. William Aiken and Hugh LaFollette (Totowa, N.J.: Littlefield, Adams, 1980), 124–53.

37. It is not clear that Rawls would count these goods as primary goods, because he does not include health among the goods he lists in *Theory of Justice.* There, Rawls briefly cites health as a natural primary good as opposed to a social primary good, e.g., wealth. Perhaps that is because, as Norman Daniels observes, much of what Rawls concerns himself with in his theory of distribution turns on goods that are connected to the fair equality of opportunity, understood in terms of the opportunity to secure jobs or offices, rather than as part of the pursuit of one's comprehensive good.

A Rawlsian might avoid this problem by arguing that health care institutions aim to provide health, much as schools aim to provide knowledge, and that each institution is instrumental to equality of opportunity and should be regulated by the general requirements of justice-as-fairness in the design of social institutions. Then the argument could subsume considerations of the good of health without complicating the theory by factoring in additional primary goods.

That move would nonetheless be complicated by the fact that Rawls's general assumptions do not adequately track the kind of institution that provides health care. As I have noted in this chapter, health care is normed by beneficence as the first virtue, contrary to Rawls's claim that "justice is the first principle of social institutions." This point seems to be missed in Daniels's attempt to secure a basis for justice in the distribution of health care. For discussions of these ideas, see Rawls, *Theory of Justice,* 1, 62; Norman Daniels, *Just Health Care* (Cambridge: Cambridge University Press, 1985), 39–48.

38. Joel Feinberg, "The Nature and Value of Rights," *Journal of Value Inquiry* 4 (1970): 255.

39. Jeffrey Blustein, *Parents and Children: The Ethics of the Family* (New York: Oxford University Press, 1982), 116–17.

40. For a discussion of primary goods, see Rawls, *Theory of Justice,* 90–95.

41. Ibid., 118. Contrast the views of Ross, who devotes little attention to specifying the content primary goods and their possible tensions. See Ross, *Children, Families,* 5–6 and passim.

42. Feinberg, "Child's Right to an Open Future," 126.

43. Ibid., 127.

44. Ibid.

45. Ibid., 140–48.

46. William F. May, "The Beleaguered Rulers: The Public Obligation of the Professional," *Kennedy Institute of Ethics Journal* 2 (1992): 38.

47. See, e.g., William M. Sullivan, *Work and Integrity: The Crisis and Promise of Professionalism in America* (New York: Basic Books, 1995).

48. May, "Beleaguered Rulers," 38.

49. Feinberg, "Child's Right to an Open Future," 126.

50. For an instructive discussion, see Shoeman, "Parental Discretion and Children's Rights." Shoeman rightly observes that formulating the tension between parental decision making and children's rights of respect does not produce a simple algorithm for settling conflicts.

51. See the National Commission for the Protection of Human Subjects of Biomedical and Behavioral Research, *Research Involving Children: Report and Recommendations* (Washington, D.C.: Government Printing Office, 1977), 5. For discussions, see Albert R. Jonsen, *The Birth of Bioethics* (New York: Oxford University Press, 1998), chap. 5, especially 153–55; Michael A. Grodin and Leonard H. Glantz, eds., *Children as Research Subjects: Science, Ethics, and Law* (New York: Oxford University Press, 1994); Leonard H. Glantz, "Research with Children," *American Journal of Law and Medicine* 24 (1988): 213–44; Loretta M. Kopelman, "Children as Research Subjects: A Dilemma," *Journal of Medicine and Philosophy* 25 (2000): 745–64.

3. PEDIATRIC PATERNALISM

1. Personal conversation, June 1998.

2. Ethics Advisory Committee Meeting at Baylin Pediatric Medical Center, November 1997.

3. Ruth Macklin, "Return to the Best Interests of the Child," in *Who Speaks for the Child? The Problems of Proxy Consent,* ed. Willard Gaylin and Ruth Macklin (New York: Plenum Press, 1982), 295.

4. Tom L. Beauchamp and James F. Childress, *Principles of Biomedical Ethics,* 5th ed. (New York: Oxford University Press, 2001), 177.

5. I place paternalism in quotation marks here because, as I will soon make plain, overriding parental autonomy does not fit the standard paradigm of paternalistic action. I describe such acts as second-party paternalism.

6. The Hegelian idea that recognition is vital to identity is developed by Charles Taylor, *Multiculturalism and "The Politics of Recognition,"* ed. Amy Gutmann (Princeton, N.J.: Princeton University Press, 1992).

7. Joel Feinberg, "Legal Paternalism," *Canadian Journal of Philosophy* 1 (September 1971): 105–24.

8. Beauchamp and Childress, *Principles of Biomedical Ethics,* 5th ed., 181.

9. Ibid.

10. For a discussion of hard and soft (but not moderate) paternalism, see Childress, *Who Should Decide? Paternalism in Health Care* (New York: Oxford University Press, 1981), 18. In their jointly authored work, Beauchamp and Childress conflate weak and soft paternalism on the one hand, and strong and hard paternalism on the other. See Beauchamp and Childress, *Principles of Biomedical Ethics,* 5th ed., 181–91. However, there is an important distinction between weak and strong paternalism on the one hand, and hard and soft paternalism on the other. Once again: The first distinction pertains to whether the act is carried out on an agent of substantial or compromised autonomy; the second distinction indicates

whether the values that are imposed are alien to or compatible with the beneficiary's own values. A weak paternalist may act according to a commitment to hard paternalism, e.g., by imposing foreign values on a patient of diminished autonomy. In *Principles of Biomedical Ethics*, 5th ed., Beauchamp and Childress defend what they call minor strong paternalism (185–87).

11. Childress, *Who Should Decide?*, 19–20.

12. See Childress, *Who Should Decide?*, 18. See also n. 19 below.

13. For a related discussion, see Donald VanDeVeer, *Paternalistic Intervention: The Moral Bounds of Benevolence* (Princeton, N.J.: Princeton University Press, 1986), 204–13. VanDeVeer uses the language of exercising first-order and second-order autonomy rather than unreflexive and reflexive paternalism. Combining his categories with mine, we can say that unreflexive paternalism ignores a patient's first-order autonomy and that reflexive paternalism is a function of a patient exercising second-order autonomy to assign decision-making authority to another party. I hasten to add that the use of the term *autonomy* in its reflexive/second-order variety is something of a misnomer, because in such cases the individual is relinquishing responsibility and leaving his or her fate to matters of chance. Kantians would judge such decisions as heteronomous.

14. Childress, *Who Should Decide?*, 16.

15. Beauchamp and Childress, *Principles of Biomedical Ethics*, 5th ed., 181.

16. Ibid.

17. For a discussion of the difference between universal and special duties, see the previous chapter.

18. For a discussion, see David J. Rothman, *Strangers at the Bedside: A History of How Law and Bioethics Transformed Medical Decision-Making* (New York: Basic Books, 1991).

19. Gerald Dworkin argues that banning the manufacturing of tobacco would be paternalistic rather than nonpaternalistic because the restriction aims to benefit individuals who smoke. Dworkin calls this "impure" paternalism because the effort to protect one group (smokers) restricts the liberty of another group (cigarette manufacturers). The fact of smokers' consent makes the restriction different from preventing industrial manufacturers from releasing pollutants into the air, because in the latter case, no one is consenting to inhaling polluted air. The difference between paternalistic and nonpaternalistic acts that restrict the liberty of nonbeneficiaries turns on whether those who benefit would consent to an unhealthy or untoward pratice.

However, it seems doubtful that smokers can be assigned the degree of volition on which Dworkin's distinction turns. Given the effects of social pressures, advertising ploys, the fact that many people begin smoking at an early age, and nicotine addiction, it seems doubtful that a ban on cigarette manufacturing would restrict a genuinely volitional activity (smoking). A better example of what Dworkin calls impure paternalism, or what Childress calls indirect paternalism, might be a ban on cigarette advertising. However, I see no advantage in calling such a restriction impure or indirect paternalism rather than nonpaternalism *simpliciter*, because the aim of the restriction would be to prevent some from enticing others into unhealthy habits. The principal party whose liberty is restricted does not benefit from the restriction. In my view, protecting some groups from the seduction of others is nonpaternalistic. See Gerald Dworkin, "Paternalism," in *Paternalism*, ed. Rolf Satorius (Minneapolis: University of Minnesota Press, 1983), 19–34, at 22; and n. 12 above.

20. President's Commission for the Study of Ethical Problems in Medicine and Biomedical and Behavioral Research, *Deciding to Forego Life-Sustaining Treatment* (Washington, D.C.: U.S. Government Printing Office, 1983), 45.

21. Angela R. Holder, *Legal Issues in Pediatrics and Adolescent Medicine* (New Haven, Conn.: Yale University Press, 1985), 127–42.

22. Walter J. Wadlington, "Consent to Medical Care for Minors," in *Children's Competence to Consent*, ed. Gary B. Melton, Gerald P. Koocher, and Michael J. Saks (New York: Plenum Press, 1983), 73.

23. Beauchamp and Childress, *Principles of Biomedical Ethics,* 5th ed., 71.

24. Ibid., 76.

25. Allen E. Buchanan and Dan W. Brock, *Deciding for Others: The Ethics of Surrogate Decision-Making* (Cambridge: Cambridge University Press, 1989), 51–52. See also Willard Gaylin, "Competence: No Longer All or None," *Who Speaks for the Child,* ed. Gaylin and Macklin, 27–54.

26. Buchanan and Brock, *Deciding for Others,* 36.

27. Ibid., 56.

28. Ibid.

29. Ibid.

30. See ibid., 82.

31. Beauchamp and Childress, *Principles of Biomedical Ethics,* 5th ed., 71.

32. Buchanan and Brock, *Deciding for Others,* 56.

33. Thomas Grisso and Linda Vierling, "Minors' Consent to Treatment: A Developmental Perspective," *Professional Psychology* 9 (August 1978): 412–27.

34. For now, I will leave aside the question of consent to nontherapeutic research. For a discussion that relies on data regarding children's capacity to consent to medical care, see Lois Weithorn and David G. Scherer, "Children's Involvement in Research Participation Decision: Psychological Considerations," in *Children as Research Subjects: Science, Ethics, and Law,* ed. Michael A. Grodin and Leonard H. Glantz (New York: Oxford University Press, 1994), 133–79.

35. Grisso and Vierling, "Minors' Consent," 416.

36. Ibid.

37. Ibid., 417.

38. Ibid.

39. Ibid., 418.

40. Ibid.

41. Ibid.

42. Ibid., 419.

43. Ibid.

44. Ibid., 420.

45. Ibid., 421.

46. Ibid., 423.

47. Ibid.

48. Ibid., 424.

49. Lois A. Weithorn and Susan B. Campbell, "The Competency of Children and Adolescents to Make Informed Treatment Decisions," *Child Development* 53 (1982): 1589–98.

50. Ibid., 1592.

51. Ibid., 1596. See also Lois A. Weithorn, "Developmental Factors and Competence to Make Informed Treatment Decisions," *Child and Youth Services* 5 (1982): 85–100.

52. Committee on Bioethics, "Informed Consent, Parental Permission, and Assent in Pediatric Practice," *Pediatrics* 95 (February 1995): 317.

53. See, e.g., Buchanan and Brock, *Deciding for Others,* 218–23; Weithorn and Campbell, "Competency," 1598; Weithorn, "Developmental Factors," 92; Gary B. Melton, "Children's Consent: A Problem in Law and Social Science"; Michael A. Grodin and Joel J. Alpert, "Informed Consent and Pediatric Care"; Gerald P. Koocher, "Competence to Consent"; Thomas Grisso, "Juveniles' Consent in Delinquency Proceedings"; Donald N. Bersoff, "Children as Participants in Psychoeducational Assessment"; Patricia Keith-Spiegel, "Children and Consent to Participate in Research"; June Louin Tapp and Gary B. Melton, "Preparing Children for Decision Making"; and Lois A. Weithorn, "Involving Children in Decisions Affecting Their Own Welfare" all in Melton, Koocher and Saks, eds., *Children's Competence to Consent;* Sanford L. Leikin, "Minors' Assent or Dissent to Medical Treatment" in *President's Commission for the Study of Ethical Problems in Medicine and Biomedical*

and Behavioral Research, Making Health Care Decisions, vol. 3 (Washington, D.C.: U.S. Government Printing Office, 1982), 179, n. 3; Lainie Friedman Ross, *Children, Families, and Health Care Decision-Making* (Oxford: Clarendon Press, 1998), 70, n. 5.

54. Weithorn and Campbell, "Competency," 1596; cf. Grisso and Vierling, "Minors' Consent," 424.

55. Weithorn and Campbell, "Competency," 1596.

56. See Carol Gilligan, *In a Different Voice: Psychological Theory and Women's Development* (Cambridge, Mass.: Harvard University Press, 1982).

57. Grisso and Vierling, "Minors' Consent," 412.

58. Committee on Bioethics, "Informed Consent," 314.

59. For one example of modeling a child's decision-making role on the adult model of informed consent, see Nancy King and Alan Cross, "Children as Decision-Makers: Guidelines for Pediatricians," *Journal of Pediatrics* 115 (July 1989): 10–16. However, King and Cross draw the parallel without reference to the role that patients' rights play in the adult model, thus making it easier to see analogies between adult informed consent and the involvement of children in pediatric medical decision-making.

60. Committee on Bioethics, "Informed Consent," 316.

61. Leikin, "Minors' Assent or Dissent," 186.

62. Ibid.

63. Ibid.

64. Ibid., 187.

65. King and Cross, "Children as Decision-Makers," 15. In contrast to my argument, King and Cross emphasize the development of autonomy rather than medical responsibility.

66. Ross's argument is marred by inconsistent statements about children's competency. Her argument is premised on the claim that "all children are incompetent to make health care decisions" (7). Ross goes on to argue that children under the age of majority can be competent decision makers, or can achieve what she calls "a threshold of competence," but she rejects the idea of assigning children veto power. In her mind, competence is "a necessary but not sufficient condition for respecting a child's health care decision-making authority" (56). But if all children are incompetent, as Ross alleges, then it is unclear why she needs to consider necessary and sufficient conditions for respecting children's decisions. She has rendered the issue of respect moot by classifying all children as incompetent.

An additional inconsistency appears if we grant Ross part of her argument, namely, that competence is a necessary but not sufficient condition for assigning children the right to make their own medical decisions. According to Ross, assigning adolescents this right would allow them to jeopardize their future autonomy. Although Ross rejects the idea that children have a "right to an open future" (48–49), her position in fact draws on a qualified version of that position: A young person's present autonomy may be overridden in order to protect his or her future autonomy.

Ross also believes that parents have an interest in protecting values intrinsic to the good of family intimacy, which adolescents might jeopardize if their medical decisions are heeded. For Ross, respect for a young person's autonomy (and veto power) when he or she reaches the age of majority may permissibly override parental interests in protecting the good of family intimacy, but not before. Assigning veto power to the age of majority, Ross heeds the legal definition of adulthood. But she fails to provide a supporting *moral* argument for drawing the line at the age of majority. It remains unclear why, on grounds of family intimacy, parents guided by Ross's argument may not maintain decision-making authority over an offspring who has reached the age of majority and who rejects their recommendation to adopt or decline medical treatment. Equally important, it is not obvious that family intimacy cannot be served by parents who respect their adolescents' (different) competent decisions. See Ross, *Children, Families,* chap. 4.

67. Joel Feinberg, "The Child's Right to an Open Future," in *Whose Child? Children's Rights, Parental Authority, and State Power,* ed. William Aiken and Hugh LaFollette (Totowa, N.J.: Littlefield, Adams, 1980), 141.

68. Hillary Rodham, "Children under the Law," *Harvard Educational Review* 43 (November 1973): 491.

69. Ibid.

4. REPRESENTING PATIENTS

1. Hanna F. Pitkin, *The Concept of Representation* (Berkeley: University of California Press, 1967), 1–13, 209.

2. Ibid., 154.

3. Ibid.

4. Ibid., 151.

5. Ibid.

6. Ibid., 146.

7. Ibid., 163.

8. Ibid., 209–10.

9. See, e.g., John Stuart Mill, *Considerations on Representative Government,* with an introduction by F. A. Hayek (Chicago: Henry Regnery, 1962), 58–59.

10. Pitkin, *Concept of Representation,* 162.

11. Ibid., chap. 7.

12. Ibid., 174.

13. Edmund Burke, "The English Constitutional System," in *Representation,* ed. Hanna F. Pitkin (New York: Atherton Press, 1969), 175–76.

14. Ibid., 169.

15. Ibid., 173–74.

16. Ibid., 172.

17. Hilaire Belloc and Cecil Chesterton, *The Party System* (London: Stephen Swift, 1911), 16.

18. Ibid., 17.

19. Ibid.

20. Pitkin, *Concept of Representation,* chap. 7.

21. There are additional features of representation that this account omits. A political representative must deliberate in an assembly comprising other representatives, and this feature is not characteristic of the duties of proxies in medical settings. Also, political representatives must reckon with diverse wishes or interests in a constituency, whereas a patient proxy is tied to one person. When political representatives think about interests, moreover, they must not only think about individual interests, but the public interest. Because I am focusing on the relation between representatives and individuals, I will not pursue these points here.

22. *In re: Quinlan,* 70 N.J. 10; 355 A.2d 647.

23. David J. Rothman, *Strangers at the Bedside: A History of How Law and Bioethics Transformed Medical Decision-Making* (New York: Basic Books, 1991), 221.

24. *In re: Quinlan,* 70 N.J. 10, at 664. For a searching critique of this idea, see Paul Ramsey, *Ethics at the Edges of Life: Medical and Legal Intersections* (New Haven, Conn.: Yale University Press, 1978), chap. 7.

25. *In re: Quinlan,* 70 N.J. 10, at 664.

26. Ibid.

27. Ibid.

28. Gerald Kelly, *Medico-Moral Problems* (St. Louis: Catholic Hospital Association of the United States, 1958), 129.

29. Richard W. Momeyer, "Medical Decisions Concerning Noncompetent Patients," *Theoretical Medicine* 4 (1983): 275–90, at 280.

30. Ibid. Momeyer prefers the language of "situationally inferrable judgment" to "substituted judgment." Under either description, the goal is to surmise what a patient would choose if he or she could choose.

31. *In re: Quinlan,* 70 N.J. 10, at 666. Momeyer errs when he writes that the *Quinlan* court "expressly directed that treatment decisions made on the basis of substituted judgment be those that the patient herself would have made—not that which the guardian may believe to be most reasonable or in the best interest of the patient, not what the patient ought to choose, but simply what the patient would choose." See Momeyer, "Medical Decisions," 279.

32. *In re: Quinlan,* 70 N.J. 10, at 664.

33. Personal communication.

34. *In re: Quinlan,* 70 N.J. 10, at 653.

35. Ibid.

36. Ibid.

37. Ibid., at 664.

38. Ibid., at 663.

39. Ibid., at 666.

40. Ibid., at 664.

41. *Superintendent of Belchertown State School v. Joseph Saikewicz,* 373 Mass. 728; 370 N.E. 2d 417 (1977).

42. The decision was formally issued a year later, in November 1977.

43. *Superintendent of Belchertown State School v. Joseph Saikewicz,* 373 Mass. 728 (1977), at 427.

44. Ibid., at 431.

45. Ibid., at 430.

46. Ibid., at 431.

47. Ibid., at 432.

48. Ibid.

49. Ibid., at 431.

50. Ibid., at 424.

51. Ibid., at 430.

52. Ibid., at 426.

53. *In the Matter of Eichner, on Behalf of Joseph Fox,* 73 A.D. 2d. 431; 426 N.Y.S.2d 517; (1980).

54. Ibid., at 525.

55. Ibid., at 526.

56. Ibid.

57. Ibid., at 530.

58. Ibid., at 546.

59. Ibid., at 547.

60. Ibid.

61. Ibid., at 548.

62. Ibid.

63. Pitkin, *Concept of Representation,* 146.

64. Bringing together these ideas, we can say that parents or caretakers of sick children must calibrate their responsibilities in one of four ways: (1) for competent (understood as sufficiently mature) children who can communicate their valid consent, parents or caretakers have no duties as proxy; (2) for inaccessible children who have competently expressed

their wishes, parents or caretakers are to function as delegates of their child's wishes to accept or refuse treatment; (3) for inaccessible children who have not competently expressed their wishes but who have provided sufficient information from which to construct valid consent or refusal, parents or caretakers are to function as representatives; (4) for children who have not crossed the threshold of competence understood as sufficient maturity, parents or caretakers are to function as guardians, deciding in behalf of the child's basic interests and seeking, when appropriate, the child's assent. Here, as with considerations of paternalism, adults are to ascertain how to treat patients as children, and when not to do so.

65. *In the Matter of Martin Seiferth, Jr.,* 309 N.Y. 80: 127 N.E. 2d 820 (1955).

66. Ibid., at 820.

67. Ibid., at 823.

68. Issues about competence and age differentiation, discussed in the previous chapter, lurk in the background of *Seiferth*. Observe that the court did not say that Martin was incompetent because his decision differed from the medical professionals' recommendations. That is, the court did not conclude that Martin's deliberative *processes* were incompetent because his *conclusions* were "misguided." Note as well that Judge Wylegala appeared to have assumed that Martin was presumptively incompetent but that, on hearing his conclusions and judgments in court chambers, shifted his procedural presumptions and allowed Martin to speak for himself. Both of those features—detaching considerations of competence from substantive assessments of a decision, and assuming a rebuttable presumption of incompetence regarding the decision-making capacities of an early adolescent—follow the contours of my argument in the previous chapter regarding paternalism, antipaternalism, and the respect owed to young patients.

69. *In the Matter of Martin Seiferth, Jr.,* 309 N.Y. 80, at 823.

70. Ibid., at 822.

71. Ibid., at 823.

72. Ibid.

73. Ibid., at 824.

74. Ibid.

75. Fuld's dissent illustrates *second-party paternalism* or *indirect paternalism,* depending on who is considered to be the decision maker in this case. Overriding Martin's father's refusal of treatment would ignore the wishes of the individual primarily responsible for Martin's welfare, exemplifying second-party paternalism. Overriding Martin's refusal of treatment would indirectly restrict his father's attempt to raise him within a certain belief system, and this exemplifies indirect paternalism. Either form of paternalism is premised on the claim that Martin's father is exercising counterfeit beneficence. For a discussion, see chap. 3.

76. *Custody of a Minor,* 375 Mass. 733; 379 N.E., 2d 1053 (1978).

77. Laetrile is a drug derived from apricot pits that contains amygdaline, a crystalline substance capable of producing cyanide. Its effectiveness in the treatment of cancer has never been established.

78. *Custody of a Minor,* 375 Mass. 733 (1978), at 1063, citing *Richards v. Forrest,* 278 Mass., 1932, at 553.

79. Ibid., at 1064.

80. Ibid., at 1054.

81. Ibid., at 1065.

82. Ibid., citing *Saikewicz,* 373 Mass. 728, 752 (1977).

83. *Custody of a Minor,* 375 Mass. 733 (1978), at 1065.

84. Ibid.

85. Ibid.

86. Ibid., cf. *Custody of a Minor,* 378 Mass. 732; 393 N.E.2d 836 (1979), at 844.

87. *Custody of a Minor,* 375 Mass. 733 (1978), at 1064.

5. BASIC INTERESTS

1. Hillary Rodham, "Children under the Law," *Harvard Educational Review* 43 (November 1973): 491.

2. *Custody of a Minor,* 375 Mass. 733; (1978), at 1063, citing *Richards v. Forrest,* 278 Mass., 1932, at 553.

3. Allen E. Buchanan and Dan W. Brock, *Deciding for Others: The Ethics of Surrogate Decision-Making* (Cambridge: Cambridge University Press, 1989), 88, 236; Ferdinand Shoeman, "Parental Discretion and Children's Rights: Background and Implications for Medical Decision-Making," *Journal of Medicine and Philosophy* 10 (1985): 45–61.

4. Ezekiel J. Emmanuel, *The Ends of Human Life: Medical Ethics in a Liberal Polity* (Cambridge, Mass.: Harvard University Press, 1991), 76.

5. Ibid., 77.

6. John Rawls, "Justice as Fairness: Political not Metaphysical," *Philosophy and Public Affairs* 14 (summer 1985): 230.

7. John Rawls, *Political Liberalism,* 2d ed. (New York: Columbia University Press, 1996), 15. Rawls's discussion of an overlapping consensus in *Political Liberalism* draws on his earlier essays, "The Idea of an Overlapping Consensus," *Oxford Journal of Legal Studies* 7 (1987): 1–27; and "The Domain of the Political and Overlapping Consensus," *New York University Law Review* 64 (May 1989): 233–55.

8. John Rawls, *A Theory of Justice* (Cambridge, Mass.: Belknap Press, 1971), 249.

9. Ibid., 92.

10. For a discussion, see Chapter 2.

11. Not all pluralistic cultures are liberal. For a discussion, see Will Kymlicka, *Multicultural Citizenship: A Liberal Theory of Minority Rights* (New York: Oxford University Press, 1995), 156–58; 183–84.

12. Emanuel, *Ends of Human Life,* 78–87.

13. Richard A. McCormick, "To Save or Let Die: The Dilemma of Modern Medicine," in McCormick, *How Brave a New World? Dilemmas in Bioethics* (Garden City, N.Y.: Doubleday, 1981), 349.

14. Ibid., 346.

15. Ibid., 349.

16. James F. Childress, *Who Should Decide? Paternalism in Health Care* (New York: Oxford University Press, 1981), 64, following Robert Nozick, *Anarchy, State, and Utopia* (New York: Basic Books, 1974), 28–35.

17. Emanuel, *Ends of Human Life,* 85.

18. McCormick, "To Save or Let Die," 346. McCormick's idea that loving relationships should be appropriately constrained by considerations of justice echoes Aquinas's understanding of the order of charity. See Thomas Aquinas, *Summa Theologiae,* 2a2ae, Q. 26.

19. Emanuel distinguishes between comparative and noncomparative conceptions of a patient's quality of life, but he fails to connect liberalism to the former or understand its resources for rejecting the latter. See Emanuel, *Ends of Human Life,* 73.

20. Tom L. Beauchamp and James F. Childress, *Principles of Biomedical Ethics,* 5th ed. (New York: Oxford University Press, 2001), 133.

21. Ibid.

22. ICU Case Conference, December 1997.

23. Ibid.

24. Ibid.

25. Ibid.

26. Family conference, April 1998.

27. ICU Case conference, April 1998.

28. Interview, April 1998.

29. For a discussion of ordinary and extraordinary means, see Chapter 4.

30. Interview, April 1998.

31. *In the Matter of Kevin Sampson,* 65 Misc. 2d 658; 317 N.Y.S. 2d 641; (1970).

32. Ibid., at 642.

33. Ibid., at 644.

34. Ibid., at 654.

35. Ibid., at 642.

36. Ibid., at 644.

37. Ibid.

38. Ibid., at 645.

39. Ibid., at 649.

40. *In the Matter of Martin Seiferth, Jr.,* 309 N.Y. 80 (1955), at 823.

41. Ibid.

42. *In the Matter of Kevin Sampson,* 65 Misc. 2d (1970), at 656, citing *In the Matter of Martin Seiferth, Jr.,* 309 N.Y. 80 (1955), at 824.

43. *In the Matter of Kevin Sampson,* 65 Misc. 2d (1970), at 655.

44. Personal correspondence, July 18, 2000.

45. McCormick, "To Save or Let Die," 349.

46. Childress, *Who Should Decide?,* 64.

6. A FIGHTER, DOING GOD'S WILL

1. William F. May, *The Physician's Covenant: Images of the Healer in Medical Ethics* (Philadelphia: Westminster Press, 1983), 64.

2. Personal interview, January 1998.

3. Ibid.

4. Personal interview, March 1998(a).

5. Personal interview, January 1998.

6. Ibid.

7. Personal interview, March 1998(a).

8. Team meeting, February 1998.

9. Personal interview, March 1998(a).

10. Ibid.

11. Personal interview, March 1998.

12. Ibid.

13. Ibid.

14. John Calvin, *Institutes of the Christian Religion* (Philadelphia: Westminster Press, 1960), 1:17, 1.

15. Personal interview, March 1998(a).

16. Ibid.

17. Ibid.

18. Baylin ICU Ethics rounds, June 1998.

19. Personal interview, March 1998(b).

20. Baylin ICU Ethics rounds, June 1998.

21. Ibid.

22. Calvin, *Institutes of the Christian Religion,* 1:16, 6–9.

23. Thomas Aquinas, *Summa Theologiae,* 2a–2ae, Q. 26.

24. Ibid., article 5.

25. I am grateful to Nancy Hiller for calling this point to my attention in a discussion of Aquinas.

7. RESPECTING JACKSON BALES'S RELIGIOUS REFUSAL

1. David J. Rothman, *Strangers at the Bedside: A History of How Law and Bioethics Transformed Medical Decision-Making* (New York: Basic Books, 1991), 243.

2. Personal interview, March 1998.

3. Michael J. Sandel, *Democracy's Discontent: America in Search of a Public Philosophy* (Cambridge, Mass.: Harvard University Press/Belknap Press, 1996), 64.

4. Ibid., 65.

5. Ibid.

6. Thomas Jefferson, "Bill for Establishing Religious Freedom," cited in Sandel, *Democracy's Discontent,* 65.

7. Sandel, *Democracy's Discontent,* 66.

8. Ibid.

9. Ibid.

10. Ibid., 70.

11. For a discussion, see Charles Taylor, *Multiculturalism and "The Politics of Recognition,"* ed. Amy Gutmann (Princeton, N.J.: Princeton University Press, 1992).

12. Ibid.

13. Baylin Core Conference Rounds, March 1998.

14. For a discussion, see Chapter 4.

15. Albert R. Jonsen, "Blood Transfusions and Jehovah's Witnesses: The Impact of the Patient's Unusual Beliefs in Critical Care," *Critical Care Clinics* 2 (January 1986): 97.

16. Ibid., 98.

17. Personal interview, March 1998.

18. Ibid.

19. In that respect, Jackson's story resembles Billy Richardson's: In both cases, what Christians call the good of redemption overrides their respect for the good of creation.

20. Jonsen, "Blood Transfusions," 97.

21. Personal interview, May 1998.

22. Ibid.

23. Ibid.

24. Kathleen Lawry, Jacquelyn Slomka, and Johanna Goldfarb, "What Went Wrong: Multiple Perspectives on an Adolescent's Decision to Refuse Blood Transfusions," *Clinical Pediatrics* (June 1996): 317–21.

25. Ibid., 319–20.

26. Ibid.

27. See Dena S. Davis, "Legal Trends in Bioethics," *Journal of Clinical Ethics* 11 (summer 2000): 184–91.

28. Baylin Core Conference Rounds, March 1998.

29. Personal interview, May 1998.

8. ERICKA'S SEPSIS, LIA'S CONVULSIONS, AND CULTURAL DIFFERENCES

1. Charles Taylor, *Multiculturalism and "The Politics of Recognition,"* ed. Amy Gutmann (Princeton, N.J.: Princeton University Press, 1992), 25.

2. Michael Walzer, *Spheres of Justice: A Defense of Pluralism and Equality* (New York: Basic Books, 1983), 273.

3. Anne Fadiman, *The Spirit Catches You and You Fall Down: A Hmong Child, Her American Doctors, and the Collision of Two Cultures* (New York: Farrar, Strauss, and Giroux, 1997).

4. Chester Randle, "Unconventional Medicine in the Pediatric Intensive Care Unit" (unpublished paper).

5. Jane Brody, "Americans Gamble on Herbs as Medicine," *New York Times,* February 9, 1997, D1, D7.

6. See, e.g., Nancy Slifman et al., "Contamination of Botanical Dietary Supplements by *Digitalis lanata,*" *New England Journal of Medicine* 339 (September 17, 1998): 806–11.

7. Denise Grady, "Articles Question Safety of Dietary Supplements," *New York Times,* September 17, 1998, A25.

8. Brody, "Americans Gamble," D7.

9. William F. May, "The Beleaguered Rulers: The Public Obligation of the Professional," *Kennedy Institute of Ethics Journal* 2 (1992): 38.

10. I discuss this point in "Love and Death in a Pediatric Intensive Care Unit," *Annual of the Society of Christian Ethics* 14 (1994): 21–39.

11. Taylor, *Multiculturalism,* 25.

12. I lay out these differences in *Casuistry and Modern Ethics: A Poetics of Practical Reasoning* (Chicago: University of Chicago Press, 1996), chap. 9.

13. Charles Taylor, "To Follow a Rule," in Taylor, *Philosophical Arguments* (Cambridge, Mass.: Harvard University Press, 1992).

14. Fadiman, *Spirit Catches You,* 100.

15. Ibid.

16. Ibid., 90.

17. Ibid., 111.

18. Ibid., 150.

19. Ibid., 210.

20. Ibid., 276.

21. For a discussion, see Taylor, *Multiculturalism,* 67–70.

22. Fadiman, *Spirit Catches You,* 261.

23. Ibid., 255.

24. Ibid.

25. Ibid., 256.

26. Ibid., 259.

27. Ibid., 148, 260.

28. Ibid., 150; cf. 252.

29. Richard A. McCormick, "To Save or Let Die: The Dilemma of Modern Medicine," in McCormick, *How Brave a New World? Dilemmas in Bioethics* (Garden City, N.Y.: Doubleday, 1981), 349.

30. Ibid., 346.

31. Ibid., 349.

32. Fadiman, *Spirit Catches You,* 210–11.

33. *Prince v. Massachusetts,* 321 U.S. 158 (1944).

34. Code of Federal Regulations, Title 45, Section 1340.1–2(b)(1).

35. See P. Monopoli, "Allocating Costs of Parental Free Exercise: Striking a New Balance between Sincere Religious Beliefs and a Child's Right to Medical Treatment," *Pepperdine Law Review* 18 (1991): 319–52.

36. Seth M. Asser and Rita Swan, "Child Fatalities from Religion-Motivated Medical Neglect," *Pediatrics* 101 (1998): 625–29.

37. Ibid., 625. See also Committee on Bioethics of the American Academy of Pediatrics, "Religious Exemptions from Child Abuse Statutes," *Pediatrics* 81 (January 1988): 169–71; "Religious Objections to Medical Care," *Pediatrics* 99 (February 1997): 279–81.

38. Taylor discusses these temptations in *Multiculturalism,* 72–73.

39. Fadiman, *Spirit Catches You,* 261.

9. (PROPERLY) MARGINALIZED ALTRUISM

1. Thomas Aquinas, *Summa Theologiae,* 2-2, Q. 26, a. 6.

2. Personal interview, October 1999.

3. For a discussion, see Robert Bellah, Richard Madsen, William M. Sullivan, Ann Swidler, and Steven M. Tipton, *The Good Society* (New York: Alfred A. Knopf, 1991), 3–18.

4. Personal interview, October 1999.

5. Ibid.

6. Denise Grady, "The New Organ Donors Are Living Strangers," *New York Times,* September 20, 1999, A1.

7. Abe Aamidor, "Wait of Her Life," *Indianapolis Star,* February 13, 2000, 1. Ms. Foster died in February 2002. See Abe Aamidor, "Celebrating a Life Filled with Courage," *Indianapolis Star,* 6 February 2002. I am grateful to Jennifer Girod for calling my attention to this case and for providing me with background information.

8. *Indianapolis Star,* April 13, 2000, A19.

9. Arthur J. Matas et al., "Nondirected Donation of Kidneys from Living Donors," *New England Journal of Medicine* 343 (August 10, 2000): 433–36.

10. Paul Ramsey, *The Patient as Person* (New Haven, Conn.: Yale University Press, 1970), 194–97. Ramsey's discussion was prompted in part by his thoughts on *Masden v. Harrison,* No. 68651 Eq., Mass. Sup. Jud. Ct., June 12, 1957, in which physicians extracted a kidney from Leonard Masden and transplanted it into his twin brother. Although this case does not involve organ donations by strangers, it poses the general question of whether physicians may harm a person without compensatory medical benefit to that person. I suspect that Ramsey would settle the case of donations from strangers along the same lines he charted in response to the case of donations from relatives.

In any event, Ramsey was correct to claim that *Masden* is a case regarding the ethics of mutilation and that the principle of totality, duly broadened to include moral wholeness and well-being, would justify transplanting an organ from one sibling to another. Ramsey sought to produce a rule that would specify what ought to count as a basis for reasonable self-sacrifice, using the idea of moral wholeness as the background consideration.

11. I borrow the phrase from Timothy P. Jackson, "Love in a Liberal Society," *Journal of Religious Ethics* 22 (spring 1994): 36.

12. Matas et al., "Nondirected Donation," 433.

13. Personal conversation, February 1998.

14. Thomas J. O'Donnell, *Morals in Medicine* (Westminster, Md.: Newman Press, 1956), 70.

15. Gerald Kelly, *Medico-Moral Problems* (St. Louis: Catholic Hospital Association of the United States, 1958), 11.

16. Ibid.

17. Gerald Kelly, "The Morality of Mutilation: Towards a Revision of the Treatise," *Theological Studies* 17 (September 1956): 332–41.

18. Warren Reich, *Medico-Moral Problems and the Principle of Totality: A Catholic Viewpoint* (Washington, D.C.: Veterans' Administration Hospitals, 1967), 34–36, 40.

19. Personal interview, May 13, 1998.

20. Emily Yellen, "A Teacher's Gift? Why, Most Certainly," *New York Times,* December 18, 1999, A9; Denise Grady, "Taking Risks to Save a Friend, Healthy Give Up Their Organs," *New York Times,* June 24, 2001, 1.

21. Søren Kierkegaard, *Works of Love,* trans. Howard and Edna Hong, with a preface by R. Gregor Smith (New York: Harper Torchbooks, 1962), chap. 2A.

22. That is not to suggest that something like altruistic actions cannot occur within preferential relations. Consider parenting. One can imagine parents who understandably "lose themselves" in their attention to a child's needs, especially a child who is physically or mentally challenged. Preferential relations do not rule out aspects of altruism, because attention to a near neighbor can nonetheless require considerable self-sacrifice or unconditional conduct.

This fact might seem to weaken the account of altruism I have offered by diminishing the difference between preferential and nonpreferential love. But it does not do so by making nonpreferential love seem more like preferential love. Quite the contrary: It makes preferential love more like nonpreferential love, casting our understanding of (some) special relationships on the model of unconditional care.

23. Baylin case consultation, October 15, 1997.

24. William F. May, *The Patient's Ordeal* (Bloomington: Indiana University Press, 1991), 180.

25. James F. Childress, *Practical Reasoning in Bioethics* (Bloomington: Indiana University Press, 1997), chap. 15. However, Childress focuses on cadavers and citizens' fear of poor treatment at death. His practical reservations about commercialization may not apply to live donors. In their jointly authored work, Beauchamp and Childress concur with the argument I defend here when they write, "It is appropriate for transplant teams, reflecting societal rules and values, to probe the donor's understanding and voluntariness. It is also appropriate to consider potential donors' motives, at least to the extent of investigating whether financial gain is the motivating factor." Beauchamp and Childress conclude that health care professionals should start with the presumption that living organ donation "is praiseworthy but optional." In my view, starting with the presumption against living organ donation is a more appropriate way to approach this issue. See Tom L. Beauchamp and James F. Childress, *Principles of Biomedical Ethics,* 5th ed. (New York: Oxford University Press, 2001), 50–51.

26. Edwin F. Healy, *Medical Ethics* (Chicago: Loyola University Press, 1956), 101.

27. Ibid., 112.

28. For a discussion, see my *Casuistry and Modern Ethics: A Poetics of Practical Reasoning* (Chicago: University of Chicago Press, 1996), 36–37, 163–70.

29. Personal interview, October 1999.

30. Childress, *Practical Reasoning,* 294–95.

31. Aamidor, "Wait of Her Life," 2.

32. For a discussion of this problem in research ethics, see Vanessa Merton, "Ethical Obstacles to the Participation of Women in Biomedical Research," in *Feminism and Bioethics: Beyond Reproduction,* ed. Susan M. Wolf (New York: Oxford University Press, 1996), 216–51.

33. Kierkegaard, *Works of Love,* 174.

34. Søren Kierkegaard, *Purity of Heart Is to Will One Thing,* trans. Douglas V. Steere (New York: Harper Torchbooks, 1956).

35. Kierkegaard, *Works of Love,* chap. 2B.

36. Ibid., 134.

37. Augustine, *On Christian Doctrine,* trans. and with an introduction by D. W. Robertson, Jr. (Indianapolis: Bobbs-Merrill, 1981).

38. For a discussion, see John Burnaby, *Amor Dei: A Study of the Religion of St. Augustine* (London: Hodder and Stoughton, 1938), chap. 4.

39. Charles Taylor, *Sources of the Self: The Making of Modern Identity* (Cambridge, Mass.: Harvard University Press, 1989), 4.

40. Personal conversation, October 1997.

41. Childress, *Practical Reasoning,* 270.

10. THE POLITICS AND ETHICS
OF A HOSPITAL ETHICS COMMITTEE

1. For accounts of the emergence and function of hospital committees, see John J. Paris and Frank E. Reardon, "Ethics Committees in Critical Care," in *Critical Care Clinics* 2 (January 1986): 111–21; Dennis F. Thompson, "Hospital Ethics," *Cambridge Quarterly of Healthcare Ethics* (1992): 203–15; Christine Mitchell and Robert D. Truog, "From the Files of a Pediatric Ethics Committee," *Journal of Clinical Ethics* 11 (summer 2000): 112–20.

2. See, e.g., Sanford Letkin and Jonathan D. Moreno, "Pediatric Ethics Committees," in *Pediatric Ethics: From Principles to Practice,* ed. Robert C. Cassidy and Alan R. Fleischman (Amsterdam: Harwood Academic Publishers, 1996), 56.

3. Amy Gutmann and Dennis F. Thompson, *Democracy and Disagreement* (Cambridge, Mass.: Harvard University Press, 1997), chaps. 2–4.

4. I borrow these from Michael Walzer, "Deliberation, and What Else?" in *Deliberative Politics: Essays on "Democracy and Disagreement,"* ed. Stephen Macedo (New York: Oxford University Press, 1999), 58–69.

5. Personal correspondence.

6. Meeting of Baylin's Ethics Advisory Committee, November 1997.

7. This information was shared during several meetings of Baylin's Ethics Advisory Committee during my observation period.

8. For a discussion of specifying and balancing rival norms, see Henry Richardson, "Specifying Norms as a Way to Resolve Concrete Ethical Problems," *Philosophy and Public Affairs* 19 (fall 1990): 279–310; Richard B. Miller, *Casuistry and Modern Ethics: A Poetics of Practical Reasoning* (Chicago: University of Chicago Press, 1996), 17–25; James F. Childress, "Moral Norms in Practical Ethical Deliberation," in *Christian Ethics: Problems and Prospects,* ed. Lisa Sowle Cahill and James F. Childress (Cleveland: Pilgrim Press, 1996), 196–217.

9. On moral constituency and representation, see Gutmann and Thompson, *Democracy and Disagreement,* chap. 4.

10. Dennis F. Thompson, *Political Ethics and Public Office* (Cambridge, Mass.: Harvard University Press, 1987), chap. 2.

11. Gutmann and Thompson, *Democracy and Disagreement,* chaps. 2–4.

12. Ibid., 53.

13. Ibid.

14. Quoted in ibid., 95.

15. See Immanuel Kant, "Perpetual Peace," in *Kant: Political Writings,* trans. H. B. Nisbet, ed. Hans Reiss (Cambridge: Cambridge University Press, 1991), 93–130. For discussions, see Gutmann and Thompson, *Democracy and Disagreement,* chap. 3; David Luban, "The Publicity Principle," in *The Theory of Institutional Design,* ed. Robert E. Goodin (Cambridge: Cambridge University Press, 1996), 154–98.

16. Quoted in Gutmann and Thompson, *Democracy and Disagreement,* 100–101.

17. Ibid., 128.

18. Margaret Urban Walker, "Keeping Moral Spaces Open: New Images of Ethics Consulting," *Hastings Center Report* 23 (March–April 1993): 33–40.

19. Ibid., 35.

20. Ibid., 34.

21. Ibid., 38.

22. I have argued that casuistry provides a third alternative to these approaches. See *Casuistry and Modern Ethics,* chap. 9.

23. Walker, "Keeping Moral Spaces Open," 40.

24. Ibid.

25. For discussions, see Kenneth E. Kirk, *Conscience and Its Problems: An Introduction to Casuistry,* 4th ed. (London: Longmans and Green, 1947); Albert R. Jonsen and Stephen Toulmin, *The Abuse of Casuistry: A History of Moral Reasoning* (Berkeley: University of California Press, 1988); Miller, *Casuistry and Modern Ethics.*

26. Robert Nozick, "Moral Complications and Moral Structures," *Natural Law Forum* 12 (1969): 1–50.

11. ETHICAL ISSUES IN PEDIATRIC RESEARCH

1. Personal interview, June 2001.

2. American Academy of Pediatrics, "Guidelines for the Ethical Conduct of Studies to Evaluate Drugs in Pediatric Populations (RE9503)." Available at: http://www.aap.org/policy/00655.html. Accessed May 6, 2002.

3. Personal conversation, June 2001.

4. American Academy of Pediatrics, "Guidelines."

5. U.S. Department of Health and Human Services. Food and Drug Administration. Regulations Requiring Manufacturers to Assess the Safety and Effectiveness of New Drugs and Biological Products in Pediatric Patients; proposed rule. *Federal Register* 62, no. 158 (August 1997): 43899–43916. For final rule, see n. 8 below.

6. Loretta M. Kopelman, "Children as Research Subjects: A Dilemma," *Journal of Medicine and Philosophy* 25 (2000): 745–64, at 745–46.

7. H. C. Shirkey, "Therapeutic Orphans," *Journal of Pediatrics* 72 (1968): 119–20.

8. U.S. Department of Health and Human Services. Food and Drug Administration. Regulations Requiring Manufacturers to Assess the Safety and Effectiveness of New Drugs and Biological Products in Pediatric Patients; Final Rule. *Federal Register* 63, no. 231 (December 1998): 66631–72.

9. Sheryl Gay Stolberg, "Children Test New Medicines Despite Doubts," *New York Times,* February 11, 2001, A1.

10. U.S. National Institutes of Health, "NIH Policy and Guidelines on the Inclusion of Children as Participants in Research Involving Human Subjects." Release date, March 6, 1998. Available at: http://www.nih.gov/grants/guide/notice-files/not98-024.html. Accessed May 15, 2002.

11. For an overview, see Jennifer Rosato, "The Ethics of Clinical Trials: A Child's View," *Journal of Law, Medicine and Ethics* 28 (winter 2000): 362–78.

12. See also Donald VanDeVeer, "Experimentation on Children and Proxy Consent," *Journal of Medicine and Philosophy* 6 (1981): 281–93; Robert J. Levine, *Ethics and Regulation of Clinical Research,* 2d ed. (New Haven, Conn.: Yale University Press, 1986), chap. 10, and the many references cited in Levine's bibliography (365–91).

13. Paul Ramsey, *The Patient as Person* (New Haven, Conn.: Yale University Press, 1970), 35. My comments here draw from my essay "Religion, Ethics, and Clinical Immersion: An Appraisal of Three Pioneers," in *Caring Well: Religion, Narrative, and Health Care Ethics,* ed. David H. Smith (Louisville: Westminster/John Knox Press, 2000), 17–42. © 2000 Westminster John Knox Press. Used by permission of Westminster John Knox Press.

14. Albert R. Jonsen, *The Birth of Bioethics* (New York: Oxford University Press, 1998), 50.

15. See Susan E. Lederer and Michael A. Grodin, "Historical Overview: Pediatric Experimentation," in *Children as Research Subjects: Science, Ethics, and Law,* ed. Michael A. Grodin and Leonard H. Glantz (New York: Oxford University Press, 1994), 3–25.

16. Ramsey, *Patient as Person*, 5.

17. Ibid., 11. Later Ramsey argues that autonomy is only a relative right in cases of medical care. But to the best of my knowledge, he never wavers about the restrictions that autonomy imposes in cases of medical experimentation. See Paul Ramsey, *Ethics at the Edges of Life: Medical and Legal Intersections* (New Haven, Conn.: Yale University Press, 1978), 156.

18. Ramsey, *Patient as Person*, 12.

19. Ibid., 13.

20. Paul Ramsey, "The Enforcement of Morals: Non-Therapeutic Research on Children," *Hastings Center Report* 6 (1976): 24.

21. Ramsey, *Patient as Person*, 14.

22. "Nuremberg Code: Directives for Human Experimentation." Available at: http://ohsr.od.nih.gov/nuremberg.php3. Accessed July 10, 2002.

23. "World Medical Association Declaration of Helsinki." Available at: http://www.wma.net/e/policy/17-c_e.html. Accessed July 10, 2002.

24. Ramsey, *Patient as Person*, 11–12.

25. Ibid., 13.

26. I am not suggesting that beneficence is the only relevant norm in pediatric ethics; my critique of Ramsey is internal to his own logic.

27. For a similar line of argument, drawing on Rawlsian ideas, see Dan W. Brock, "Ethical Issues in Exposing Children to Risks in Research," in *Children as Research Subjects*, ed. Grodin and Glantz, 81–101.

28. My views should be contrasted with two other contributions, by Richard A. McCormick and Thomas H. Murray. McCormick sought to rebut Ramsey by arguing that a child "would choose [nontherapeutic research] if he were capable of choice because he *ought* to do so." Parental permission to enroll a child in research "is morally valid precisely as it is a reasonable presumption of the child's wishes." Drawing on a theory of the natural law, McCormick holds that there are "certain identifiable values that we *ought* to support, attempt to realize, and never directly suppress because they are definitive of our flourishing and well-being." Sharing burdens of health care and research is good for us as humans, something we ought to do. "And to the extent that we *ought* to do so, it is a reasonable construction of our wishes to say that we would do so." The reasonableness of such a presumption justifies the idea of vicarious or proxy consent. See Richard A. McCormick, "Proxy Consent in the Experimentation Situation," in McCormick, *How Brave a New World? Dilemmas in Bioethics* (Garden City, N.J.: Doubleday, 1981), 51–71.

For Murray, McCormick's views are too sanguine. McCormick holds that a child "would choose [to volunteer] if he were capable of choice because he *ought* to do so" (61). As Murray notes, "the move from 'ought' to 'would' is an interminable battle fought between parents and children as well as within every person's psyche." Eschewing arguments about vicarious consent, Murray defends low-risk nontherapeutic research if the risks are small and the benefits to the community are great. See Thomas H. Murray, *The Worth of the Child* (Berkeley: University of California Press, 1996), 81.

My view is similar to McCormick's and Murray's in that it focuses on sharing burdens. But my view is justified by principles of fairness rather than by duties that attach to human flourishing or proportionality.

29. U.S. 45 CRF46.404-7 (2001).

30. Baylin Ethics retreat, June 2001.

31. See the U.S. Food and Drug Administration Pediatric Ethics Working Group Consensus Statement on the use of placebos. Available at: http://www.fda.gov/cder/pediatric/ethics-statement-2000.htm. Accessed May 7, 2002.

32. J. Janofsky and B. Starfield, "Assessment of Risk in Research on Children," *Journal of Pediatrics* 98 (1981): 759–60.

33. See Esther H. Wender, "Assessment of Risk to Children," in *Children as Research Subjects,* ed. Grodin and Glantz, 181–92.

34. Personal interview, June 2001.

35. This standard of risk comes close to Terence F. Ackerman's proposal for a standard of minimal risk. However, unlike Ackerman, I would exclude spanking a child as an appropriate form of parental intervention. See Terence F. Ackerman, "Moral Duties of Parents and Nontherapeutic Clinical Research Procedures Involving Children," *Bioethics Quarterly* 2 (summer 1980): 94–111, at 107.

36. Contrast my argument with Ross's, who justifies minimal-risk nontherapeutic pediatric research on the model of constrained parental autonomy. According to Ross, parents are permitted to enroll a child in minimal risk nontherapeutic research, even against the child's wishes, because doing so "is one way in which parents can attempt to steer their child's development into a socially responsible adult." The rationale is largely moral and pedagogical: "The model of constrained parental autonomy permits parents to override their child's dissent in minimal risk research if they believe that it will serve to guide his development according to their vision of the good life, realizing that their child may ultimately reject this conception of the good." The problem with this view is that there are other, less coercive ways for parents to impart their vision of the good life than forcing a child to participate in medical research. Heeding a child's dissent can be followed up with discussions about why choosing otherwise would have honored morally important values. My view, in contrast, is premised on the fairness of turn-taking and would not require children to participate against their objections. See Lainie Friedman Ross, *Children, Families, and Health Care Decision-Making* (Oxford: Clarendon Press, 1998), 93.

37. A related question is motivational: Why would parents volunteer children for nontherapeutic research? Recall from Chapter 9 that medical professionals have no grounds for harming patients without a commensurate prospect of benefit. Yet as we saw in that chapter, benefits can be construed in more than physiological terms. How I handle motivational questions in that chapter is applicable to this one as well.

38. Personal interview, June 2001.

39. Stolberg, "Children Test New Medicines," A1.

40. Personal interview, June 2001.

41. Stolberg, "Children Test New Medicines," A1.

42. Personal interview, June 2001.

43. Baylin Ethics retreat, June 2001

44. On "moral constituencies," see Amy Gutmann and Dennis F. Thompson, *Democracy and Disagreement* (Cambridge, Mass.: Harvard University Press, 1997), chap. 4.

45. American Academy of Pediatrics, "Guidelines."

46. Michael J. Sandel, *Democracy's Discontent: America in Search of a Public Philosophy* (Cambridge, Mass.: Harvard University Press/Belknap Press, 1996), 64.

47. Stolberg, "Children Test New Medicines," A1.

48. Personal interview, June 2001.

49. The "Best Pharmaceuticals for Children Act," signed into law on January 4, 2002, established a publicly funded program to award contracts to study off-patent drugs in pediatric patients, but Congress failed to authorize expenditures to finance such studies in FY 2002. See http://www.fda.gov/cder/pediatric/index.htm. Accessed July 15, 2002.

50. Md. 29, 782 A.2d. 807 (2001).

51. "Lead-Based Paint Study." Available at: http://www.hopkinsmedicine.org/press/2001/SEPTEMBER/leadfactsheet.htm. Accessed May 4, 2002.

52. See Tamar Lewin, "U.S. Investigating Johns Hopkins Study of Lead Paint Hazard," *New York Times,* August 24, 2001, A11.

53. *Grimes v. Kennedy Krieger Institute, Inc.; Myron Higgins, a minor, etc., et al., v. Kennedy Krieger Institute, Inc.,* 366 Md. 29, 782 A.2d., at 850.

54. Ibid., at 855.

55. Ibid., at 825.

56. Ibid., at 843.

57. Ibid.

58. Ibid., at 814.

59. See also Loretta Kopelman, "Pediatric Research Regulations under Legal Scrutiny: *Grimes* Narrows Their Interpretation," *Journal of Law, Medicine and Ethics* 30 (spring 2002): 38–49; Lainie Friedman Ross, "In Defense of the Hopkins Lead Abatement Studies," *Journal of Law, Medicine and Ethics* 30 (spring 2002): 50–57.

60. *Grimes v. Kennedy Krieger Institute, Inc.; Myron Higgins, a minor, etc., et al., v. Kennedy Krieger Institute, Inc.,* 366 Md. 29, 782 A.2d., at 850.

61. Ibid., at 848.

62. Ibid., at 812.

63. Ibid., at 821.

64. Ibid., at 815.

65. Ibid., at 814.

66. Ibid., at 843.

67. See n. 22.

68. *Grimes v. Kennedy Krieger Institute, Inc.; Myron Higgins, a minor, etc., et al., v. Kennedy Krieger Institute, Inc.,* 366 Md. 29, 782 A.2d., at 814.

69. Ibid., at 817.

70. Ibid., at 814.

71. Ibid., at 832.

72. Ibid., at 814.

73. Ibid., at 850.

74. Ramsey, *Patient as Person,* 12.

75. The Ethics Advisory Group for the Center for Drug Evaluation and Research in the U.S. Food and Drug Administration took up several of these issues in November 1999, but no changes in the federal regulations have materialized. See "Ethical Issues in Pediatric Pharmaceutical Research Where There Is No Primary Intention of Direct Benefit." Available at: http://www.fda.gov/cder/pediatric/pedethics-1199.htm. Accessed May 7, 2002

CONCLUSION

1. Consider the analogy with sovereign states: A despotic regime might violate basic rights, thus justifying internal dissent, agitation, reform movements, perhaps revolution. But the right to dissent is not the same as the right of others to intervene. Groups within a regime have greater liberties to reform or revolt than outsiders have to intrude. For a discussion, see Michael Walzer, "The Moral Standing of States: A Response to Four Critics," *Philosophy and Public Affairs* 9 (spring 1980): 209–29.

2. John Rawls, *A Theory of Justice* (Cambridge, Mass.: Belknap Press, 1971), 7, 464. See also John Rawls, *Justice as Fairness: A Restatement,* ed. Erin Kelly (Cambridge, Mass.: Harvard University Press, 2001), 10, 162–66.

3. In a similar spirit, Susan Moller Okin develops what she calls the "positive potential" of Rawls's views for a humanist theory of gender justice in *Justice, Gender, and the Family* (New York, Basic Books, 1989). My arguments will focus less on gender than on children and social justice.

4. John Rawls, "The Idea of Public Reason Revisited," in *Collected Papers,* ed. Samuel Freeman (Cambridge, Mass.: Harvard University Press, 1999), 596. See also n. 2 above. Rawls's account refutes the idea, widely held by antiliberals, that liberal doctrine ignores the family.

5. For Rawls on a "sense of justice," see *Theory of Justice,* 46, 312, 454, 505–10.

6. For a discussion that traces parallels between Piaget and Rawls, see Samantha Brennan and Robert Noggle, "Rawls's Neglected Childhood: Reflections on the Original Position, Stability, and the Child's Sense of Justice," in *The Idea of a Political Liberalism: Essays on Rawls,* ed. Victoria Davion and Clark Wolf (Lanham, Md.: Rowman and Littlefield, 2000), 46–72.

7. Rawls, *Theory of Justice,* 463.

8. Ibid., 464.

9. Ibid., 465.

10. Ibid., 464.

11. Ibid., 467–72.

12. Ibid., 469.

13. Ibid., 470.

14. Ibid., 469.

15. Ibid.

16. Ibid., 472–79.

17. Ibid., 476.

18. Ibid., 475.

19. Ibid., 494.

20. Ibid., 471.

21. Michael J. Sandel, *Liberalism and the Limits of Justice,* 2d ed. (Cambridge: Cambridge University Press, 1998), 31.

22. Ibid., 32.

23. Rawls, *Theory of Justice,* 3.

24. Sandel, *Liberalism and the Limits of Justice,* 2d ed., 33.

25. Ibid., 32.

26. Aristotle, *Nicomachean Ethics,* 1155a25.

27. Sandel, *Liberalism and the Limits of Justice,* 2d ed., 32.

28. Ibid.

29. Okin rightly argues that Sandel fails to understand what Rawls means by saying that justice is the first virtue of social institutions. As Okin notes, to say that justice is the primary virtue of social institutions does not imply that justice is the supreme virtue. Okin's main charge against Sandel is that he romanticizes the family and fails to address how families must be seen in a nonideal light. My complaint is different: Sandel fails properly to understand that the good of care requires distributive mechanisms given the conditions of human finitude, conditions that are relevant to families that operate on even the best of terms. See Okin, *Justice, Gender, and the Family,* 27–33.

30. Rawls, *Theory of Justice,* 465.

31. Ibid., 440.

32. Ibid.

33. Ibid., 178.

34. For a discussion, see Okin, *Justice, Gender, and the Family,* 14–24.

35. Rawls, *Justice as Fairness,* 166. Ross's argument appears to picture the family as a prepolitical sphere and thus more immune from social criticism than I am arguing for here. Liberal justice along Rawlsian lines, duly developed to apply to domestic affairs, provides greater grounds for scrutinizing the justice of child-rearing than Ross's account of liberalism suggests. See Lainie Friedman Ross, *Children, Families, and Health Care Decision-Making* (Oxford: Clarendon Press, 1998), 3–8, 23, 49, 152–53, 158, 163–64, 172.

36. Rawls, *Theory of Justice,* 7.

37. Ibid., 15.

38. Rawls, "Idea of Public Reason Revisited," 598.

INDEX

Richard B. Miller is a Professor in the Department of Religious Studies at Indiana University, where he serves as departmental chair. He is the author of *Interpretations of Conflict: Ethics, Pacifism, and the Just-War Tradition* (1991) and *Casuistry and Modern Ethics: A Poetics of Practical Reasoning* (1996). He has edited *War in the Twentieth Century: Sources in Theological Ethics* (1993) and has written numerous articles in moral philosophy and religious ethics.